# Drug Resistance: Clinical Aspects

# Drug Resistance: Clinical Aspects

Edited by Casey Hammond

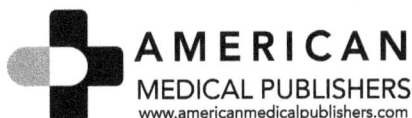

**AMERICAN**
MEDICAL PUBLISHERS
www.americanmedicalpublishers.com

American Medical Publishers,
41 Flatbush Avenue,
1st Floor, New York,
NY 11217, USA

Visit us on the World Wide Web at:
www.americanmedicalpublishers.com

ISBN: 978-1-63927-210-5

**Cataloging-in-Publication Data**

Drug resistance : clinical aspects / edited by Casey Hammond.
    p. cm.
Includes bibliographical references and index.
ISBN 978-1-63927-210-5
1. Drug resistance. 2. Pharmacology. 3. Clinical pharmacology.
4. Immunopharmacology. I. Hammond, Casey.
QR177 .D78 2022
616.904 1--dc23

# Table of Contents

**Permissions**

**List of Contributors**

**Index**

# Preface

The reduction in the effectiveness of a medication such as antimicrobial or antineoplastic to treat a disease is known as drug resistance. The term is used to denote the resistance that pathogens have acquired. The resistance that a microbe has developed to resist the effects of an antimicrobial medication that could treat it, is known as antimicrobial resistance. Antineoplastic resistance is the resistance of cancerous or neoplastic cells to survive and grow without getting affected by cancer therapies. The microbes acquire resistance to both chemicals as well as physical factors such as temperature, radiation, sound, magnetism or exposure to a chemical. The four mechanisms through which the microorganisms manifest resistance to antimicrobials are the alteration of the target site, drug inactivation and modification, alteration of the metabolic pathways and reduced drug accumulation. This book provides comprehensive insights into the field of drug resistance. It will also provide interesting topics for research which interested readers can take up. The extensive content of this book provides the readers with a thorough understanding of the subject.

This book is a result of research of several months to collate the most relevant data in the field.

When I was approached with the idea of this book and the proposal to edit it, I was overwhelmed. It gave me an opportunity to reach out to all those who share a common interest with me in this field. I had 3 main parameters for editing this text:

1. Accuracy – The data and information provided in this book should be up-to-date and valuable to the readers.

2. Structure – The data must be presented in a structured format for easy understanding and better grasping of the readers.

3. Universal Approach – This book not only targets students but also experts and innovators in the field, thus my aim was to present topics which are of use to all.

Thus, it took me a couple of months to finish the editing of this book.

I would like to make a special mention of my publisher who considered me worthy of this opportunity and also supported me throughout the editing process. I would also like to thank the editing team at the back-end who extended their help whenever required.

**Editor**

# High rates of multidrug resistance among uropathogenic *Escherichia coli* in children and analyses of ESBL producers from Nepal

Narayan Prasad Parajuli[1,3*], Pooja Maharjan[1], Hridaya Parajuli[1], Govardhan Joshi[1], Deliya Paudel[1], Sujan Sayami[2] and Puspa Raj Khanal[3]

## Abstract

**Background:** Emergence of Extended-spectrum beta-lactamase producing *Escherichia coli* causing urinary tract infections (UTI) among pediatric patients is an increasing problem worldwide. However, very little is known about pediatric urinary tract infections and antimicrobial resistance trend from Nepal. This study was conducted to assess the current antibiotic resistance rate and ESBL production among uropathogenic *Escherichia coli* in pediatric patients of a tertiary care teaching hospital of Nepal.

**Methods:** A total of 5,484 urinary tract specimens from children suspected with UTI attending a teaching hospital of Nepal over a period of one year were processed for the isolation of bacterial pathogens and their antimicrobial susceptibility testing. *Escherichia coli* ($n = 739$), the predominant isolate in pediatric UTI, was further selected for the detection of ESBL-production by phenotypic combination disk diffusion test.

**Results:** Incidence of urinary tract infection among pediatric patients was found to be 19.68% and *E coli* (68.4%) was leading pathogen involved. Out of 739 *E coli* isolates, 64.9% were multidrug resistant (MDR) and 5% were extensively drug resistant (XDR). Extended spectrum beta lactamase (ESBL) was detected in 288 (38.9%) of the *E coli* isolates.

**Conclusion:** Alarming rate of drug resistance among pediatric uropathogens and high rate of ESBL-producing *E. coli* was observed. It is extremely necessary to routinely investigate the drug resistance among all isolates and formulate strict antibiotics prescription policy in our country.

**Keywords:** Urinary tract infection, Children, *E coli*, ESBL, Nepal

## Background

Urinary tract infection (UTI) is among the most common causes of febrile illness in children requiring antimicrobial treatment [1]. Worldwide, an estimated 8% of girls and 2% of boys experience at least one episode of UTI by the age of seven years and recurrence occurs in 12-30% of them within a year [2]. Pediatric UTI in many instances, remain under-diagnosed because of the absence of specific symptoms and signs, particularly in infants and young children [2, 3]. Therefore, accurate diagnosis and appropriate use of antimicrobials for treatment and prevention of urinary tract infections (UTIs) is vital to reduce the burden and also to prevent the possible long-term consequences [4].

*Escherichia coli* have been recognised as the most common pathogen accounting for majority of urinary tract infections in children [5]. Antimicrobial therapy, usually of traditional antibiotics, is commonly prescribed to treat urinary tract infections in pediatric patients. However, increased rates acquired resistance in *E. coli* has made usual antibiotics less acceptable choice for empirical therapy in recent years [1]. The most common mechanism associated with acquired resistance in *E. coli* and other *Enterobacteriaceae* is the production of hydrolytic enzymes called β-lactamases [6, 7]. Extended-spectrum β-lactamase (ESBL), a major beta lactamase enzyme,

* Correspondence: narayan.parajuli@iom.edu.np
[1]Department of Clinical Laboratory Services, Manmohan Memorial Medical College and Teaching Hospital, P.O.B.: 15201 Swayambhu, Kathmandu, Nepal
[3]Department of Laboratory Medicine, Manmohan Memorial Institute of Health Sciences, Kathmandu, Nepal
Full list of author information is available at the end of the article

has the ability to hydrolyze oxyimino-cephalosporins, and monobactams but not cephamycins or carbapenems and inhibited in-vitro by inhibitors such as clavulanic acid, sulbactam and tazobactam [8]. Since their evolution in 1983, more than 300 types of ESBLs have been identified in various members of the family *Enterobacteriaceae* and other non-enteric organisms [3, 6]. The infections associated with these ESBL producing isolates are difficult to treat because of their resistance towards beta lactam agents and also due to the emergence of co-existing resistance determinants such as aminoglycosides and fluoroquinolones [7]. Moreover, emergence of ESBL producing bacteria, particularly *E. coli* and *K. pneumoniae* causing pediatric urinary tract infections is a worldwide concern [9]. Options for the treatment of such multidrug resistant (MDR) gram negative bacterial infections are generally limited, and very few antibiotics are approved for use in children [10].

In Nepal, pediatric UTIs are usually treated empirically because of the unavailability of standard therapeutic guidelines and local susceptibility data [11, 12]. Knowledge of the etiological agent of UTIs and their antimicrobial resistance patterns in our setting may help clinicians in choosing the appropriate antimicrobial treatment. Moreover, most of the studies on pediatric urinary tract infections caused by multidrug resistant and ESBL producing bacteria have been reported from western world [10, 13], but the same from South Asian region including Nepal are scarce on the published literature [14]. In this perspective, the present study was designed to investigate the clinical isolates of multi-drug resistant and ESBL producing *Escherichia coli* causing urinary tract infections in children visiting a tertiary care teaching hospital in Nepal.

## Methods
### Study design and setup
A cross-sectional study was carried out for 1 year (June 2015 - May 2016) in the department of Microbiology and Pediatric Medicine, Manmohan Memorial Medical College and Teaching Hospital (MMCTH), a tertiary care hospital with 500 patient beds in Kathmandu, the capital city of Nepal. Study hospital is a referral center with medical, surgical, gynecological, pediatric, geriatric and other specialties.

### Inclusion and exclusion criteria
During the study period, children up to 14 years of age presented to the pediatric outpatient department or admitted to pediatric inpatient ward with a clinical diagnosis of UTI were included. The clinical diagnosis of UTI was made by respective unit pediatrician in the presence of fever and/or any of the symptoms such painful micturition, increased frequency, burning micturition, or suprapubic pain/flank pain. Those children who had previous known history of antimicrobial therapy within 48 h prior to attending the

hospital and samples which grew more than one type of organism was considered as contaminated and hence, excluded from the study.

### Laboratory methods
A total of 5,484 non-repetitive urine specimens (Midstream, Suprapubic, Catheter aspirated and Clean catch) representing urinary tract infections in pediatric patients (0-14 years) were processed semi-quantitatively by inoculating 0.001 ml of the specimen (by using a calibrated wire loop) onto the cystine lactose electrolyte deficient (CLED) agar for the isolation and identification of significant uropathogens [15]. The inoculated plates were incubated for 24 h at 37 °C in aerobic atmosphere. Growth of a single organism with a count of $\geq 10^5$ colony-forming units (CFU)/ml were considered to represent the infection and were identified using appropriate routine identification methods including colony morphology, Gram-stain, and an in-house set of biochemical tests [15]. *Escherichia coli*, the predominant uropathogen, was selected for the determination of antimicrobial susceptibility as well as identification of the multidrug resistant (MDR), extensively drug resistant (XDR) and extended spectrum beta lactamase (ESBL) producing isolates.

### Antimicrobial susceptibility testing
The susceptibility of bacterial isolates against different antibiotics was tested by the disk diffusion method [modified Kirby-Bauer method] on Mueller Hinton agar (Hi-Media, India) following standard procedures recommended by the Clinical and Laboratory Standards Institute (CLSI), Wayne, USA [16]. Antibiotics that were tested in our study include Ampicillin (AMP 25 µg), Amoxycillin clavulanate (AMC20/10 µg), Aztreonam (30 µg) Gentamycin (GEN10µg), Ciprofloxacin (CIP5µg), Levofloxacin (LEV5µg) trimethoprim sulfamethoxazole/cotrimoxazole (COT30µg), Cephalexin (CN30 µg), Cefixime (CFM5µg), Ceftriaxone (CTR30µg), Ceftazidime (CAZ30µg), Piperacillin tazobactam (PIT 100/10 µg), Imipenem (IMP 10 µg), Meropenem (MRP 10 µg) Tigecycline (TGC30µg), and Colistin sulphate (CT10µg) (HiMedia Laboratories, India). Interpretations of antibiotic susceptibility results were made according to the zone size interpretative standards of CLSI [16]. *Escherichia coli* ATCC 25922 was used as a control organism for antibiotic susceptibility testing.

### Identification of Multidrug Resistant (MDR), Extensive Drug Resistant (XDR) and potential ESBL *Escherichia coli*
MDR and XDR isolates were identified according to the combined guidelines of the European Centre for Disease Prevention and Control (ECDC) and the Centers for Disease Control and Prevention (CDC) [17]. In this study, the isolate resistant to at least one antimicrobial from three different group of first line drugs tested was

regarded as multidrug resistant (MDR). Extensively drug resistant (XDR) isolates were identified when the isolates are resistant to at least one agent in all but two or fewer antimicrobial categories (i.e., bacterial isolates remain susceptible to only one or two categories).

Isolates of *E. coli* were examined for their susceptibility to third generation cephalosporins by using Ceftazidime (30 μg) and Cefotaxime (30 μg) disks. If the zone of inhibition (ZOI) was ≤25 mm for Ceftriaxone, ≤22 mm for Ceftazidime and/or ≤27 mm for Cefotaxime, the isolate was considered a potential ESBL producer as recommended by CLSI and further tested by confirmatory methods [16].

### Confirmatory test of ESBL
Isolates considered potential ESBL producers by initial screening were emulsified with nutrient broth to adjust the inoculum density equal to that of 0.5 Mac Farland turbidity standards. Combination Disk test (CDT), as recommended by the CLSI, was performed in all isolates presumed to be ESBL producers. In this test, Ceftazidime (30 μg) disks alone and in combination with clavulanic acid (Ceftazidime + clavulanic Acid, 30/10 μg) disks, were applied onto a plate of Mueller Hinton Agar (MHA) which was inoculated with the test strain and then incubated in ambient air for 16-18 h of incubation at 35 ± 2 °C. Isolate that showed increase of ≥ 5 mm in the zone of inhibition of the combination discs in comparison to that of the Ceftazidime disk alone was considered an ESBL producer [16].

### Data analysis
The information regarding patient's profile and the results were entered into a computer program. Data analysis was carried out using the Statistical Package for Social Sciences [SPSS$^{TM}$] version 20.0 [IBM, Armonk, NY, USA] and presented in percentage base distribution. Data with p value of less than 0.05 (CI-95%) was regarded as significant.

### Ethical consideration
Written approval was taken from Institutional Review Committee of Manmohan Memorial Institute of Health Sciences (MMIHS) after submitting and presenting research proposal. Written informed consent was taken from every patient or their guardians before enrollment into the study.

## Results
### Patient demographics
During the study period, a total of 5,484 representative specimens of urinary tract from pediatric patients suspected with urinary tract infections were processed. Among total clinical specimens, 1079 (19.68%) were found with growth of at least one significant pathogen confirming urinary tract infection (UTI). Female (659, 61.0%) were most affected group of patients in both inpatient and outpatient department ($p < 0.005$). Maximum number of cases was found in the children of age group 1 to 4 years (Table 1). *Escherichia coli* ($n$ =739, 68.5%) was the most common organism isolated from urinary tract infections in pediatric group in this study.

### Antimicrobial resistance pattern of *E. coli*
High level of drug resistance was noted in *E. coli* isolates. Among 739 *E. coli* isolated, highest resistance (87% each) were to ampicillin and cephalexin, followed by ciprofloxacin (78%), cefixime (71%) and levofloxacin (67%) respectively. Very few isolates (5%) were resistant to imipenem whereas entire strains revealed high susceptibility (100% each) towards colistin and tigecycline (Table 2).

### Multidrug resistant (MDR) and Extensive drug resistant (XDR) isolates
Among total 739 *E. coli* isolates subjected for antimicrobial susceptibility testing, 480 (64.9%) isolates were found multidrug resistant (MDR) and 37 (5.0%) isolates were extensive drug resistant (XDR). MDR isolates were resistant to ampicillin (100%), amoxicillin clavulanate (84.7%), cephalexin (81.6%) and ciprofloxacin (80.6%) respectively. However, MDR isolates were susceptible towards amikacin (87%), imipenem (92%) and piperacillin tazobactam (81%). Although the number of XDR isolates was low, they were completely resistant to all antibiotics except colistin and tigecycline (Table 2).

**Table 1** Pediatric patients with Urinary tract infections ($N = 1079$)

| Patients with Urinary tract infections | | | | | | | |
|---|---|---|---|---|---|---|---|
| Age Group | Male (%) | Female (%) | p | Outpatient (%) | Inpatient (%) | p | Cc |
| <1 | 87 | 129 | 0.352 | 54 | 162 | 0.001 | 0.014 |
| 1 to 4 | 129 | 141 | 0.001 | 119 | 151 | 0.004 | 0.104 |
| 5 to 9 | 118 | 238 | 0.004 | 248 | 108 | 0.007 | 0.083 |
| 10 to 14 | 86 | 151 | 0.193 | 151 | 86 | 0.001 | 0.029 |
| Total | 420 | 659 | | 572 | 507 | | |

Cc Contingency coefficient

**Table 2** Antibiotic susceptibility of MDR, XDR and ESBL *E coli* isolates

| Antibiotics | No. of resistant isolates (%) | | | |
|---|---|---|---|---|
| | Total isolates (%) | MDR (n = 480)% | XDR (n = 37)% | ESBL (n = 288)% |
| Ampicillin | 645(87) | 480(100) | 37(100) | 288(100) |
| Amoxicillin-clavulanate | 355(48) | 407(84.7) | 37(100) | 288(100) |
| Piperacillin-tazobactam | 244(33) | 91(19) | 37(100) | 78(27) |
| Cephalexin | 645(87) | 392(81.6) | 37(100) | 265(92) |
| Cefixime | 525(71) | 312(65) | 37(100) | 288(100) |
| Ceftazidime | 333(45) | 306(64) | 37(100) | 288(100) |
| Ceftriaxone | 333(45) | 306(64) | 37(100) | 288(100) |
| Aztreonam | 318(43) | 294(61) | 37(100) | 288(100) |
| Imipenem | 37(5) | 37(8) | 37(100) | 28(10) |
| Gentamycin | 244(33) | 130(27) | 37(100) | 118(41) |
| Amikacin | 103(14) | 64(13) | 37(100) | 52(18) |
| Ciprofloxacin | 576(78) | 387(80.6) | 37(100) | 225(78) |
| Levofloxacin | 495(67) | 245(51) | 37(100) | 155(54) |
| Cotrimoxazole | 310(42) | 158(33) | 37(100) | 141(49) |
| Tigecycline | 0(0) | 0(0) | 0(0) | 0(0) |
| Colistin | 0(0) | 0(0) | 0(0) | 0(0) |

### ESBL *E coli* and their susceptibility pattern

Extended spectrum beta lactamase (ESBL) enzyme was detected in 288(38.9%) *E. coli* isolates. Penicillins, cephalosporins and monobactam group of antibiotics were appeared completely ineffective (100% resistance) against ESBL producers. However, ESBL producing *E coli* strains were susceptible to reserve class of antibiotics including imipenem (90%), colistin (100%) and tigecycline (100%) (Table 2).

### Discussion

To the best of our knowledge, this report represents the first description of ESBL producing uropathogenic *E. coli* involved in pediatric cases of urinary tract infections from our country, Nepal. Urinary tract infections are the most common infections in children and *E. coli* being leading pathogenic agent in these infections; it was our matter of interest. There was no previous report before this study to estimate the most common pathogen and its resistant pattern in pediatrics patients with urinary tract infection in our hospital.

The incidence of urinary tract infection based on significant bacterial growth among pediatric patients in this study was 19.6% and *E. coli* (68.5%) was the predominant pathogen. Similar rates have been previously reported from nearby hospitals [11, 12] and from studies of other countries [18–22]. Concurrently, significantly more females (61.0%) were found with UTI corroborating with other similar studies [12, 19, 20]. In our study, children of age group 1-4 years were found with highest number of UTI cases (contingency coefficient 0.104). Similar study

from nearby hospital also reported that children less than six years of age were found UTI prone [11]. Urinary tract infection was significantly more prevalent in the female children of age group 1-4 and 5-9 years and also, more inpatients were found with UTI ($p < 0.05$). The higher rates of UTI in this age group might be due to immune status, sanitation, and ascending infection with fecal flora.

The high prevalence of ESBL-producing uropathogenic *E. coli* (38.9%) among children is reported in this study. In addition, this study also documents the enhanced resistance of ESBL producing *E. coli* to other antimicrobial groups like aminoglycosides and fluoroquinolones. Indeed, variations in the prevalence rates of ESBL-producing *E. coli* isolates in children around the globe and even among different hospitals within a country have been reported. Our prevalence rate of ESBL producing *E coli* (38.9%) is close to the findings reported by other studies in different parts of Asian region including Shettigar et al. (37.7%) from India [22], Pourakbari et al. (37%) and Rezai et al. (30.5%) from Iran [21, 23], Moore et al. (44%) from Cambodia [19] and Kizilca et al. (41.4%) from Turkey [24]. Extremely higher rates of ESBL *E coli* have also been reported, notably by Chinnasami et al. (83%) from India [25], Masud et al. (53.8%) from Bangladesh [20] and Shah et al. (50.9%) from Pakistan [18]. The increased rate of ESBL-producing bacteria causing infection in community as well as hospital settings constitutes an undeniable trend. Worldwide, pediatric UTIs due to ESBL-producing bacteria are an important part of this problem because they limit therapeutic choices and increases morbidity of infection [26]. However, lower rates of ESBL-producing *E.*

*coli* were also reported, particularly from developed countries including 9.3% from USA [27], 10.2% from Korea [28], 14% from Taiwan [26], 14.1% from Lebanon [5] and 20.2% from Turkey [29]. These variations in the rate of ESBL producing strains of *E coli* among UTI cases might be attributable to the geographical difference, local antibiotic prescribing policy, the extensive use of broad spectrum antibiotics especially third generation cephalosporins and endemicity of drug resistance pathogens in the locality.

ESBL producing bacteria causing infections in children may have various complications and adverse outcomes [30]. ESBL producers are non susceptible to aminopenicillins and ureidopenicillins as well as extended-spectrum β-lactam agents like second- and third-generation cephalosporins. Use of these agents as the first choice for the treatment of urinary tract infections may lead to the inappropriate treatment and predispose to long term renal complications [24]. Therefore, antimicrobial therapy in infections with ESBL producing organism is really challenging. Published reports showed that ESBL- producing strains causing UTI in children associated with prior hospitalization, beta-lactam therapy, catheterization, underlying co-morbidity and infancy [24].

In this study, multidrug resistant (MDR) and extensively drug resistant *E coli* were found 64.9% and 5.0% respectively. Increasing pattern of resistance of urinary tract pathogens against common antibiotics in Nepal have also been reported by other researchers [12, 31] but MDR rates and drug resistance pattern among pediatric isolates from Nepal was not available. It is observed that ampicillin, cephalexin, ciprofloxacin and cefixime were poorly effective against uropathogenic *E coli*. Only 13% of the isolates were found susceptible to all the antibiotics tested. Cephalosporin, the commonly prescribed antibiotic as empirical therapy in pediatric and adults, resistance to this group of antibiotics was found high. Almost 45% of *E coli* isolates were resistant to at least one cephalosporin and monobactam. Similar rates of antimicrobial resistance was documented in the study from Bangladesh [20], Iran [32] and India [14]. However, compared to previous reports from Nepal, we observed a considerable increase in resistance against penicillins, aminoglycosides, quinolones and ceftriaxone [12, 31]. Lower rates of resistance among the pediatric isolates causing UTI have been documented in western countries [33].

Higher resistance to penicillins third generation cephalosporins in this study has been attributable to ESBL production among gram negative isolates. In ESBL producing isolates, augumentins (combined with beta lactamase inhibitor) such as amoxicillin clavulanate or piperacillin tazobactam can be used as alternative antimicrobials [34]. However, in this study, alarming state of resistance was observed among ESBL producers towards amoxicillin clavulanate (100%) and piperacillin tazobactam (27%). In the case when UTI is caused by an ESBL producing bacteria in children, the broadest-spectrum antibiotic agents such as carbapenems are recommended [35] but they are only useful in hospitalized patients. In this study, too, carbapenems were found effective to the ESBL isolates. Nevertheless, for pediatric UTIs in our setting, cotrimoxazole, amoxicillin clavulanate, ciprofloxacin and amikacin can still be used as first line therapy. Furthermore, other non carbapenem groups of antibiotics in UTIs due to ESBL-producing strains have also been described [36, 37]. ESBL stable cephamycins, fosfomycin and nitrofurantoin were shown effective for UTIs caused by ESBL-producing strains but their clinical utility as monotherapy is controversial [38–40]. In addition, ESBLs usually confer resistance to other classes of antibiotics, such as quinolones and trimethoprim/sulfamethoxazole, therefore susceptibility testing of these agents is important [23]. In this study, entire MDR isolates were resistant to ampicillin and 33% isolates were resistant to cotrimoxazole, 19% to piperacillin tazobactam and 8% to imipenem whereas no isolates were found to be resistant to colistin and tigecycline. Similarly, all XDR isolates were resistant to most of the antimicrobials tested whereas colistin and tigecycline were the most effective regimens against XDR isolates. Similar rate of resistance has been documented by Ansari et al. [41] but their study included *E coli* isolates from all age groups.

The level of drug resistance in uropathogenic *E coli* among pediatric patient in this study is a serious issue. Previous reports have suggested that higher resistance is likely to be occurring in the communities with higher proportion of young children and high antibiotic consumption [42]. In Nepal, higher antimicrobial pressure for community infections and inappropriate therapeutic guidelines for pediatric patients might be attributable to this menacing scenario [12, 31]. Resistance to the broad spectrum cephalosporins, fluoroquinolones and aminoglycosides among the ESBL producing *E.coli* isolates in this study necessitates the use of carbapenem as alternative choice for pediatric UTIs. Although we found carbapenems as the most effective agent against the ESBL but the high rate of resistance from similar studies is of special concern [41]. Furthermore, the genes associated with antibiotic resistance usually reside in plasmid and may transfer antibiotic resistance to other wild strains of bacteria [20]. Therefore, evidence based therapy with broad spectrum antibiotics for serious or critical cases to prevent bacterial resistance is extremely needful. Aminoglycosides, amoxicillin clavulanate and trimethoprim sulfamethoxazole/cotrimoxazole would be useful alternatives as empirical antibiotics for children suspected with UTIs in our scenario.

## Limitations of the study

This study has a number of limitations. We could not evaluate the risk factors and outcome of pediatric UTI cases in our setting. Further cohort studies with antimicrobial therapy and outcome would generate more significant results. Antimicrobial susceptibility testing by dilution methods and determination of minimum inhibitory concentration (MIC) of therapeutic antibiotics would be helpful for treatment and monitoring of the drug resistant infections. Due to unavailability of resources, we could not detect the genotype of ESBLs among E coli isolates. Further investigations with larger patient population and multiple centers would generate more significant ideas.

## Conclusion

We found the menacing state of drug resistance in almost all of the E coli isolates included in this study. Childhood UTIs caused by ESBL-producing E. coli has been emerged as a serious problem in our setting. Aminoglycosides and carbapenems can be used as alternative regimens for serious infections caused by MDR E coli. Furthermore, it is extremely necessary to formulate a strict antibiotics prescription policy and prudent use antibiotics in our country.

### Abbreviation

ASM: American Society for Microbiology; ATCC: American Type Culture Collection; CDT: Combined Disk Test; CLSI: Clinical and Laboratory Standard Institute; E coli: Escherichia coli; ESBL: Extended spectrum beta-lactamases; MDR: Multidrug resistant; MHA: Mueller Hinton Agar; MIC: Minimum inhibitory concentration; UTI: Urinary tract infection; XDR: Extensive drug resistant

### Acknowledgements

We are deeply thankful to all the patients participating in this study. Our special thanks go to all the laboratory staffs, management and officials of Manmohan Memorial Teaching Hospital Kathmandu for providing the opportunity to carry out this research work.

### Funding

No monetary funding support has been received for this study.

### Authors' contributions

NPP conceived the design of the study, reviewed the literature and performed the laboratory investigations. PM, HP and GJ performed the laboratory tests and helped in manuscript preparation. SS identified the clinical cases, DP and PRK guided the necessary laboratory tests. NPP prepared the manuscript with the guidance of PRK. All authors read the manuscript and approved.

### Competing interests

The authors declare that they have no competing interests.
Nepal. Letter of approval (Ref No: 005/MMIHS/2071) was obtained after submitting and presenting the proposal to the committee. Informed consent was taken from the patients or their parents before participating to the study. Data regarding personal information and infectious disease were coded and kept confidential.

### Author details

[1]Department of Clinical Laboratory Services, Manmohan Memorial Medical College and Teaching Hospital, P.O.B.: 15201Swayambhu, Kathmandu, Nepal. [2]Department of Pediatrics, Manmohan Memorial Medical College and Teaching Hospital, Kathmandu, Nepal. [3]Department of Laboratory Medicine, Manmohan Memorial Institute of Health Sciences, Kathmandu, Nepal.

### References

1. Zorc JJ, Kiddoo DA, Shaw KN. Diagnosis and management of pediatric urinary tract infections. Clin Microbiol Rev. 2005;18(2):417–22.
2. Desai DJ, Gilbert B, McBride CA. Paediatric urinary tract infections: Diagnosis and treatment. Aust Fam Physician. 2016;45(8):558–63.
3. Robinson JL, Le Saux N. Management of urinary tract infections in children in an era of increasing antimicrobial resistance. Expert Rev Anti Infect Ther. 2016;14(9):809–16.
4. Hay AD, Sterne JA, Hood K, Little P, Delaney B, Hollingworth W, Wootton M, Howe R, MacGowan A, Lawton M, et al. Improving the Diagnosis and Treatment of Urinary Tract Infection in Young Children in Primary Care: Results from the DUTY Prospective Diagnostic Cohort Study. Ann Fam Med. 2016;14(4):325–36.
5. Hanna-Wakim RH, Ghanem ST, El Helou MW, Khafaja SA, Shaker RA, Hassan SA, Saad RK, Hedari CP, Khinkarly RW, Hajar FM, et al. Epidemiology and characteristics of urinary tract infections in children and adolescents. Front Cell Infect Microbiol. 2015;5:45.
6. Paterson DL, Bonomo RA. Extended-spectrum beta-lactamases: a clinical update. Clin Microbiol Rev. 2005;18(4):657–86.
7. Livermore DM. Current epidemiology and growing resistance of gram-negative pathogens. Korean J Intern Med. 2012;27(2):128–42.
8. Bradford PA. Extended-spectrum beta-lactamases in the 21st century: characterization, epidemiology, and detection of this important resistance threat. Clin Microbiol Rev. 2001;14(4):933–51. table of contents.
9. Sedighi I, Arabestani MR, Rahimbakhsh A, Karimitabar Z, Alikhani MY. Dissemination of extended-spectrum beta-lactamases and quinolone resistance genes among clinical isolates of uropathogenic escherichia coli in children. Jundishapur J Microbiol. 2015;8(7):e19184.
10. Uyar Aksu N, Ekinci Z, Dundar D, Baydemir C. Childhood urinary tract infections caused by ESBL-producing bacteria: Risk factors and empiric therapy. Pediatr Int. 2016. 0.1111/ped.13112. (Epub ahead of print).
11. Rai GK, Upreti HC, Rai SK, Shah KP, Shrestha RM. Causative agents of urinary tract infections in children and their antibiotic sensitivity pattern: a hospital based study. Nepal Med Coll J. 2008;10(2):86–90.
12. Singh SD, Madhup SK. Clinical profile and antibiotics sensitivity in childhood urinary tract infection at Dhulikhel Hospital. KUMJ. 2013;11(44):319–24.
13. Flokas ME, Detsis M, Alevizakos M, Mylonakis E. Prevalence of ESBL-producing Enterobacteriaceae in paediatric urinary tract infections: A systematic review and meta-analysis. J Infect. 2016;73(6):547–57.
14. Sharma S, Kaur N, Malhotra S, Madan P, Ahmad W, Hans C. Serotyping and antimicrobial susceptibility pattern of escherichia coli isolates from urinary tract infections in pediatric population in a tertiary care hospital. J Pathog. 2016;2016:2548517.
15. Isenberg HD. Clinical Microbiology Procedures Handbook. 2nd edition. Washington DC: ASM press; 2004.
16. Performance Standards for Antimicrobial Disk Susceptibility Tests.2012. Clinical and Laboratory Standards Institute. 2012, M02-A11 (Approved Standard—Eleventh Edition).
17. Magiorakos AP, Srinivasan A, Carey RB, Carmeli Y, Falagas ME, Giske CG, Harbarth S, Hindler JF, Kahlmeter G, Olsson-Liljequist B, et al. Multidrug-resistant, extensively drug-resistant and pandrug-resistant bacteria: an international expert proposal for interim standard definitions for acquired resistance. Clin Microbiol Infect. 2012;18(3):268–81.
18. Shah Samin Ullah AAG. Islam Rehman Gohar: etiology and antibiotic resistance pattern of community-acquired urinary tract infections in children. KJMS. 2015;8(3):428.
19. Moore CE, Sona S, Poda S, Putchhat H, Kumar V, Sopheary S, Stoesser N, Bousfield R, Day N, Parry CM. Antimicrobial susceptibility of uropathogens isolated from Cambodian children. Paediatr Int Child Health. 2016:1–5. [Epub ahead of print].
20. Masud MR, Afroz H, Fakruddin M. Prevalence of extended-spectrum beta-lactamase positive bacteria in radiologically positive urinary tract infection. Springer Plus. 2014;3:216.

21. Pourakbari B, Ferdosian F, Mahmoudi S, Teymuri M, Sabouni F, Heydari H, Ashtiani MT, Mamishi S. Increase resistant rates and ESBL production between E. coli isolates causing urinary tract infection in young patients from Iran. Braz J Microbiol. 2012;43(2):766–9.

22. Shettigar SCG, Roche R, Nayak N, Anitha KB, Soans S. Bacteriological profile, antibiotic sensitivity pattern, and detection of extended-spectrum β-lactamase in the isolates of urinary tract infection from children. J Child Health. 2016;3(1):5.

23. Rezai MS, Salehifar E, Rafiei A, Langaee T: Characterization of Multidrug Resistant Extended-Spectrum Beta-Lactamase-Producing Escherichia coli among Uropathogens of Pediatrics in North of Iran. 2015, 2015:309478

24. Kizilca O, Siraneci R, Yilmaz A, Hatipoglu N, Ozturk E, Kiyak A, Ozkok D. Risk factors for community-acquired urinary tract infection caused by ESBL-producing bacteria in children. Pediatr Int. 2012;54(6):858–62.

25. Balaji Chinnasami SS. Kanimozhi Sadasivam, Sekar Pasupathy Pathogens Causing Urinary Tract Infection in Children and their in vitro Susceptibility to Antimicrobial Agents- A Hospital Based Study. Biomed Pharmacol J. 2016;9(1):7.

26. Wu CT, Lee HY, Chen CL, Tuan PL, Chiu CH. High prevalence and antimicrobial resistance of urinary tract infection isolates in febrile young children without localizing signs in Taiwan. J Microbiol Immunol Infect=Wei mian yu gan ran za zhi. 2016;49(2):243–8.

27. Degnan LA, Milstone AM, Diener-West M, Lee CK. Extended-spectrum beta-lactamase bacteria from urine isolates in children. J Pediatr Pharmacol Ther. 2015;20(5):373–7.

28. Han SB, Lee SC, Lee SY, Jeong DC, Kang JH. Aminoglycoside therapy for childhood urinary tract infection due to extended-spectrum beta-lactamase-producing Escherichia coli or Klebsiella pneumoniae. BMC Infect Dis. 2015;15:414.

29. Dotis J, Printza N, Marneri A, Gidaris D, Papachristou F. Urinary tract infections caused by extended-spectrum betalactamase-producing bacteria in children: a matched casecontrol study. Turk J Pediatr. 2013;55(6):571–4.

30. Lee B, Kang SY, Kang HM, Yang NR, Kang HG, Ha IS, Cheong HI, Lee HJ, Choi EH. Outcome of antimicrobial therapy of pediatric urinary tract infections caused by extended-spectrum beta-lactamase-producing enterobacteriaceae. Infect Chemother. 2013;45(4):415–21.

31. Sharma A, Shrestha S, Upadhyay S, Rijal P. Clinical and bacteriological profile of urinary tract infection in children at Nepal Medical College Teaching Hospital. Nepal Med Coll J. 2011;13(1):24–6.

32. Mirsoleymani SR, Salimi M, Shareghi Brojeni M, Ranjbar M, Mehtarpoor M. Bacterial pathogens and antimicrobial resistance patterns in pediatric urinary tract infections: a four-year surveillance study (2009-2012). Int J Pediatr. 2014;2014:126142.

33. Stultz JS, Doern CD, Godbout E. Antibiotic resistance in pediatric urinary tract infections. Curr Infect Dis Rep. 2016;18(12):40.

34. Ramphal R, Ambrose PG. Extended-spectrum beta-lactamases and clinical outcomes: current data. Clin Infect Dis. 2006;42 Suppl 4:S164–172.

35. Dalgic N, Sancar M, Bayraktar B, Dincer E, Pelit S. Ertapenem for the treatment of urinary tract infections caused by extended-spectrum beta-lactamase-producing bacteria in children. Scand J Infect Dis. 2011;43(5):339–43.

36. Park SH, Choi SM, Chang YK, Lee DG, Cho SY, Lee HJ, Choi JH, Yoo JH. The efficacy of non-carbapenem antibiotics for the treatment of community-onset acute pyelonephritis due to extended-spectrum beta-lactamase-producing Escherichia coli. J Antimicrob Chemother. 2014;69(10):2848–56.

37. Asakura T, Ikeda M, Nakamura A, Kodera S. Efficacy of empirical therapy with non-carbapenems for urinary tract infections with extended-spectrum beta-lactamase-producing Enterobacteriaceae. Int J Infect Dis. 2014;29:91–5.

38. Tasbakan MI, Pullukcu H, Sipahi OR, Yamazhan T, Ulusoy S. Nitrofurantoin in the treatment of extended-spectrum beta-lactamase-producing Escherichia coli-related lower urinary tract infection. Int J Antimicrob Agents. 2012;40(6):554–6.

39. Veve MP, Wagner JL, Kenney RM, Grunwald JL, Davis SL. Comparison of fosfomycin to ertapenem for outpatient or step-down therapy of extended-spectrum beta-lactamase urinary tract infections. Int J Antimicrob Agents. 2016;48(1):56–60.

40. Lepeule R, Ruppe E, Le P, Massias L, Chau F, Nucci A, Lefort A, Fantin B. Cefoxitin as an alternative to carbapenems in a murine model of urinary tract infection due to Escherichia coli harboring CTX-M-15-type extended-spectrum beta-lactamase. Antimicrob Agents Chemother. 2012;56(3):1376–81.

41. Ansari S, Nepal HP, Gautam R, Shrestha S, Neopane P, Gurung G, Chapagain ML. Community acquired multi-drug resistant clinical isolates of Escherichia coli in a tertiary care center of Nepal. Antimicrob Resist Infect Control. 2015;4:15.

42. Bryce A, Hay AD, Lane IF, Thornton HV, Wootton M, Costelloe C. Global prevalence of antibiotic resistance in paediatric urinary tract infections caused by Escherichia coli and association with routine use of antibiotics in primary care: systematic review and meta-analysis. BMJ. 2016;352:i939.

# 2

# Colonization of long-term care facility residents in three Italian Provinces by multidrug-resistant bacteria

Elisabetta Nucleo[1], Mariasofia Caltagirone[1], Vittoria Mattioni Marchetti[1], Roberto D'Angelo[2], Elena Fogato[2], Massimo Confalonieri[3], Camilla Reboli[3], Albert March[4], Ferisa Sleghel[4], Gertrud Soelva[4], Elisabetta Pagani[5], Richard Aschbacher[5], Roberta Migliavacca[1*], Laura Pagani[1], AMCLI – GLISTer Group and ESCMID Study Group Elderly Infections – ESGIE

### Abstract

**Background:** Rationale and aims of the study were to compare colonization frequencies with MDR bacteria isolated from LTCF residents in three different Northern Italian regions, to investigate risk factors for colonization and the genotypic characteristics of isolates. The screening included *Enterobacteriaceae* expressing extended-spectrum β-lactamases (ESβLs) and high-level AmpC cephalosporinases, carbapenemase-producing *Enterobacteriaceae*, *Pseudomonas aeruginosa* or *Acinetobacter baumannii*, methicillin-resistant *Staphylococcus aureus* (MRSA) and vancomycin-resistant enterococci (VRE).

**Methods:** Urine samples and rectal, inguinal, oropharyngeal and nasal swabs were plated on selective agar; resistance genes were sought by PCR and sequencing. Demographic and clinical data were collected.

**Results:** Among the LTCF residents, 75.0% (78/104), 69.4% (84/121) and 66.1% (76/115) were colonized with at least one of the target organisms in LTCFs located in Milan, Piacenza and Bolzano, respectively. ESβL producers (60.5, 66.1 and 53.0%) were highly predominant, mainly belonging to *Escherichia coli* expressing CTX-M group-1 enzymes. Carbapenemase-producing enterobacteria were found in 7.6, 0.0 and 1.6% of residents; carbapemenase-producing *P. aeruginosa* and *A. baumannii* were also detected. Colonization by MRSA (24.0, 5.7 and 14.8%) and VRE (20.2, 0.8 and 0.8%) was highly variable. Several risk factors for colonization by ESβL-producing *Enterobacteriaceae* and MRSA were found and compared among LTCFs in the three Provinces. Colonization differences among the enrolled LTCFs can be partially explained by variation in risk factors, resident populations and staff/resident ratios, applied hygiene measures and especially the local antibiotic resistance epidemiology.

**Conclusions:** The widespread diffusion of MDR bacteria in LTCFs within three Italian Provinces confirms that LTCFs are an important reservoir of MDR organisms in Italy and suggests that future efforts should focus on MDR screening, improved implementation of infection control strategies and antibiotic stewardship programs targeting the complex aspects of LTCFs.

**Keywords:** Long-term care facilities, Multicenter study, ESβL, AmpC, Carbapenemases, MRSA, VRE

* Correspondence: roberta.migliavacca@unipv.it; r.miglia@unipv.it
[1]Department of Clinical Surgical Diagnostic and Pediatric Sciences, Laboratory of Microbiology and Clinical Microbiology, University of Pavia, Via Brambilla 74, 27100 Pavia, Italy
Full list of author information is available at the end of the article

# Background

Life expectancy in Italy is rapidly increasing, with present values of 80.1 years for males and 84.7 for females [1]. Due to the ageing population, long-term care facilities (LTCFs), which provide ongoing skilled nursing care to residents and help meet both the medical and non-medical needs of elderly individuals with a chronic illness or disability, play an important role in the Italian healthcare system. Residents in LTCFs have a variety of risk factors for colonization with multidrug-resistant (MDR) bacteria; therefore, these facilities represent reservoirs of: i) *Enterobacteriaceae* expressing extended-spectrum β-lactamases (ESβLs), derepressed/acquired high-level AmpC cephalosporinases or carbapenemases, ii) *Pseudomonas aeruginosa* or *Acinetobacter baumannii* producing carbapenemases and iii) methicillin-resistant *Staphylococcus aureus* (MRSA) and vancomycin-resistant enterococci (VRE) [2–4].

To promote detailed studies of various microbiological aspects related to LTCFs in Italy, the Association of Italian Clinical Microbiologists (Associazione Microbiologi Clinici Italiani; AMCLI) in 2016 has set up a new working group consisting of Clinical Microbiologists (Gruppo di Lavoro per lo Studio delle Infezioni nelle Residenze Sanitarie Assistite e Strutture assimilabili; *GLISTer*); one of the main objectives of this working group is the study of the distribution and prevalence of MDR organisms in Italian LTCFs and therefore a multicenter point-prevalence survey, including the main MDR bacteria as described above, was performed in 2016 on residents of LTCFs, located in three Northern Italian cities.

# Methods

## The aim

Rationale and aims of the study were to compare colonization frequencies with MDR bacteria of LTCF residents in three different Northern Italian cities, located in different Italian regions, and to investigate their genotypic characteristics. Moreover, risk factors for colonization were compared between LTCFs and colonization prevalence was correlated with the local epidemiology of invasive MDR isolates.

## Facilities, patient characteristics and survey design

In October–November 2016, a multicenter point-prevalence screening study was conducted in four LTCFs concerning i) *Enterobacteriaceae* with ESβLs, carbapenemases or high-level AmpCs, ii) *P. aeruginosa* or *A. baumannii* with carbapenemases, iii) MRSA and VRE. The four facilities, located in the Northern Italian Provinces of Milan ($n = 1$), Piacenza ($n = 2$) and Bolzano ($n = 1$), offer high skilled 24 h nursing care.

Although the overall study was performed over a period of 2 months, the sampling interval in each facility lasted for a maximum of 1 week. All residents of the four LTCFs were eligible to participate, and the study was approved by the Ethics Committees of the three referring hospitals; informed written consent was obtained from the residents or, if they were unable to consent, from their relatives.

## Microbiological methods

Sample processing, microbial identification and antibiotic susceptibility testing were carried out in the clinical microbiology laboratories of the referral hospitals. Microbiological methods for the LTCF screening study in Bolzano were previously described [5]. Similar methods were used in the epidemiological studies of Milan and Piacenza LTCFs, with minor modifications.

For the screening of MDR bacteria from LTCF residents in Milan midstream or catheter urine samples were cultured on Oxoid Brilliance™ ESβL plates (Thermo Scientific, UK), applying a 10 µg imipenem (IMP) disc (Oxoid, Thermo Scientific, UK), and on Oxoid Brilliance™ VRE (Thermo Scientific, UK). Inguinal, oropharyngeal and rectal swabs were seeded on Oxoid Brilliance™ ESβL, applying a 10 µg IMP disc, on Oxoid Brilliance™ VRE and on CHROMagar™ MRSA (BD Diagnostics, MD). Nasal swabs were plated on CHROMagar™ MRSA. All plates were incubated at 35 ± 2 °C under aerobic conditions for 24–48 h. Isolate identification and antibiotic susceptibility testing were performed by the BD Phoenix™ System (BD Diagnostics, MD), according to European Committee on Antimicrobial Susceptibility Testing (EUCAST) criteria [6], using PHOENIX NMIC/ID402 for non-urinary Gram-negative bacteria, PHOENIX UNMIC/ID403 for Gram-negative isolates from urine cultures, and PHOENIX PMIC/ID88 for MRSA and VRE. The strains were phenotypically confirmed for β-lactamase production by the ESBL+AMPC Screen Kit and the KPC + MBL Confirm ID Kit (Rosco Diagnostica A/S, Denmark).

Similarly, for screening of MDR bacteria from LTCF residents in Piacenza, midstream or catheter urine samples were seeded on ChromID CPS agar (BioMèrieux, Marcy l'Etoile, France); rectal swabs on ChromID ESBL Agar (BioMèrieux, Marcy l'Etoile, France), on ChromID VRE Agar (BioMèrieux, Marcy l'Etoile, France) and on Mac Conkey agar applying a 10 µg meropenem (MER) disc (Oxoid, Thermo Scientific, UK); nasal swabs on Chapman Agar (Oxoid, Thermo Scientific, UK), on ChromID ESBL and on MacConkey agar applying a 10 µg MER disc; and inguinal swabs on Mannite salt agar (Oxoid, Thermo Scientific, UK). Plates were incubated at 35 ± 2 °C under aerobic conditions for 24–48 h. Isolate identification and antibiotic susceptibility testing were performed using the Vitek 2 System (BioMèrieux, Marcy l'Etoile, France), calibrated against EUCAST criteria [6], with AST-N202 cards (including an ESβL test) for Gram-negative bacteria, AST-P632 cards (with both oxacillin and cefoxitin) for MRSA and AST-P586 cards for VRE. Identification of β-lactamase types was based on Vitek 2 results and on the synergistic effects obtained by the ESβL+AMPC Screen Kit and the KPC + MBL Confirm ID Kit (Rosco Diagnostica A/S, Denmark). VRE were confirmed by vancomycin and teicoplanin Etest strips (BioMèrieux, Marcy l'Etoile, France).

### Molecular characterization of resistance genes

Molecular characterization of all MDR isolates was performed in a common reference laboratory, located at the University of Pavia. Total DNA was extracted by the automated Puro extraction system (DID, Milan, Italy), using the DNA tissue kit, according to manufacturer's instructions. The presence of ESβL and carbapenemase genes was investigated by PCR, targeting $bla_{CTX-M}$-, $bla_{SHV}$- $bla_{KPC}$-, $bla_{VIM}$-, $bla_{IMP}$-, $bla_{OXA-48}$-, $bla_{NDM}$- and $bla_{GES}$-type genes, and using published primers and conditions [7–15], summarized in Additional file 1: Table S1. *A. baumannii* isolates were screened for the presence of the following carbapenemase genes: $bla_{OXA-23}$-like, $bla_{OXA-24}$-like, $bla_{OXA-51}$-like and $bla_{OXA-58}$-like [16–18]. The presence of IS*Aba1* elements adjacent to $bla_{OXA-51}$-like genes was determined as previously described [19]; AmpC genes were detected by a multiplex PCR [20].

Bacterial isolates collected from the LTCF in Milan were screened for $bla_{KPC}$-, $bla_{VIM}$-, $bla_{OXA-48}$- and $bla_{NDM}$-type genes by the Cepheid GeneXpert System and confirmed by PCR. Check-MDR CT103 XL array (Check points Health B.V., Wageningen, The Netherlands) has been used to investigate the *bla* gene content of a carbapenem-resistant *P. aeruginosa* strain obtained from an oropharyngeal swab, which tested negative by previous molecular assays.

For gene sequencing, PCR products were purified using the quantum Wizard® SV Gel and PCR Clean-Up System (Promega, Madison, WT, USA) and subjected to double-strand Sanger sequencing. Sequences were analyzed according to the BLAST software [21].

### Statistical analysis

A significance level of $p \leq 0.05$ was used. In-house physicians reviewed hospital records and, using a standard questionnaire, recorded demographic and clinical data as follows: patient age, gender, length of stay, Barthel immobility score, coma, comorbidities (dementia, urinary incontinence, diabetes, cancer, vascular diseases, chronic obstructive pulmonary disease, decubitus ulcer), presence of infection, antibiotic treatment in the preceding 3 months and the presence of indwelling medical devices. The significance of differences in risk factors and colonization proportions was calculated using the proportion comparison test. Logistic regression analyses were developed to investigate colonization of at least

one site with ESβL producers and MRSA as dependent variables, first as univariate and then as multivariate models, including predictors with $p < 0.05$ in the univariate analysis, comprising the specific LTCF of residence, using stepwise logistic selection. Analysis were performed using the Medcalc® software version 15.11.4 (MedCalc software, Ostend, Belgium).

### Results

A variable percentage of LTCF residents, present during the point-prevalence survey in the four LTCFs, agreed to participate: 104/310 (34%) in Milan, 121/326 (37%) in Piacenza (2 LTCFs, with 71/216 and 50/110 participating residents, respectively), and all 115 (100%) residents in the LTCF in Bolzano; no specific LTCF resident selection criteria were used in Milan and Piacenza and resident characteristics of enrolled and not-enrolled residents were similar. The median age of LTCF residents in Milan, Piacenza and Bolzano was 82 years (range: 65–96 years), 86 years (range: 63–102 years) and 77 years (range: 30–94 years) for males, and 90 years (range: 71–102 years), 88 years (69–105 years) and 84 years (24–96 years) for females, respectively. The median length of stay of residents in the LTCFs in Milan, Piacenza and Bolzano was 23 months (range: 1–199 months), 34 months (range: 1–172 months) and 19 months (range: 1–174 months), respectively. Various healthcare staff/resident ratios were found in the LTCFs in Milan (ratio: 0.62; 193/310), Piacenza (ratio: 0.61; 201/326; corresponding to 73/110 and 128/216 in the two enrolled LTCFs, respectively) and Bolzano (ratio: 0.79; 91/115). Demographic and clinical details of the enrolled LTCF residents are summarized in Table 1.

Isolation frequencies and molecular characterization of the antibiotic resistance determinants are shown in Table 2. A high percentage of LTCF residents were colonized with at least one of the target MDR organisms in Milan (75.0%; 78/104), Piacenza (69.4%; 84/121) and Bolzano (66.1%; 76/115); moreover, many residents from Milan (37.5%; 39/104), Piacenza (19.8%; 24/121) and Bolzano (30.4%; 35/115) were colonized with more than one MDR organism.

ESβL-producing *E. coli* expressing $bla_{CTX-M}$-like genes were highly predominant in Milan (80.4%), Piacenza (97.0%) and Bolzano (80.3%) and CTX-M-type determinants were also identified in *Proteus mirabilis*, *Klebsiella pneumoniae*, *Citrobacter koseri*, *Enterobacter cloacae complex* and *Serratia marcescens*. Most $bla_{CTX-M}$- genes belonged to group-1 (72.4%), followed by group-9 (14.8%) and other groups (12.8%). A $bla_{BEL}$-like gene was detected in a *P. aeruginosa* strain from the LTCF in Milan.

In total, ten carbapenemase-producing *Enterobacteriaceae* were detected: $n = 7$ KPC-producing *K. pneumoniae* and $n = 1$ VIM-1-producing *E. cloacae*

**Table 1** Demographic and clinical details of LTCF residents from three Italian Provinces

| | Milan (M), % (n = 104) | Piacenza (P), % (n = 121) | Bolzano (B), % (n = 115) | Significant differences (p-value) |
|---|---|---|---|---|
| Male sex | 30.7 | 26.4 | 43.4 | M vs. B (0.05); P vs. B (0.006) |
| Age ≥ 86 years | 58.7 | 60.3 | 35.6 | M vs. B (< 0.001); P vs. B (< 0.001) |
| Antibiotics in preceding 3 months | 24.0 | 50.4 | 23.4 | M vs. P (< 0.001); P vs. B (< 0.001) |
| Fluoroquinolones | 8.6 | 7.4 | 5.2 | |
| Penicillins | 2.8 | 1.6 | 12.1 | M vs. B (0.01); P vs. B (0.001) |
| Cephalosporins | 5.7 | 24.8 | 1.7 | M vs. P (< 0.001); P vs. B (< 0.001) |
| Dementia | 42.3 | 79.3 | 68.7 | M vs. P (< 0.001); M vs. B (< 0.001) |
| Peripheral vascular disease | 59.6 | 47.1 | 71.3 | P vs. B (< 0.001) |
| Urinary incontinence | 74.0 | 84.3 | 85.2 | M vs. P (0.05); M vs. B (0.04) |
| Diabetes | 19.2 | 16.5 | 20.8 | |
| Cancer | 8.6 | 8.2 | 9.5 | |
| Decubitus ulcer | 6.7 | 5.7 | 11.3 | |
| Chronic obstructive pulmonary disease | 11.5 | 9.1 | 18.2 | P vs. B (0.04) |
| Physical disability (Barthel immobility score of 0) | 10.4 | 41.3 | 67.8 | M vs. P (< 0.001); M vs. B (< 0.001); P vs. B (< 0.001) |
| Coma | 0.0 | 0.0 | 17.4 | M vs. B (< 0.001); P vs. B (< 0.001) |
| Any medical device | 10.5 | 23.9 | 38.2 | M vs. P (0.009); M vs. B (< 0.001); P vs. B (0.01) |
| Percutaneous enteral gastrostomy tube | 2.8 | 11.5 | 20.8 | M vs. P (0.01); M vs. B (< 0.001); P vs. B (0.05) |
| Tracheostomy tube | 0.0 | 1.6 | 9.5 | M vs. B (0.001); P vs. B (0.007) |
| Urinary catheter | 8.6 | 6.6 | 18.2 | M vs. B (0.04); P vs. B (0.006) |
| Nasogastric tube | 0.0 | 9.1 | 1.7 | M vs. P (0.001); P vs. B (0.01) |
| Length of stay in LTCF < 6 months | 17.7 | 8.2 | 17.3 | M vs. P (0.03); P vs. B (0.03) |
| Hospital admission in previous 12 months, any department | 22.3 | 15.8 | 38.2 | M vs. B (0.01); M vs. P (< 0.001) P vs. B (< 0.001) |
| Geriatrics | 0.0 | 1.6 | 9.5 | M vs. B (p = 0.001); P vs. B (p = 0.007) |
| Medicine | 4.8 | 5.7 | 6.0 | |
| Orthopedics | 3.8 | 3.3 | 4.3 | |
| Infection | 3.8[a] | 5.7[b] | 0.8[c] | P vs. B (0.03) |

[a]Urinary tract infection - UTI (2), respiratory tract infection - RTI (1), infected prosthesis (1)
[b]RTI (6), UTI (1), skin and soft tissue infection (1)
[c]UTI (1)

*complex* were isolated from LTCF residents in Milan, and n = 2 VIM-1 producers (one *E. coli* and one *Citrobacter amalonaticus*) from residents in Bolzano. Two carbapenemase-positive *P. aeruginosa* were isolated from LTCF residents in Piacenza: in one case a $bla_{GES-5}$ and in the other a $bla_{VIM}$-like gene were identified. Moreover, two *P. aeruginosa* isolates collected in Milan and Piacenza presented a $bla_{GES-1}$ ESβL. Nine $bla_{OXA-23}$-positive *A. baumannii* were isolated from two and seven LTCF residents in Milan and Piacenza, respectively.

MRSA strains were most frequently isolated from LTCF residents in Milan and Bolzano, whereas VRE isolates were highly prevalent in Milan (n = 21 *Enterococcus faecalis*), but rare in Piacenza (n = 1 *E. faecalis*) and Bolzano (n = 1 *Enterococcus faecium*).

Colonization of LTCF residents with ESβL-producing enterobacteria and MRSA was associated with several risk factors in univariate and multivariate analysis (Table 3). In multivariate analysis, the LTCF of residence was an independent risk factor for ESβL ($p \leq 0.03$ for all comparisons, except $p = 0.53$ for the comparison of Milan vs. Piacenza) and MRSA ($p \leq 0.02$ for all comparisons) colonization. Risk factors for MRSA colonization were also associated with resident's gender; for the following risk factors significant differences between male (n = 226) and female (n = 114) residents were found: age > 85 years (M: 34.5%; F: 20.4%; $p < 0.001$), hospitalization within the previous 12 months (M: 35.0%; F: 20.4%; $p = 0.03$), administration of any antibiotic within the previous 3 months (M: 40.3%; F: 29.6%; $p = 0.04$) and coma (M: 10.5%; F: 3.5%; $p = 0.009$).

**Table 2** Colonization percentages in residents from LTCFs of three Italian Provinces

| | % of LTCF residents colonized with specific resistance phenotype and genotype and significant differences ($p \leq 0.05$) | | | |
| --- | --- | --- | --- | --- |
| | Milan (*n* = 104) | Piacenza (*n* = 121) | Bolzano (*n* = 115) | Significant differences ($p \leq 0.05$) |
| All resistance groups (MRSA; VRE; ESβL-/AmpC-producing enterobacteria; carbapenemase-producing enterobacteria, *Pseudomonas aeruginosa* and *Acinetobacter baumannii*) | 75.0 | 69.4 | 66.1 | |
| All ESβL-positive enterobacteria | 60.5 | 66.1 | 53.0 | P vs. B (0.04) |
| *Escherichia coli*, ESβL-positive | 48.0 | 55.3 | 45.2 | |
| *bla*CTX-M-group-1 | 33.6 | 41.3 | 28.7 | P vs. B (0.04) |
| *bla*CTX-M-group-9 | 6.7 | 5.7 | 9.5 | |
| *bla*CTX-M-group, other than 1 or 9 | 4.8 | 9.9 | 0.0 | P vs. B (< 0.001) |
| *Proteus mirabilis*, ESβL-positive | 14.4 | 9.1 | 7.0 | |
| *bla*CTX-M-group-1 | 3.8 | 4.1 | 0.0 | M vs. B (0.04); P vs. B (0.03) |
| *bla*CTX-M-group-9 | 1.9 | 0.0 | 0.0 | |
| *Klebsiella pneumoniae*, ESBL-positive | 6.7 | 5.7 | 6.1 | |
| *bla*CTX-M-group-1 | 5.7 | 4.1 | 1.7 | |
| *bla*CTX-M-group-9 | 0.9 | 0.8 | 0.0 | |
| *bla*CTX-M-group, other than 1 or 9 | 0.0 | 0.0 | 2.7 | |
| *Morganella morganii*, ESβL-positive | 1.9 | 1.6 | 2.6 | |
| *Citrobacter koseri*, ESβL-positive | 0.0 | 3.3 | 0.8 | |
| *bla*CTX-M-group other than 1 or 9 | 0.0 | 3.3 | 0.0 | |
| *Enterobacter cloacae complex*, ESβL-positive | 0.9 | 0.8 | 0.0 | |
| *bla*CTX-M-group-1 | 0.0 | 0.8 | 0.0 | |
| *bla*CTX-M-group other than 1 or 9 | 0.9 | 0.0 | 0.0 | |
| *Serratia marcescens*, ESβL-positive | 0.0 | 0.8 | 0.0 | |
| *bla*CTX-M-group-1, *bla*CTX-M-15-like | 0.0 | 0.8 | 0.0 | |
| *Providencia stuartii* | 1.9 | 0.0 | 0.0 | |
| All high-level AmpC-positive enterobacteria | 5.7 | 3.3 | 25.2 | M vs. B (< 0.001); P vs. B (< 0.001) |
| *Enterobacter cloacae complex*, high-level AmpC | 0.0 | 0.8 | 0.0 | |
| *Morganella morganii*, high-level AmpC | 3.8 | 0.8 | 24.3 | M vs. B (< 0.001); P vs. B (< 0.001) |
| *bla*DHA-type | 3.8 | 0.8 | 8.7 | P vs. B (0.004) |
| *Citrobacter freundii*, high-level AmpC | 0.0 | 0.8 | 0.0 | |
| *Proteus mirabilis*, high-level AmpC | 1.9 | 0.0 | 0.8 | |
| *bla*CMY-type | 0.0 | 0.0 | 0.8 | |
| *Serratia marcescens*, high-level AmpC | 0.0 | 0.8 | 0.0 | |
| *Providencia rustigianii*, high-level AmpC | 0.9 | 0.0 | 0.0 | |
| All carbapenemase-positive enterobacteria | 7.6 | 0.0 | 1.6 | M vs. P (0.002); M vs. B (0.03) |
| *Klebsiella pneumoniae*, *bla*KPC-type | 6.7 | 0.0 | 0.0 | M vs. P (0.004); M vs. B (0.05) |
| *Escherichia coli*, *bla*VIM-1 | 0.0 | 0.0 | 0.8 | |
| *Enterobacter cloacae complex*, *bla*VIM-1 | 0.9 | 0.0 | 0.0 | |
| *Citrobacter amalonaticus*, *bla*VIM-1 | 0.0 | 0.0 | 0.8 | |
| Carbapenemase-positive *Pseudomonas aeruginosa* | 0.0 | 1.6 | 0.0 | |
| *bla*VIM-type | 0.0 | 0.8 | 0.0 | |
| *bla*GES-5 | 0.0 | 0.8 | 0.0 | |
| Carbapenemase-positive *Acinetobacter baumannii* | 1.9 | 5.8 | 0.0 | P vs. B (0.009) |
| *bla*OXA-23-like | 1.9 | 5.8 | 0.0 | P vs. B (0.009) |

**Table 2** Colonization percentages in residents from LTCFs of three Italian Provinces *(Continued)*

|  | % of LTCF residents colonized with specific resistance phenotype and genotype and significant differences ($p \leq 0.05$) | | | |
|  | Milan ($n = 104$) | Piacenza ($n = 121$) | Bolzano ($n = 115$) | Significant differences ($p \leq 0.05$) |
|---|---|---|---|---|
| MRSA | 24.0 | 5.7 | 14.8 | M vs. P ($< 0.001$); P vs. B (0.02) |
| VRE | 20.2[a] | 0.8[a] | 0.8[b] | M vs. P ($< 0.001$); M vs. B ($< 0.001$) |

Notes: [a]*Enterococcus faecalis*; [b]*Enterococcus faecium*

## Discussion

The study evaluated the degree of colonization with drug-resistant bacteria among residents of LTCFs located in three Northern Italian Provinces, finding high colonization of residents in Milan (75.0%), Piacenza (69.4%) and Bolzano (66.1%). Many residents had more than one target organism, underscoring the role of LTCFs as a reservoir for these isolates [2–4].

Colonization of LTCF residents with ESβL-producing enterobacteria was highly prevalent in all the surveyed LTCFs (60.5% in Milan, 66.1% in Piacenza and 53.0% in Bolzano), and group-1 CTX-M-type enzymes were highly predominant, especially in *E. coli* (80–97% of isolates). Notably, about 82% of *K. pneumoniae* and 32% of *P. mirabilis* isolates also harbored a $bla_{CTX-M}$-type gene. In the same Bolzano LTCF, here screened for ESβL-producing enterobacteria, high colonization percentages, equal to 64.0 and 49.0%, were previously found in 2008 [22] and 2012 [23], respectively; the latter survey also screened a second LTCF in the Province of Bolzano, showing a colonization prevalence of 56.0%. In an Italian study carried out in 2006, a colonization prevalence of 54.0% was found in LTCF residents bearing a urinary catheter [24], while a more recent multicenter study, performed in 2015 and involving 12 Italian LTCFs, reported a mean ESβL colonization of 57.3% (range: 32.8–81.5%) [25]. In all these Italian studies, CTX-M enzymes were the predominantly produced ESβLs. The high ESβL colonization rates of > 50% in Italian LTCF residents are paralleled by high ESβL prevalence in invasive *E. coli* isolates [26]. Generally, ESβL carriage in most European countries is strikingly lower than that found in Italy [4], with exceptions reported from Ireland [27, 28] and Portugal [29].

In our screening study, high-level AmpC-producing *Enterobacteriaceae* were rarely isolated in LTCF residents in Milan and Piacenza, but 24.3% of LTCF residents in Bolzano were colonized by *M. morganii* expressing a high-level DHA-AmpC phenotype; $bla_{DHA}$-type genes in LTCF isolates have previously been found in a few *E. coli* and *K. pneumoniae* strains from Korea [30], but to our knowledge have not yet been reported in Italian LTCFs.

Carbapenemase-producing enterobacteria were not found in LTCF residents in Piacenza, rarely in Bolzano (1.6%) and more frequently in Milan (7.6%). As found in previous studies of carbapenemase-producing *Enterobacteriaceae* from Bolzano [22, 23, 31], the VIM-1-producing *E. coli* and *C. amalonaticus* isolates from residents in this study were also positive for $bla_{SHV-12}$. In the present study, all carbapenemase producers from Milan, except an *E. cloacae complex* isolate expressing a $bla_{VIM-1}$ gene, had KPC-type enzymes; similar results have been reported by other Italian studies in LTCF residents [25, 32, 33]. Carbapenemase-producing enterobacteria, especially KPC-producing *K. pneumoniae*, are epidemically spread in Italy [34] and the emergence of this MDR phenotype in LTCFs is worrying, expanding the reservoir of this health care threat. Nevertheless, as previously summarized [4], carbapenemase-producing *Enterobacteriaceae* are still rare in Italian LTCF residents; the reasons are probably multifactorial, comprising clinical characteristics of the enrolled residents [35] and the low carbapenem selective pressure in LTCFs. On average, only 1.1% of residents enrolled in our screening study received carbapenems within the previous 3 months (data not shown). Nevertheless, a carbapenemase-producing enterobacteria prevalence of 7.6% (mainly KPC-producing *K. pneumoniae*), reported here for the LTCF in Milan, gives rise to concern and has to be addressed by future hygiene and antibiotic stewardship measures.

This study shows the emergence of carbapenemase-producing *P. aeruginosa* in LTCF residents in Piacenza, identifying single isolates with $bla_{VIM}$-type and $bla_{GES-5}$ determinants. *P. aeruginosa* expressing $bla_{VIM}$-type determinants is widely spread in Italy [36], and an outbreak of GES-5-producing *P. aeruginosa* was reported from a LTCF in Japan [37]. Moreover, the ESβL genes $bla_{GES-1}$ and $bla_{BEL}$-like were found in two and one *P. aeruginosa* isolates, respectively; the latter rarely detected β-lactamase was previously recovered in *P. aeruginosa* strains from Belgium [18]. *A. baumannii* producing OXA-23 carbapenemases have an epidemic diffusion in Italy [38], reflected in the present study by the isolation of this resistance type from LTCF residents in Milan (1.9%) and Piacenza (5.8%).

MRSA colonization prevalence here reported ranged widely in the surveyed LTCFs (5.7, 14.8 and 24.0% in Milan, Piacenza and Bolzano, respectively), similar to other Italian studies [25, 39, 40]. Varying MRSA

**Table 3** Resident's risk factors for ESβL and MRSA colonization (cumulative data: Milan, Piacenza, Bolzano)

| | ESBL, % (n = 203) | No ESBL, % (n = 137) | Univariate analysis OR (CI 95%) | p | Multivariate analysis OR (CI 95%) | p | MRSA, % (n = 45) | No MRSA, % (n = 295) | Univariate analysis OR (CI 95%) | p | Multivariate analysis OR (CI 95%) | p |
|---|---|---|---|---|---|---|---|---|---|---|---|---|
| Male sex | 34.9 | 31.3 | 1.17 (0.74–1.86) | 0.49 | | | 51.1 | 30.8 | 2.34 (1.24–4.42) | 0.008 | 2.31 (1.16–4.59) | 0.01 |
| Age ≥ 86 years | 52.7 | 49.2 | 1.15 (0.74–1.78) | 0.53 | | | 39.0 | 53.0 | 0.56 (0.29–1.10) | 0.09 | | |
| Antibiotics in preceding 3 months | 39.9 | 23.3 | 2.17 (1.34–3.54) | 0.001 | 1.74 (1.02–2.98) | 0.04 | 37.7 | 32.5 | 1.25 (0.65–2.41) | 0.48 | | |
| Fluoroquinolones | 7.8 | 5.8 | 1.38 (0.57–3.32) | 0.47 | | | 15.5 | 5.7 | 3.01 (1.17–7.73) | 0.02 | 3.59 (1.26–10.25) | 0.01 |
| Penicillins | 7.3 | 2.9 | 2.65 (0.86–8.17) | 0.09 | | | 11.1 | 4.7 | 2.50 (0.85–7.34) | 0.09 | | |
| Cephalosporins | 14.2 | 6.5 | 2.37 (1.08–5.18) | 0.03 | | | 4.4 | 12.2 | 0.33 (0.07–1.44) | 0.14 | | |
| Dementia | 63.0 | 66.4 | 0.86 (0.54–1.36) | 0.52 | | | 62.2 | 64.7 | 0.89 (0.47–1.71) | 0.74 | | |
| Peripheral vascular disease | 62.5 | 59.1 | 1.15 (0.74–1.80) | 0.52 | | | 62.2 | 61.0 | 1.05 (0.55–2.00) | 0.87 | | |
| Urinary incontinence | 83.2 | 78.8 | 1.33 (0.77–2.31) | 0.30 | | | 82.2 | 81.3 | 1.06 (0.46–2.40) | 0.89 | | |
| Diabetes | 18.7 | 18.9 | 0.98 (0.56–1,71) | 0.30 | | | 26.6 | 17.6 | 1.69 (0.82–3.51) | 0.15 | | |
| Cancer | 11.8 | 4.3 | 2.92 (1.16–7.36) | 0.02 | 3.47 (1.32–9.16) | 0.01 | 4.4 | 9.5 | 0.44 (0.10–1.93) | 0.27 | | |
| Decubitus ulcer | 9.8 | 5.1 | 2.03 (0.83–4.94) | 0.12 | | | 6.6 | 8.1 | 0.80 (0.23–2.79) | 0.73 | | |
| Chronic obstructive pulmonary disease | 11.8 | 14.6 | 0.78 (0.41–1.48) | 0.45 | | | 15.5 | 12.5 | 1.28 (0.53–3.08) | 0.57 | | |
| Physical disability (Barthel immobility score of 0) | 47.7 | 32.3 | 1.91 (1.21–3.02) | 0.005 | 2.10 (1.15–3.83) | 0.01 | 37.7 | 41.0 | 0.87 (0.45–1.66) | 0.67 | | |
| Coma | 6.9 | 4.3 | 1.61 (0.60–4.31) | 0.33 | | | 6.6 | 5.7 | 1.16 (0.32–4.15) | 0.81 | | |
| Any medical device | 32.5 | 13.1 | 3.18 (1.79–5.66) | < 0.001 | 2.81 (1.44–5.47) | 0.002 | 33.3 | 23.3 | 1.63 (0.83–3.21) | 0.15 | | |
| Percutaneous enteral gastrostomy tube | 15.7 | 6.5 | 2.66 (1.22–5.77) | 0.01 | | | 11.1 | 12.2 | 0.89 (0.33–2.42) | 0.83 | | |
| Tracheostomy tube | 4.9 | 2.1 | 2.31 (0.62–8.56) | 0.21 | | | 4.4 | 3.7 | 1.20 (0.25–5.60) | 0.81 | | |
| Urinary catheter | 15.7 | 4.3 | 4.08 (1.66–10.06) | 0.002 | | | 20.0 | 9.8 | 2.29 (1.00–5.23) | 0.04 | 2.61 (0.06–6.43) | 0.03 |
| Nasogastric tube | 5.9 | 0.7 | 8.54 (1.09–66.49) | 0.04 | | | 4.4 | 3.7 | 1.20 (0.25–5.60) | 0.81 | | |
| Length of stay in LTCF < 6 months | 15.6 | 11.9 | 1.36 (0.71–2.61) | 0.34 | | | 16.6 | 13.7 | 1.25 (0.51–3.00) | 0.61 | | |
| Hospital admission in previous 12 months | 24.2 | 27.0 | 0.87 (0.53–1.43) | 0.58 | | | 37.7 | 23.4 | 1.97 (1.02–3.81) | 0.04 | | |
| Infection | 5.4 | 2.9 | 1.90 (0.59–6.11) | 0.27 | | | 8.8 | 3.7 | 2.51 (0.76–8.28) | 0.12 | | |

ND: not determined; factors included in multivariate analysis are in italics. For multivariate analysis only significant values are shown

colonization prevalence, ranging from close to zero up to levels higher than 37%, has been reported in European studies [4].

Colonization by VRE in the present study was highly variable, ranging from 0.8 to 20.2%. VRE-carriage in European LTCF residents was found to be low, ranging from 0.0–3% [28, 41, 42].

For *Enterobacteriaceae* significant differences in colonization frequencies of LTCF residents were found: i) for CTX-M-type ESβL-producing *E. coli* between Piacenza (highest prevalence) and Bolzano, ii) for high-level AmpC-producing *M. morganii* (highest prevalence in Bolzano), iii) for carbapenemase producers, with highest prevalence in Milan, iv) for carbapenemase-producing *A. baumannii*, showing highest prevalence in Piacenza, and v) for MRSA and VRE, most prevalent in Milan. Therefore, no clear picture of general colonization differences can be deduced from overall colonization prevalence data.

A variety of risk factors for MRSA and ESβL colonization have previously been reported [4]; many of these have also been analyzed in the present survey. Interestingly, male residents carried a more than double risk for MRSA carriage when compared with female residents, probably because of the higher frequencies of other risk factors in males (administration of any antibiotic within the previous 3 months, hospitalization within the previous 12 months and coma), predisposing men rather than women to MRSA acquisition. Moreover, in our study the trend for an inverse correlation ($p = 0.09$) between age > 85 years and MRSA prevalence was associated with a significantly lower percentage of male residents > 85 years, compared to females; similar results have been found by other authors [43]. In the present survey, administration of cephalosporins during the previous 3 months resulted to be an independent risk factor for ESβL colonization; the LTCFs in Piacenza registered the highest consumption of cephalosporins, correlating with highest ESβL prevalence in LTCF residents from Piacenza. Other independent risk factors for ESβL colonization were physical disability, the presence of any invasive medical device and cancer. Whereas no significant differences were found between residents in the three Provinces for cancer as risk factor, physical disability and the presence of any medical device showed highest prevalence in the LTCF in Bolzano; nonetheless, LTCF residents in Bolzano had the lowest ESβL prevalence in the present screening study.

Therefore, further factors may have contributed to the observed differences, comprising staff/resident ratio and practiced hygiene and infection control measures [44]. The LTCF in Bolzano showed the highest staff/resident ratio, and understaffing has been shown to be a risk factor for colonization of LTCF residents by MDR organisms [2]. All of the surveyed LTCFs in the present study

follow hygiene, infection prevention and control measures according to guidelines of The Society for Healthcare Epidemiology of America (SHEA) and The Association for Professionals in Infection Control and Epidemiology (APIC) [45]. Nonetheless, the Bolzano LTCF had introduced enforced hygiene measures, according to the World Health Organization guidelines [46], after the 2008 screening study, showing an ESβL colonization prevalence of 64.0% in LTCF residents [22]; colonization frequency decreased significantly to 49.0% ($p = 0.02$) in 2012 [23], arriving at a slightly higher percentage of 53.0% in 2016, but other factors such as changed case mixes and risk factors may also have contributed to this decrease in ESβL prevalence [23].

Significant differences in antibiotic resistance epidemiology of blood culture isolates, used as a proxy for the general local antibiotic resistance epidemiology, were registered, as derived from European Antimicrobial Resistance Surveillance Network (EARS-Net) data for 2016 [26]. Specifically, we found the following antibiotic resistance data referred to the geographic regions of Milan, Piacenza and Bolzano, respectively: *E. coli* third generation cephalosporin-resistant: 22.1% (29/131), 29.4% (71/259) and 17.8% (56/314); *K. pneumoniae* carbapenem-resistant: 29.2% (7/24), 13.5% (10/74) and 6.2% (4/64); *A. baumannii* carbapenem-resistant: 50.0% (1/2,) 100.0% (24/24) and 0.0% (0/2); MRSA: 36.0% (18/50), 49.7% (82/165) and 14.6% (20/137); *E. faecalis* VRE: 0.0% (0/20), 2.4% (2/83) and 0.0% (0/41); *E. faecium* VRE: 10.0% (1/10), 22.2% (6/27) and 8.0% (2/25). This data for blood culture isolates, compared with our LTCF screening data, correlates well for ESβL-producing *E. coli*, carbapenem-resistant *K. pneumoniae* and *A. baumannii*; on the other hand, no correlation for MRSA and VRE can be derived. Patient transfer between acute-care facilities and LTCFs contribute to the diffusion of MDR organisms in both settings; such bi-directional movement of MDR bacteria, related to acute systemic infections, might be more significant for *Enterobacteriaceae* and *A. baumannii* than for MRSA and VRE.

Moreover, the snapshot approach used in this study might lead to the sudden increase in prevalence of a specific resistance phenotype, as shown for high-level AmpC-producing *M. morganii* detected in 2016 from Bolzano LTCF residents [5], which could be a transient phenomenon. Similarly, the high prevalence of VRE in LTCF residents from Milan could be due to a transitory local epidemic event.

Finally, the local circulation of highly transmissible clones, for example ESβL-producing *E. coli*, KPC-producing *K. pneumoniae* and OXA-23-producing *A. baumannii* could contribute to the explanation of the here reported screening results [38, 47].

This study has some limitations. First, it has been done in only four LTCFs, located in three different Provinces in Northern Italy, and therefore data may not be extrapolated to other Italian LTCFs with differing characteristics. Second, the number of LTCF residents participating in the study was variable, ranging from 34% in Milan up to 100% in Bolzano. Third, we did not use an enrichment step during the laboratory analysis; this limitation is partially compensated by using 4–5 different specimen types for the screening of MDR bacteria. Fourth, different sample types, types of media and laboratory methodologies have been used in the three laboratories processing the samples from the different LTCFs. Fifth, molecular characterization and typing of isolates in the 2016 study was limited, not including pulsed-field gel electrophoresis (PFGE) and sequence typing (ST) of isolates and therefore not permitting the identification of epidemic clusters. Finally, screening of healthcare workers has been done only in one of the enrolled LTCFs [5], but not in the other surveyed facilities. Despite these limitations, the strength of our study is the comparison of colonization prevalence between LTCFs located in three different Provinces, comparing it also with differences in risk factors for colonization and in the local epidemiology of invasive isolates.

## Conclusions

We performed a multicenter point-prevalence study in LTCFs located in three different Provinces in Northern Italy and found high colonization prevalence of LTCF residents for MDR organisms, especially ESβL-producing *E. coli*. Variability between the different facilities was noticeable also for other MDR organisms. Differences can be partially explained by i) differences in risk factors for colonization by MDR organisms, ii) changes in resident populations and staff/resident ratios, iii) applied hygiene measures and iv) differences in the local epidemiology of antibiotic resistance of clinical isolates. This widespread diffusion of MDR bacteria in LTCFs of three Italian Provinces confirms that these healthcare facilities are an important reservoir for MDR organisms. Future efforts should focus on screening activities, infection control strategies tailored on the complex aspects of LTCFs and implementation of antibiotic stewardship programs.

## Abbreviations

AMCLI: Association of Italian Clinical Microbiologist; APIC: The Association for Professionals in Infection Control and Epidemiology; CTX-M: Cefotaximase-Munich type Extended-Spectrum β-Lactamase; EARS-Net: European Antimicrobial Resistance Surveillance Network; ESβL: Extended-Spectrum β-Lactamase; EUCAST: European Committee on Antimicrobial Susceptibility Testing; GLISTer: Gruppo di Lavoro per lo Studio delle Infezioni nelle Residenze Sanitarie Assistite e Strutture Assimilabili; KPC: *Klebsiella Pneumoniae* Carbapenemase; LTCF: Long-Term Care Facility; MBL: Metallo-β-Lactamase; MDR: Multidrug-Resistant; MRSA: Methicillin-Resistant *Staphylococcus aureus*; PCR: Polymerase Chain Reaction; PFGE: Pulsed-Field Gel Electrophoresis; SHEA: The Society for Healthcare Epidemiology of America; ST: Sequence Typing; VIM: Verona Integron-Encoded Metallo-β-Lactamase; VRE: Vancomycin-Resistant Enterococci

## Acknowledgements

We wish to thank the residents and their relatives who agreed to participate in this study, the managements and staff of the long-term care facilities and the microbiology laboratories for excellent advice and technical assistance. We are grateful to Dr. Francesco Luzzaro, Lecco, for providing regional EARS-Net antimicrobial resistance data from the geographic region of Milan.
Members of the GLISTer group are kindly acknowledged: Laura Pagani, Massimo Confalonieri, Richard Aschbacher, Claudio Farina, Paolo Fazii, Francesco Luzzaro, Pier Giorgio Montanera.
Prof. Roberta Migliavacca is a member of the European Society of Clinical Microbiology and Infectious Diseases - Study Group for Infections in the Elderly (ESGIE) and would like to thank ESGIE members for their stimulating support to write this manuscript.

## Funding

The microbiological work was partially funded by a research grant of the "Fondo Ricerca e Giovani 2016" -University of Pavia and by an unconditional grant of Cepheid.

## Authors' contributions

EN, [1]MC, VMM, RM performed molecular analysis; RDA, [3]MC, EP, AM, FS, GS provided patient's sample data; EF, CR, RA performed and interpreted phenotypic investigations; RA, RM, LP analyzed and interpreted results; RA was a major contributor in writing the manuscript. All authors read and approved the final manuscript.

## Competing interests

The authors declare that they have no competing interests.

## Author details

[1]Department of Clinical Surgical Diagnostic and Pediatric Sciences, Laboratory of Microbiology and Clinical Microbiology, University of Pavia, Via Brambilla 74, 27100 Pavia, Italy. [2]Laboratory of Clinical Microbiology, ASP "Golgi-Redaelli", via Bartolomeo d'Alviano 78, 20146 Milan, Italy. [3]O.U. of Microbiology, Azienda Sanitaria Locale di Piacenza, Piacenza, Italy. [4]Geriatric Unit, Comprensorio Sanitario di Bolzano, Bolzano, Italy. [5]Microbiology and Virology Laboratory, Comprensorio Sanitario di Bolzano, Bolzano, Italy.

## References

1. Istituto nazionale di statistica. http://www.istat.it/. Accessed 24 July 2017.
2. Moro ML, Gagliotti C. Antimicrobial resistance and stewardship in long-term care settings. Future Med. 2013;8:1011–25.
3. Cassone M, Mody L. Colonization with multi-drug resistant organisms in nursing homes: scope, importance, and management. Curr Geriatr Rep. 2015;4:87–95.
4. Aschbacher R, Pagani E, Confalonieri M, Farina C, Fazii P, Luzzaro F, et al. Review on colonization of residents and staff in Italian long-term care facilities by multidrug-resistant bacteria compared with other European countries. Antimicrob Resist Infect Control. 2016;5:33.
5. March A, Aschbacher R, Sleghel F, Soelva S, Kaczor M, Migliavacca R, et al. Colonization of residents and staff of an Italian long-term care facility and an adjacent acute-care hospital geriatric unit by multidrug-resistant bacteria. New Microbiol. 2017;40:258–63.
6. The European Committee on Antimicrobial Susceptibility Testing. Breakpoint tables for interpretation of MICs and zone diameters. Version 6.0, 2016. http://www.eucast.org
7. Pagani L, Dell'Amico E, Migliavacca R, D'Andrea MM, Giacobone E, Amicosante G, et al. Multiple CTX-M-type extended-spectrum-lactamases in nosocomial isolates of *Enterobacteriaceae* from a hospital in Northern Italy. J Clin Microbiol. 2003;41:4264–9.
8. Eckert C, Gautier V, Arlet G. DNA sequence analysis of the genetic environment of various blaCTX-M genes. J Antimicrob Chemother 2006; 57:14–23.
9. Perilli M, Dell'Amico E, Segatore B, De Massis RR, Bianchi C, Luzzaro F, et al. Molecular characterization of extended-spectrum β-lactamases produced by nosocomial isolates of *Enterobacteriaceae* from an Italian nationwide survey. J Clin Microbiol. 2002;40:611–4.

10. Rasheed JK, Jay C, Metchock B, Berkowitz F, Weigel L, Crellin J, et al. Evolution of extended-spectrum beta-lactam resistance (SHV-8) in a strain of *Escherichia coli* during multiple episodes of bacteremia. Antimicrob Agents Chemother. 1997;41:647–53.

11. Yigit H, Queenan AM, Anderson GJ, Domenech-Sanchez A, Biddle JW, Steward CD, et al. Novel carbapenem-hydrolyzing-lactamase, KPC-1, from a carbapenem-resistant strain of *Klebsiella pneumoniae*. Antimicrob Agents Chemother. 2001;45:1151–61.

12. Poirel L, Walsh TR, Cuvillier V, Nordmann P. Multiplex PCR for detection of acquired carbapenemase genes. Diagn Microbiol Infect Dis. 2011;70:119–23.

13. Migliavacca R, Docquier JD, Mugnaioli C, Amicosante G, Daturi R, Lee K. Simple microdilution test for detection of metallo-beta-lactamase production in *Pseudomonas aeruginosa*. J Clin Microbiol. 2002;40:4388–90.

14. Lagatolla C, Tonin EA, Monti-Bragadin C, Dolzani L, Gombac F, Bearzi C, et al. Endemic carbapenem-resistant *Pseudomonas aeruginosa* with acquired metallo-β-lactamase determinants in European hospital. Emerg Infect Dis. 2004;10:535–8.

15. Poirel L, Le Thomas I, Naas T, Karim A, Nordmann P. Biochemical sequence analyses of GES-1, a novel class a extended-spectrum β-lactamase, and the class 1 integron In52 from *Klebsiella pneumoniae*. Antimicrob Agents Chemother. 2000;44:622–32.

16. Woodford N, Ellington MJ, Coelho JM, Turton JF, Ward ME, Brown S, et al. Multiplex PCR for genes encoding prevalent OXA carbapenemases in *Acinetobacter spp.* Int J Antimicrob Agents. 2006;27:351–3.

17. Poirel L, Docquier J-D, De Luca F, Verlinde A, Ide L, Rossolini GM, et al. BEL-2, an extended-Spectrum β-lactamase with increased activity toward expanded-Spectrum Cephalosporins in *Pseudomonas aeruginosa*. Antimicrob Agents Chemother. 2010;54:533–5.

18. Higgins PG, Lehmann M, Seifert H. Inclusion of OXA-143 primers in a multiplex polymerase chain reaction (PCR) for genes encoding prevalent OXA carbapenemases in *Acinetobacter* spp. Int J Antimicrob Agents. 2010;35:305.

19. Turton JF, Ward ME, Woodford N, Kaufmann ME, Pike R, Livermore DM, et al. The role of ISAba1 in expression of OXA carbapenemase genes in *Acinetobacter baumannii*. FEMS Microbiol Lett. 2006;258:72–7.

20. D'Andrea MM, Nucleo E, Luzzaro F, Giani T, Migliavacca R, Vailati F. CMY-16, a novel acquired AmpC-type β-lactamase of the CMY/LAT lineage in multifocal monophyletic isolates of *Proteus mirabilis* from northern Italy. Antimicrob Agents Chemother. 2006;50:618–24.

21. National Center for Biotechnology Information (NCBI). Basic Local Alignment Search Tool (BLAST). http://blast.ncbi.nlm.nih.gov/Blast.cgi. Accessed 24 July 2017.

22. March A, Aschbacher R, Dhanji H, Livermore DM, Böttcher A, Sleghel F, et al. Colonization of residents and staff of a long-term-care facility and adjacent acute-care hospital geriatric unit by multiresistant bacteria. Clin Microbiol Infect. 2010;16:934–44.

23. March A, Aschbacher R, Pagani E, Sleghel F, Soelva G, Hopkins KL, et al. Changes in colonization of residents and staff of a long-term care facility and an adjacent acute-care hospital geriatric unit by multidrug-resistant bacteria over a four-year period. Scand J Infect Dis. 2014;46:114–22.

24. Arnoldo L, Migliavacca R, Regattin L, Raglio A, Pagani L, Nucleo E, et al. Prevalence of urinary colonization by extended spectrum-beta-lactamase *Enterobacteriaceae* among catheterised inpatients in Italian long-term care facilities. BMC Infect Dis. 2013;13:124.

25. Giufrè M, Ricchizzi E, Accogli M, Barbanti F, Monaco M, Pimentel de Araujo F, et al. Colonization by multidrug-resistant organisms in long-term care facilities in Italy: a point-prevalence study. Clin Microbiol Infect. 2017;23:961–7.

26. European Centre for Disease Prevention and Control. https://ecdc.europa.eu/. Accessed 24 July 2017.

27. Rooney PJ, O'Leary MC, Loughrey AC, McCalmont M, Smyth B, Donaghy P, et al. Nursing homes as a reservoir of extended-spectrum beta-lactamase (ESBL)-producing ciprofloxacin-resistant *Escherichia coli*. J Antimicrob Chemother. 2009;64:635–41.

28. Ludden C, Cormican M, Vellinga A, Johnson JR, Austin B, Morris D. Colonisation with ESBL-producing and carbapenemase-producing *Enterobacteriaceae*, vancomycin-resistant enterococci, and meticillin-resistant *Staphylococcus aureus* in a long-term care facility over one year. BMC Infect Dis. 2015;15:168.

29. Rodrigues C, Mendes AC, Sima F, Bavlovič J, Machado E, Novais Â, et al. Long-term care facility (LTCF) residents colonized with multidrug-resistant (MDR) *Klebsiella pneumoniae* lineages frequently causing infections in Portuguese clinical institutions. Infect Control Hosp Epidemiol. 2017;38:1127–30.

30. Yoo JS, Byeon J, Yang J, Yoo JI, Chung GT, Lee YS. High prevalence of extended-spectrum beta-lactamases and plasmid-mediated AmpC beta-lactamases in *Enterobacteriaceae* isolated from long-term care facilities in Korea. Diagn Microbiol Infect Dis. 2010;67:261–5.

31. Carattoli A, Aschbacher R, March A, Larcher C, Livermore DM, Woodford N. Complete nucleotide sequence of the IncN plasmid pKOX105 encoding VIM-1, QnrS1 and SHV-12 proteins in *Enterobacteriaceae* from Bolzano, Italy compared with IncN plasmids encoding KPC enzymes in the USA. J Antimicrob Chemother. 2010;65:2070–5.

32. Del Franco M, Paone L, Novati R, Giacomazzi CG, Bagattini M, Galotto C, et al. Molecular epidemiology of carbapenem resistant *Enterobacteriaceae* in Valle d'Aosta region, Italy, shows the emergence of KPC-2 producing *Klebsiella pneumoniae* clonal complex 101 (ST101 and ST1789). BMC Microbiol. 2015;15:260.

33. Piazza A, Caltagirone M, Bitar I, Nucleo E, Spalla M, Fogato E, et al. Emergence of *Escherichia coli* sequence type 131 (ST131) and ST3948 with KPC-2, KPC-3 and KPC-8 carbapenemases from a long-term care and rehabilitation facility (LTCRF) in northern Italy. Adv Exp Med Biol. 2016;901:77–89.

34. Giani T, Pini B, Arena F, Conte V, Bracco S, Migliavacca R, et al. Epidemic diffusion of KPC carbapenemase-producing *Klebsiella pneumoniae* in Italy: results of the first countrywide survey, 15 may to 30 June 2011. Euro Surveill. 2013;18(22)

35. Prasad N, Labaze G, Kopacz J, Chwa S, Platis D, Pan CX, et al. Asymptomatic rectal colonization with carbapenem-resistant *Enterobacteriaceae* and *Clostridium difficile* among residents of a long-term care facility in New York City. Am J Infect Control. 2016;44:525–32.

36. Rossolini GM, Luzzaro F, Migliavacca R, Mugnaioli C, Pini B, De Luca F, et al. First countrywide survey of acquired metallo-beta-lactamases in gram-negative pathogens in Italy. Antimicrob Agents Chemother. 2008;52:4023–9.

37. Kanayama A, Kawahara R, Yamagishi T, Goto K, Kobaru Y, Takano M, Morisada K, et al. Successful control of an outbreak of GES-5 extended-spectrum β-lactamase-producing *Pseudomonas aeruginosa* in a long-term care facility in Japan. J Hosp Infect. 2016;93:35–41.

38. Principe L, Piazza A, Giani T, Bracco S, Caltagirone MS, Arena F, et al. Epidemic diffusion of OXA-23-producing *Acinetobacter baumannii* isolates in Italy: results of the first cross-sectional countrywide survey. J Clin Microbiol. 2014;52:3004–10.

39. Brugnaro P, Fedeli U, Pellizzer G, Buonfrate D, Rassu M, Boldrin C, et al. Clustering and risk factors of methicillin-resistant *Staphylococcus aureus* carriage in two Italian long-term care facilities. Infection. 2009;37:216–21.

40. Monaco M, Bombana E, Trezzi L, Regattin L, Brusaferro S, Pantosti A, et al. Methicillin-resistant *Staphylococcus aureus* colonizing residents and staff members in a nursing home in northern Italy. J Hosp Infect. 2009;73:182–4.

41. Jans B, Schoevaerdts D, Huang TD, Berhin C, Latour K, Bogaerts P, et al. Epidemiology of multidrug-resistant microorganisms among nursing home residents in Belgium. PLoS One. 2013;8:e64908.

42. Hogardt M, Proba P, Mischler D, Cuny C, Kempf VA, Heudorf U. Current prevalence of multidrug-resistant organisms in long-term care facilities in the Rhine-main district, Germany, 2013. Euro Surveill. 2015;20(26)

43. Nillius D, von Müller L, Wagenpfeil S, Klein R, Herrmann M. Methicillin-resistant *Staphylococcus aureus* in Saarland, Germany: the long-term care facility study. PLoS One. 2016; https://doi.org/10.1371/journal.pone.0153030.

44. Dyar OJ, Pagani L, Pulcini C. Strategies and challenges of antimicrobial stewardship in long-term care facilities. Clin Microbiol Infect. 2015;21:10–9.

45. Smith PW, Bennett G, Bradley S, Drinka P, Lautenbach E, Marx J, et al. SHEA/APIC guideline: infection prevention and control in the long-term care facility. Infect Control Hosp Epidemiol. 2008;29:785–814.

46. http://apps.who.int/iris/bitstream/10665/44102/1/9789241597906_eng.pdf. Accessed 24 July 2017.

47. Mathers AJ, Peirano G, Pitout JD. The role of epidemic resistance plasmids and international high-risk clones in the spread of multidrug-resistant *Enterobacteriaceae*. Clin Microbiol Rev. 2015;28:565–91.

# 3

# Impact of single room design on the spread of multi-drug resistant bacteria in an intensive care unit

Teysir Halaby[1][*] (ID), Nashwan al Naiemi[1,2,3], Bert Beishuizen[4], Roel Verkooijen[1], José A. Ferreira[5], Rob Klont[1,4] and Christina vandenbroucke-Grauls[2]

## Abstract

**Background:** Cross-transmission of nosocomial pathogens occurs frequently in intensive care units (ICU). The aim of this study was to investigate whether the introduction of a single room policy resulted in a decrease in transmission of multidrug-resistant (MDR) bacteria in an ICU.

**Methods:** We performed a retrospective study covering two periods: between January 2002 and April 2009 (old-ICU) and between May 2009 and March 2013 (new-ICU, single-room). These periods were compared with respect to the occurrence of representative MDR Gram-negative bacteria. Routine microbiological screening, was performed on all patients on admission to the ICU and then twice a week. Multi-drug resistance was defined according to a national guideline. The first isolates per patient that met the MDR-criteria, detected during the ICU admission were included in the analysis. To investigate the clonality, isolates were genotyped by DiversiLab (*bioMérieux*, France) or Amplified Fragment Length Polymorphism (AFLP). To guarantee the comparability of the two periods, the 'before' and 'after' periods were chosen such that they were approximately identical with respect to the following factors: number of admissions, number of beds, bed occupancy rate, per year and month.

**Results:** Despite infection prevention efforts, high prevalence of MRD bacteria continue to occur in the original facility. A marked and sustained decrease in the prevalence of MDR-GN bacteria was observed after the migration to the new ICU, while there appear to be no significant changes in the other variables including bed occupancy and numbers of patient admissions.

**Conclusion:** Single room ICU design contributes significantly to the reduction of cross transmission of MRD-bacteria.

## Background

Cross-transmission of nosocomial pathogens has been shown to occur frequently in intensive care units (ICU) [1]. It may be promoted by several factors including environmental source [2], invasive procedures, and understaffing [3]. Bacterial cross-transmissions account for a significant part of ICU-acquired infections [4], the majority of which are associated with Gram-negative (GN) microorganisms [5]. GN-infections in turn lead to substantial morbidity, mortality and costs [6]. Interventions aimed at reducing the spread of nosocomial pathogens

include contact precautions and isolation of patients, especially when multi-drug resistant (MDR) organisms are involved [7] and hand hygiene [8], which has been considered the most important control measures [9]. Despite evidence that transmission of pathogens by way of health care workers' hands is a major cause of nosocomial infections [10], compliance with policies and procedures for infection control has been uniformly poor [11]. Nursing patients in single-patient rooms can improve hand washing compliance and facilitate cleaning and decontamination and thereby contribute to infection control [12].

In this retrospective study we describe the long-term persistence and transmission of MDR-GN organisms in an ICU despite extensive infection control precautions.

* Correspondence: t.halaby@labmicta.nl
[1]Laboratory for Medical Microbiology and Public Health, Boerhaavelaan 59, 7555, BB, Hengelo, The Netherlands
Full list of author information is available at the end of the article

We present evidence for the role of the single room design of the new facility to which the ward was eventually moved in their control.

## Methods

### Setting

The study covered two periods: a first period between January 2002 and April 2009 (old-ICU) and a second between May 2009 and March 2013 (new-ICU, single-room). In the first period patients were nursed in an ICU with 21 beds: five in single ventilated rooms and with ante-room, four in two double rooms without ante-rooms, and 12 in an open bay (Fig. 1). The total number of beds in use was 18, since a maximum of nine out of the 12 open bay beds was used for admissions at any given time.

This ICU was closed on two occasions: from January through May 2003 because of an ongoing outbreak with ESBL-producing *Klebsiella pnumoniae* (ESBL-Kp) which started in 2001 [13], and between January and March 2008 because of an outbreak with multi-drug resistant *Acinetobacter baumannii* (MDR-Ab). Because of these outbreaks and because there was evidence of persistent colonization and spread of other MDR-GN among patients in the ICU despite extensive infection control efforts, it was ultimately decided to transfer the ICU in May 2009 to a newly built ICU, which consisted of a two-floor unit, each with 9 single rooms with controlled ventilation and ante-room (Fig. 2). The two floors were identical regarding treatment facilities and casemix. Initially only 16 beds were used. In January 2011 the number beds in use was increased to 18. Only new patients were admitted to the new ICU and no patients we transferred from the old ICU during migration.

### Surveillance

Routine microbiological screening started in February 2002 and continued through the whole study period. Screening was performed on all patients on admission to the ICU and then twice a week. Screening was done by culture of throat and rectal-swab specimens and, in intubated patients, of tracheal fluid samples. When clinically indicated, samples were also obtained from relevant body sites, such as wounds. MDR-GN strains were stored at –70 °C.

### Bacteriological methods

From January 2002 until April 2010, species identification was routinely performed by classical biochemical methods and the API 20E system. Antimicrobial susceptibility testing was performed by the agar dilution method according to the National Committee on Clinical Laboratory Standards (NCCLS), now called Clinical and Laboratory Standards Institute (CLSI) [14]. From April 2010 on, the Vitek 2 Advanced Expert System (bioMérieux, France) was used to identify strains, to determine antimicrobial susceptibility using the EUCAST breakpoints [15], and to perform phenotypic screening for ESBL. ESBL confirmation was performed by the double disk synergy test with cefotaxime and/or ceftazidime, and clavulanic acid [16].

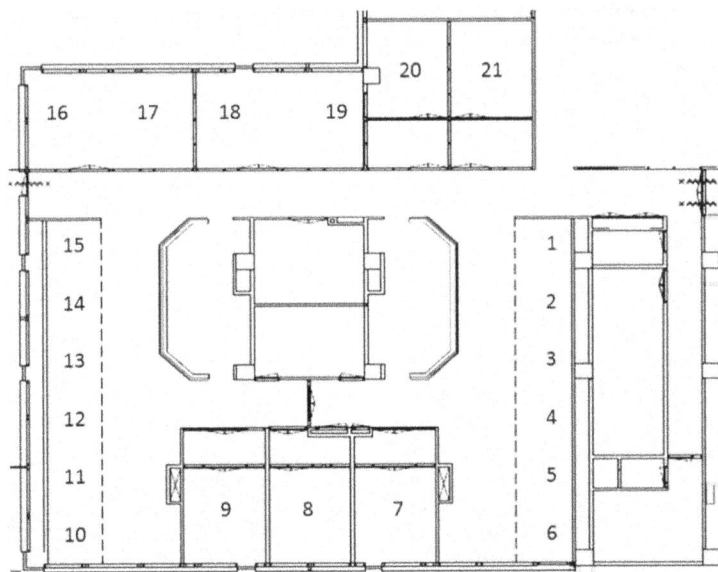

**Fig. 1** Floor plan of the ICU before conversion: 1–6 and 10–15: beds situated in the open bay; 7–9 and 20–21: single rooms with controlled ventilation and with anteroom; 16/17 and 18/19: rooms without controlled ventilation an without anteroom

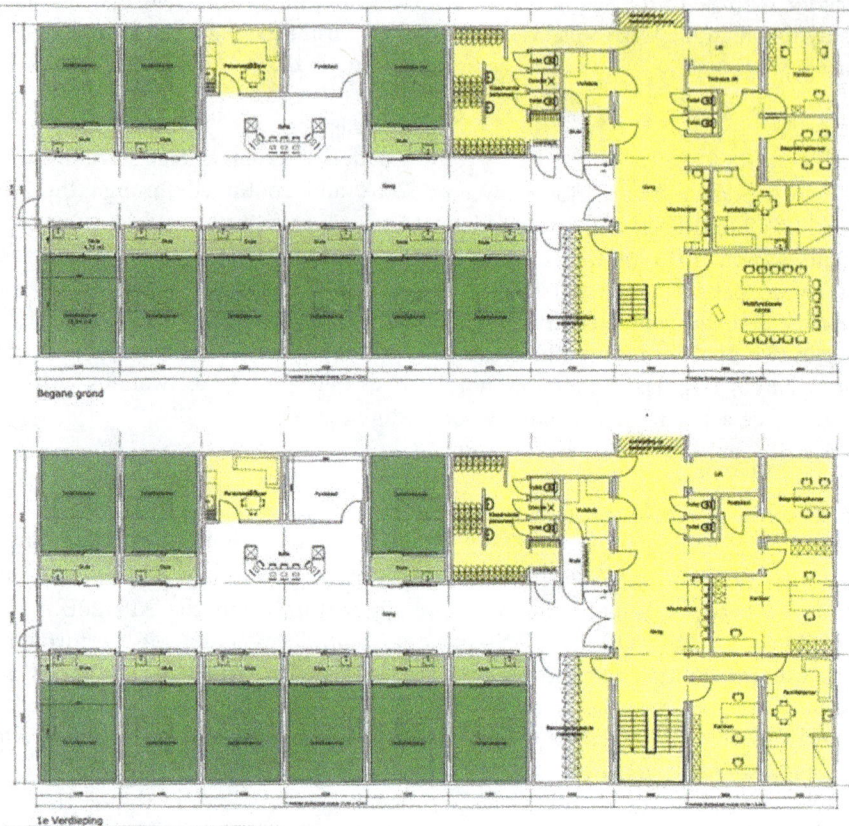

**Fig. 2** Plan of the new ICU consisting of two identical floors with 9 patient rooms each. Single patient rooms with anteroom are indicated by dark green and light green, respectively

## Infection control

Before the outbreak, infection control measures in the ICU were implemented according to a national guideline [17]. Infection prevention measures were mainly based on the so-called "work island" principle, which means contact precautions in the area surrounding the ventilated patient bed, including cleaning and disinfection and hand hygiene before entering and by leaving the patient area.

When an increase in the number of patients colonized with ESBL-Kp was noticed in August 2001, an outbreak management team was formed, including an infection control nurse, an ICU medical officer, a consultant microbiologist, and an ICU nurse. Infection control practices were reinforced, including labelling and isolation of ESBL-Kp-positive patients in the single-patient rooms, cohort nursing of ESBL-Kp-colonised patients to the two-bedded rooms when more patients were found colonized, and disinfection of hospital equipment and high-touch surfaces. Since the outbreak remained uncontrolled despite these measures (Fig. 3), an intensified infection control programme was started. This included from September 2002, the use of a 'short stay' four-bedded unit outside the ICU area for patients expected

to be admitted to the ICU for fewer than 72 h. Secondly, from October 2002 onwards, patients admitted to the ICU received selective decontamination of the digestive tract (SDD). The aim of the SDD treatment in this setting was to reduce colonization of the digestive tract with resistant bacteria [18]. SDD was given as topical mixture of nonabsorbable antibiotics including tobramycin, colistin and Amphotericin B (respective doses: 80, 100, and 500 mg), applied on the buccal mucosa and as a suspension administered via a nasogastric tube in the gastrointestinal tract, four times a day [19].

Finally, the ICU was temporarily closed from January through May 2003 for thorough cleaning and disinfection, during which period patients were admitted to a temporary, 16-bed ICU. The same infection control policy from the closed ICU was continued. No new patients with ESBL-Kp were detected during this period, until one week before moving the ICU back to the main location. After the ICU was moved back to the main location, an increase in the incidence of ESBL-Kp positive patients was noted (Fig. 3). In 2005 a decrease in the incidence was observed; however, the outbreak remained uncontrolled. In 2007, it was concluded that radical facility changes in design and infection control policy were

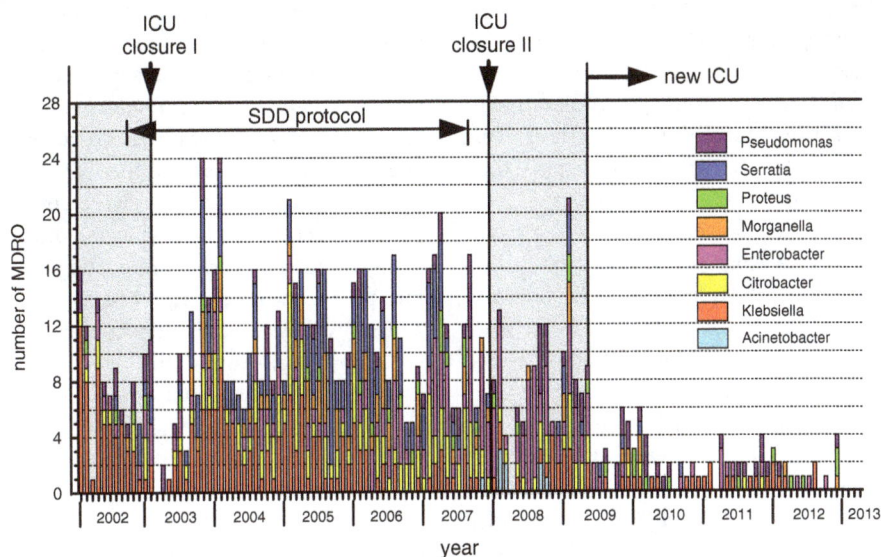

**Fig. 3** Occurrence of MDR-resistant bacteria (each counted once per patient) between January 2002 and March 2013 with indication of the main infection control measures that were taken on the ICU. ICU closure I: during January–May 2003 for thorough cleaning and disinfection; ICU closure II: temporary closure for new admissions because of an outbreak with multi-drug resistant *A. baumannii*. After all beds became available through discharges the unit including equipment was decontaminated with vaporized hydrogen peroxide; new ICU opened with single-bed rooms

needed for optimal infection control practices. Short-term changes that followed within the following year included SDD discontinuation (April 2007), the appointment of additional infection control practitioners, and the promotion of a high level of compliance with infection control measures.

Between January and March 2008 the ward was closed due to an outbreak with MDR-Ab. Rigorous infection control measures were implemented including the grouping of MDR-Ab-positive patients in single rooms with controlled ventilation, education of staff, enforcement of hand hygiene and surface decontamination. In addition, the ward was temporarily closed for new admissions. After all beds became available through discharges, the unit including equipment was decontaminated with vaporized hydrogen peroxide (VHP), according to manufacturer's instructions (Infection Control BV, Eemnes, the Netherlands). Short-term changes were implemented, including the reduction of the number of beds to 16, and the unit was re-opened on April the 3rd 2008. In April 2009 the ICU was moved to a semi-permanent (http://www.cadolto.com/en/products/healthcare_buildings/hospitals) single-room unit (Fig. 2). Nurse-to-patient ratio (0,66) did not change. The same infection control protocols were maintained. In the single-room unit, a hand washing sink was located in each ante-room and an alcohol-based hand rub dispenser in each ante-room and at the bedside.

### Retrospective microbiological analysis

In 2014, a retrospective study was undertaken on existing laboratory databases to collect data on the occurrence of MDR-GN, including ESBL-Kp, *Citrobacter* spp., *Proteus* spp., *Enterobacter* spp., *Serratia* spp., *Morganella* spp., *Pseudomonas* spp. and *Acinetobacter* spp. Multi-drug resistance among Gram-negative bacteria was defined according to a national guideline (Table 1) [20].

**Table 1** Definition of MDR Gram-negative bacteria [20]

|  | ESBL | carbapenems | fluoroquinolons | aminoglycosides | ceftazidime | piperacillin | cotrimoxazole |
|---|---|---|---|---|---|---|---|
| *K. pneumonia* | A | A | B | B |  |  |  |
| other Enterobacteriaceae[a] |  |  | B | B |  |  | B |
| *P. aeruginosa* |  | C | C | C | C | C |  |
| *A. baumannii* |  | A | B | B | B |  |  |

*MDR* multi-drug resistant
[a] Proteus, Morganella, Serratia, Citrobacter, Enterobacter spp.
A: presence of ESBL production or resistance against this antibacterial agent or group is sufficient to define the microorganism as being MDR
B: resistance against 2 antibacterial agents or against at least 2 of the indicated groups is required to define the microorganism as being MDR
C: resistance against 3 antibacterial agents or against antimicrobial agents from at least 3 of the indicated groups is required to define the microorganism as being MDR

The first isolates per patient, that met the MDR-criteria, detected during the ICU admission were included in the analysis.

Since the dilutions values of antimicrobial agents that were tested in the agar dilution method were available in the Laboratory Information System (LIS), it was possible to compensate for the change from CLSI to EUCAST by retrospectively redefining the breakpoints of the tested isolates to meet the MDR-criteria. During the whole study period, ESBL identification was performed on *K. pneumonia*, *K. oxytoca* and bacteriemic *P. mirabilis* isolates that screened suspected [14]. Bacteriemic *P. mirabilis* isolates were not detected [21], hence, no ESBL confirmation was performed. So, from the ESBL-positive Enterobacteriaceae only *K. pneumonia* isolates were included in the analysis. The other Enterobacteriaceae were included not as whether or not carrying ESBL but when meeting the HRMO criteria.

Clonality of stored ESBL-Kp isolates obtained between 2002 and 2007 was retrospectively investigated by DiversiLab (bioMérieux, France) [21]. Available data from typing of *Enterobacter*, *Acinetobacter*, *P. aeruginosa*, *Citorbacter freundii*, *E. coli* and ESBL-Kp isolates obtained after 2007, prospectively investigated by DiversiLab or AFLP [22], were also included in this study. Frequency distribution of the MDR Gram-negative bacteria that were used for genotyping is shown in Fig. 4.

### Statistical analysis

Our objective was to investigate whether the introduction of a single room policy resulted in a decrease in the number of transmissions of MDR within the ICU. For this purpose we compared a period before the introduction of the policy and a period following it with respect to the occurrence of representative MDR isolates of the species *Citrobacter*, *Enterobacter*, *Morganella*, *Proteus*, *Serratia* and *Pseudomonas*. To guarantee the comparability of the two periods, the 'before' and 'after' periods were chosen such that they were approximately identical with respect to the following factors: number of admissions, number of beds, bed occupancy rate, per year and month (the average length of stay per month can be dispensed with since it is determined by the average number of admissions and the occupancy rate). A data set derived from the NICE database (National Intensive Care Evaluation, https://www.stichting-nice.nl) was combined with the laboratory data and upon examination of the monthly figures related to numbers of admissions, number of beds and bed occupancy it was decided to compare the periods from April 2008 to April 2009 and from May 2009 to December 2010, during the whole length of which the number of beds was kept at 16, as the 'before' and 'after' periods for the main part of the analysis. A third period (a second 'after' period) from January 2011 to March 2012, in which the capacity of the ICU was increased to 18 beds, was used for subsidiary analyses.

The two periods were compared with respect to a single variable (e.g. number of transmissions of a given bacterium or bed occupancy) by a permutation test with month as a 'block factor' based on a so-called *sum statistic* [23]. This is the sum, over the available months, of the monthly differences in the average values of the variable in the two periods. The blocking by month should correct for eventual seasonal patterns in the number of

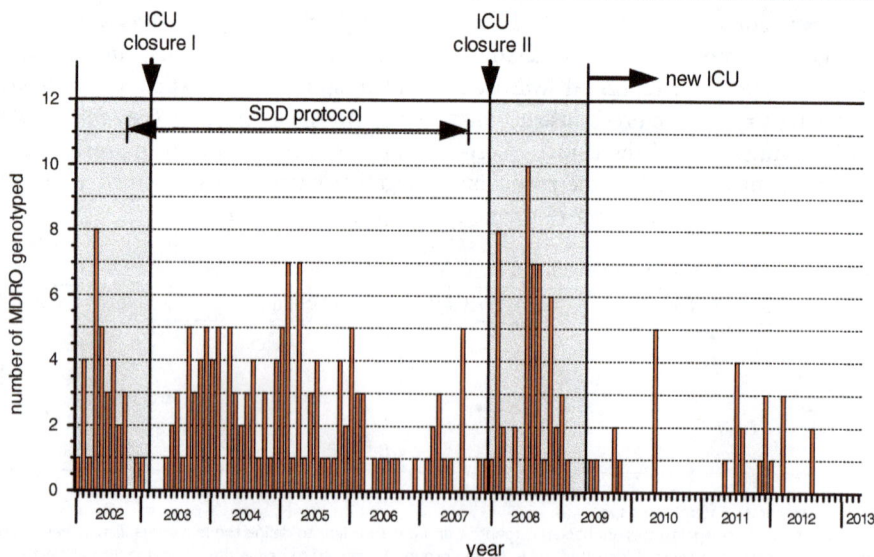

**Fig. 4** Frequency distribution of the MDR Gram negative bacteria that were used for genotyping

transmissions. In order to compare the two periods with respect to the transmissions of the six different species *simultaneously* we used a generalization of the permutation test based on the sum of the six sum statistics corresponding to the six bacteria. The rationale for using this test was the "principle of coherence" [24]: if the intervention does have a positive (or at least non-negative) effect then that effect consists of a decrease (or at least non-increase) in the number of all the bacteria. All the tests were two-sided. Despite several tests being carried out, no multiple testing corrections are presented because, by the nature of the data and of the hypotheses tested, the *p*-values are either unequivocally large or unequivocally small. Statistical analyses were carried out with programs written in R [25], which may be obtained from the authors upon request.

## Results

The numbers of patients carrying MDR-*Citrobacter* spp., *Proteus* spp., *Enterobacter* spp., *Serratia* spp., *Morganella* spp. and *Pseudomonas* spp. and ESBL-Kp are shown in Fig. 3.

### ESBL-Producing *K. pneumoniae*

Between January 2002 and March 2013, 225 patients with ESBL-Kp were identified (Fig. 3). Typing of 163 isolates (one isolate per patient) by REP-PCR revealed that the majority was clonally related. Of these isolates 121, obtained between January 2002 and July 2007, were found to be identical [21], while 42 appeared unrelated to the major clone. Typing of 10 out of the 17 ESBL-Kp isolates obtained between March 2008 and April 2009 (after disinfection of the old ICU with VHP and before the move to the new ICU), showed no clonal relation of these isolates to the outbreak strain. However, two clusters of strains were identified: one of two strains (isolated on 3/11/2008 and 11/12/2008), and the other of three strains (isolated on 18/12/2008, 29/12/2008 and 3/1/2009). The remaining five isolates had different patterns.

### A. Baumannii

In October 2007, a patient known to harbour MDR-Ab was transferred from a Turkish hospital to the ICU and was directly placed in a separate room in strict isolation. During his admission, which lasted three weeks, and after discharge, no spread of the MDR-Ab was seen, until early in January 2008, when two patients were found to carry a strain of MDR-Ab. The patients were placed in separate rooms with controlled ventilation in strict isolation. During the following two weeks, MDR-Ab was detected in three more patients. Genotyping showed clonal relationship between strains from the five patients, one strain from the index patient and seven

from the ICU environment. The unit was closed in the third week of January and re-opened in March 2008.

### Other MDR-gram negative organisms

Between March 2008 and April 2009, 46 patients carrying MDR *E. cloacae* were identified. Typing of 23 isolates obtained between April and August 2008, with Diversilab [26] revealed two clusters: one of 7 and one of 13 strains. The remaining three strains had different patterns.

After the old ICU was reopened in March 2008, cross transmission of new microorganisms re-emerged and persisted as evidenced by genotyping of ESBL-Kp (unrelated to the major clone) and MDR *E. cloacae* (Fig. 5).

### New ICU period

After the migration to the new ICU, a marked decrease in the prevalence of MDR-GN was observed (Fig. 6). Available data from typing of *Enterobacter*, *Acinetobacter*, *P. aeruginosa*, *C. freundii*, *E. coli* and ESBL-Kp isolates obtained after the migration showed no transmission (Fig. 7).

The test comparing the 'before' (April 2008 to April 2009) and 'after' (May 2009 to December 2010) periods regarding the numbers of transmissions of the six bacteria jointly yielded a *p*-value of 0.001. With respect to the number of admissions, the comparison between the 'before' and 'after' periods and between the 'after' period and *the second* 'after' period (January 2011 to March 2012) no significant changes were observed (*p*-values of 0.17, and 0.34).

With respect to bed occupancy, testing for differences between the 'before' and 'after' periods yields a p-value of 0.99. In contrast, there was evidence for a difference between the 'after' period and *the second* 'after' period (increase in the capacity of the ICU from 16 to 18 beds), with a p-value of 0.007.

Comparing the 'before' and 'after' periods with regard to each species one at a time, p-values of 0.0015, 0.0005, 0.37, 0.99, 0.25, and 0.39 for *Citrobacter*, *Enterobacter*, *Morganella*, *Proteus*, *Serratia* and *Pseudomonas*, respectively, were found.

## Discussion

Our results provided strong evidence that the single room policy as an infection control strategy has contributed significantly to the control of cross transmission of resistant pathogens in the ICU.

In this study we analysed the history of an ICU which was affected by a protracted clustered occurrence of MDR bacteria despite extensive infection control precautions. Control was ultimately achieved by closing the ward and moving it into a new single room designed facility.

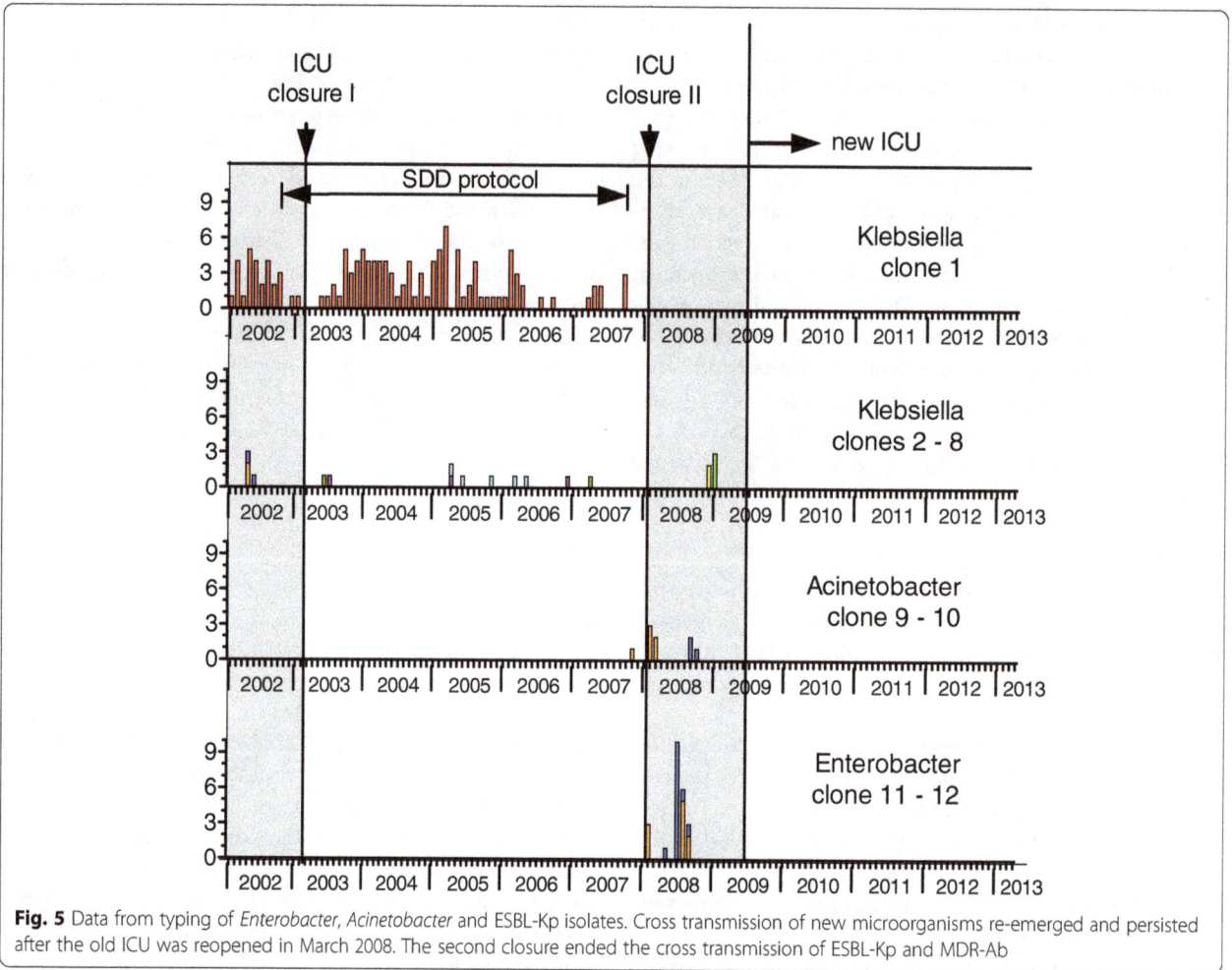

**Fig. 5** Data from typing of *Enterobacter*, *Acinetobacter* and ESBL-Kp isolates. Cross transmission of new microorganisms re-emerged and persisted after the old ICU was reopened in March 2008. The second closure ended the cross transmission of ESBL-Kp and MDR-Ab

Despite combined interventions, including education to improve adherence to hand hygiene practices, use of contact precautions, isolation of ESBL-Kp positive patients and temporary ward closure in early 2003, the colonization by endemic ESBL-Kp, as evidenced by

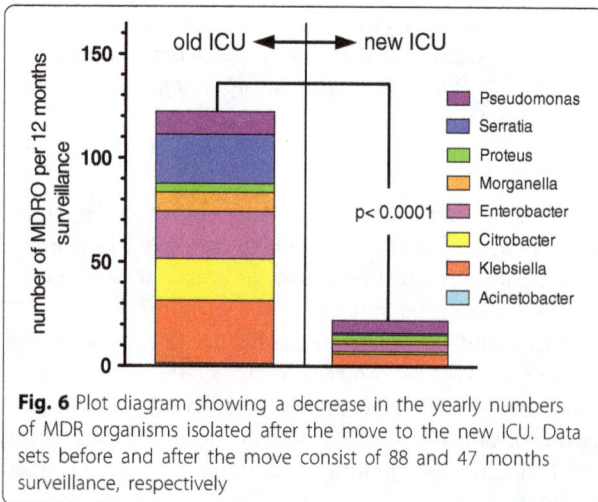

**Fig. 6** Plot diagram showing a decrease in the yearly numbers of MDR organisms isolated after the move to the new ICU. Data sets before and after the move consist of 88 and 47 months surveillance, respectively

genotyping with DiversiLab, and by other MDR-Gram negative bacteria was observed soon after the unit was re-opened. Educational meetings were held and hand hygiene was emphasized on several occasions. Recorded observations about hand hygiene performance, and adherence to hygiene protocols were not part of the experimental design, hence could not be described during the study period. Even if lack of adherence to hand washing protocols alone may not explain the failure to halt transmission [27], breaches in hand hygiene may have promoted it [28].

Although the importance of colonization pressure in transmission of MDR-GN bacteria has not fully been estimated [29], our data suggest that the increased number of colonized patients has contributed to the persistence of MDR-bacteria. Not only was the proportion of colonized patients high, patients were also colonized with multiple MDR-GN bacteria. Selection of these bacteria may have been facilitated by the start and the prolonged use of SDD. Prior to the introduction of SDD, most ESBL-Kp isolates were resistant to tobramycin, and upon exposure to colistin,

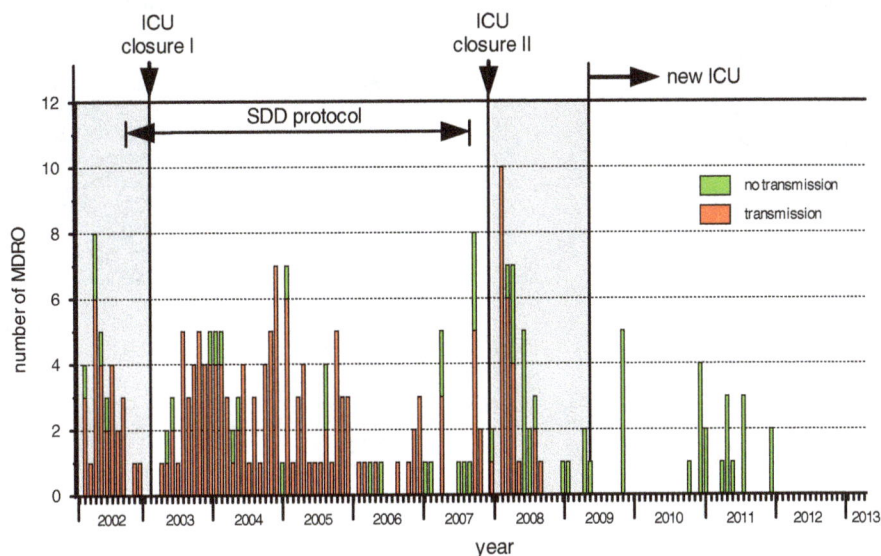

**Fig. 7** Pooled data from typing of *Enterobacter*, *Acinetobacter*, *P. aeruginosa*, *C. freundii*, *E. coli* and ESBL-Kp isolates. In the new ICU no transmission was observed

heteroresistant subpopulations may have been selected for. In addition, the proportion of tobramycin resistance among pathogens intrinsically resistant to colistin (*Proteus*, *Morganella*, and *Serratia* spp.) increased under the use of SDD, and decreased after stopping SDD [21]. Abundant carriage of these MDR-bacteria under SDD, i.e. colonization pressure [30] may have enhanced the risk of their spread and acquisition.

Although temporary ward closure has been shown to control ESBL-Kp outbreaks adequately [31], in our case the ESBL-Kp outbreak persisted after closure of the ICU early in 2003. The reason for this is not clear; no common environmental source was identified, and cultures obtained from the hands of nursing and medical staff performed on one occasion were negative. After the second ward closure and decontamination with HPV early in 2008, clonal spread of the ESBL-Kp or MDR-Ab was not observed again. However, transmission and persistence of new MDR-GN bacteria after the ward was reopened continued to occur, as evidenced by typing of ESBL-Kp and *E. cloacae* strains.

Single-bed room design has been shown beneficial in reducing contact transmission and acquisition of resistant bacteria in several studies [32–36]. It enables the separation of patients upon admission and prevents transmission from unrecognized carriers of pathogens. By design, single rooms are furnished with a conveniently located sink in each, provided by sufficient and accessible alcohol-based hand-rub dispensers. Affecting staff behavior by single-room design has in one study been found a possible element that contributed to higher hand hygiene

compliance, compared to an open plan ICU [32]. Another study showing a substantial reduction in transmission of some microorganisms after converting the ICU to private rooms, has attributed the observed reduction to better hand hygiene by hospital staff, rather than to the move to a new and uncontaminated enviromnemt [33]. The results from our study supports these findings. Although adherence to hand hygiene practice was not measured, ending of cross-transmission occurred only after the move to the new ICU (Fig. 6).

In this study, after the move to the single room unit, a clear and sustained decrease in the prevalence of the MDR-GN bacteria was observed, except for MDR-*P. aeruginosa* which, however, could not be explained by cross transmission since the genotyping of five isolates between July and October 2009 revealed no similarities. Statistical analysis testing for differences between the periods before and after the move to the single room unit showed good evidence that the single room policy was very effective in controlling the cross transmission of the MDR bacteria in this ICU.

## Conclusion

Protracted clustered occurrence of MDR bacteria in an ICU despite extensive infection control precautions, including temporary ward closure on two occasions, was ended only by the transformation of the unit into a single-room unit. Single room ICU design significantly contributed to the reduction of cross transmission of MRD-bacteria.

**Acknowledgments**
Not applicable.

**Funding**
None.

**Authors' contributions**
Conception and design of the study: TH, NN, CG. Acquisition of data: AB, RK, TH. Analysis and interpretation of data: RV, JF. Drafting and revising the manuscript: all authors. Final approval of the manuscript: all authors.

**Competing interests**
The authors declare that they have no competing interests.

**Author details**
[1]Laboratory for Medical Microbiology and Public Health, Boerhaavelaan 59, 7555, BB, Hengelo, The Netherlands. [2]Department of Medical Microbiology & Infection Control, VU University Medical Center, Amsterdam, The Netherlands. [3]Medical Microbiology and Infection Control, Ziekenhuisgroep Twente, Almelo, The Netherlands. [4]Department of intensive care, Medisch Spectrum Twente, Enschede, The Netherlands. [5]Department of Statistics, Informatics and Modelling, National Institute for Public Health and the Environment, RIVM, Bilthoven, The Netherlands.

**References**
1. Weist K, Pollege K, Schulz I, Rüden H, Gastmeier P. How many nosocomial infections are associated with cross-transmission? A prospective cohort study in a surgical intensive care unit. Infect Control Hosp Epidemiol. 2002; 23:127–32.
2. Crnich CJ, Safdar N, Maki DG. The role of the intensive care unit environment in the pathogenesis and prevention of ventilator-associated pneumonia. Respir Care. 2005;50:813–36. discussion 36–8
3. Halwani M, Solaymani-Dodaran M, Grundmann H, Coupland C, Slack R. Cross-transmission of nosocomial pathogens in an adult intensive care unit: incidence and risk factors. J Hosp Infect. 2006;63:39–46.
4. Kola A, Schwab F, Bärwolff S, Eckmanns T, Weist K, Dinger E, et al. Is there an association between nosocomial infection rates and bacterial cross transmissions? Crit Care Med. 2010;38:46–50.
5. Weinstein RA. Epidemiology and control of nosocomial infections in adult intensive care units. Am J Med. 1991;91(suppl. 3B):179S–84S.
6. Vincent JL, Rello J, Marshall J, Silva E, Anzueto A, Martin CD, et al. International study of the prevalence and outcomes of infection in intensive care units. JAMA. 2009;302:2323–9.
7. Siegel JD, Rhinehart E, Jackson M, Chiarello L. Management of multidrug-resistant organisms in health care settings, 2006. Am J Infect Control. 2007; 35(Suppl 2):S165–93.
8. Pittet D. Improving compliance with hand hygiene in hospitals. Infect Control Hosp Epidemiol. 2000;21:381–6.
9. Stewardson A, Allegranzi B, Sax H, Kilpatrick C, Pittet D. Back to the future: rising to the Semmelweis challenge in hand hygiene. Future Microbiol. 2011;6:855–76.
10. Pittet D, Allegranzi B, Sax H, Dharan S, Pessoa-Silva CL, Donaldson L, et al. Evidence-based model for hand transmission during patient care and the role of improved practices. Lancet Infect Dis. 2006;6:641–52.
11. Erasmus V, Daha TJ, Brug H, Richardus JH, Behrendt MD, Vos MC, et al. Systematic review of studies on compliance with hand hygiene guidelines in hospital care. Infect Control Hosp Epidemiol. 2010;31:283–94.
12. Ulrich RS, Zimring C, Zhu X, DuBose J, Seo HB, Choi YS, et al. A review of the research literature on evidence-based healthcare design. HERD. 2008;1: 61–125.
13. Mazzariol A, Roelofsen E, Koncan R, Voss A, Cornaglia G. Detection of a new SHV-type extended-Spectrum β-lactamase, SHV-31, in a *Klebsiella pneumoniae* strain causing a large nosocomial outbreak in The Netherlands. Antimicrob Agents Chemother. 2007;51:1082–4.
14. National Committee for Clinical Laboratory Standards. Methods for antimicrobial susceptibility tests for bacteria that grow aerobically. Approved standard M7-A5. NCCLS: Wayne; 2000.
15. The European Committee on Antimicrobial Susceptibility Testing. Breakpoint tables for interpretation of MICs and zone diameters. Version. 2010;1:0. http://www.eucast.org
16. Livermore DM, Brown DF. Detection of beta-lactamase-mediated resistance. J Antimicrob Chemother. 2001;48(Suppl 1):59–64.
17. Infection Prevention Working Party. Infection Prevention in the intensive care unit. Guideline 39. Mededelingen en bekendmakingen. Nieuwe richtlijn van de Werkgroep Infectiepreventie. Ned Tijdschr Geneeskd. 1999;143:2077–8.
18. van der Spoel JI, Gerritsen RT. SDD for the prevention and control of outbreaks. In: van der Voort PHJ, van Saene HKF, editors. Selective digestive tract decontamination in intensive care medicine: a practical guide to controlling infection. Springer-Verlag Italia. Italy: Milan; 2008. p. 141–54.
19. Rommes HJ. The concept of SDD. In: van der Voort PHJ, van Saene HKF, editors. Selective digestive tract decontamination in intensive care medicine: a practical guide to controlling infection. Springer-Verlag Italia, Milan, Italy. 2008. P. 37–45.
20. Kluytmans-Vandenbergh MF, Kluytmans JA, Voss A. Dutch guideline for preventing nosocomial transmission of highly resistant microorganisms (HRMO). Infection. 2005;33:309–13.
21. Halaby T, Al Naiemi N, Kluytmans J, van der Palen J, Vandenbroucke-Grauls CM. Emergence of colistin resistance in Enterobacteriaceae after the introduction of selective digestive tract decontamination in an intensive care unit. Antimicrob Agents Chemother. 2013;57:3224–9.
22. Savelkoul PH, Aarts HJ, de Haas J, Dijkshoorn L, Duim B, Otsen M, Rademaker JL, Schouls L, Lenstra JA. Amplified-fragment length polymorphism analysis: the state of an art. J Clin Microbiol. 1999;37:3083–91.
23. Rosenbaum, Rosenbaum, P.R. (2002). Observational Studies. Second edition. Springer, section. 2:4.
24. Rosenbaum, Rosenbaum, P.R. (2002). Observational studies. Second edition. Springer.,chapter 9.
25. Core Team R. R: a language and environment for statistical computing. In: R foundation for statistical computing. Vienna: Austria. URL; 2017. https://www.R-project.org.
26. Fluit AC, Terlingen AM, Andriessen L, Ikawaty R, van Mansfeld R, Top J, et al. Evaluation of the DiversiLab system for detection of hospital outbreaks of infections by different bacterial species. J Clin Microbiol. 2010;48:3979–89.
27. Silvestri L, Petros AJ, Sarginson RE, de la Cal MA, Murray AE, van Saene HK. Handwashing in the intensive care unit: a big measure with modest effects. J Hosp Infect. 2005;59:172–9.
28. Burke JP. Infection control - a problem for patient safety. N Engl J Med. 2003;348:651–6.
29. Harris AD, McGregor JC, Furuno JP. What infection control interventions should be undertaken to control multidrug-resistant gram-negative bacteria? Clin Infect Dis. 2006;43(Suppl. 2):S57–61.
30. Bonten MJ, Slaughter S, Ambergen AW, Hayden MK, van Voorhis J, Nathan C, Weinstein RA. 1998. The role of colonization pressure" in the spread of vancomycin-resistant enterococci: an important infection control variable. Arch Intern Med 158:1127–1132.
31. Macrae MB, Shannon KP, Rayner DM, Kaiser AM, Hoffman PN, French GLA. Simultaneous outbreak on a neonatal unit of two strains of multiply antibiotic resistant Klebsiella Pneumoniae controllable only by ward closure. J Hosp Infect. 2001;49:183–92.
32. Levin PD, Golovanevski M, Moses AE, Sprung CL, Benenson S. Improved ICU design reduces acquisition of antibiotic-resistant bacteria: a quasi-experimental observational study. Crit Care. 2011;15:R211.
33. Teltsch DY, Hanley J, Loo V, Goldberg P, Gursahaney A, Buckeridge DL. Infection acquisition following intensive care unit room privatization. Arch Intern Med. 2011;171:32–8.
34. Bonizzoli M, Bigazzi E, Peduto C, Tucci V, Zagli G, Pecile P, et al. Microbiological survey following the conversion from a bay-room to single-room intensive care unit design. J Hosp Infect. 2011;77:84–6.
35. Mulin B, Rouget C, Clément C, Bailly P, Julliot MC, Viel JF, et al. Association of private isolation rooms with ventilator-associated Acinetobacter baumanii pneumonia in a surgical intensive-care unit. Infect Control Hosp Epidemiol. 1997;18:499–503.
36. Detsky ME, Etchells E. Single-patient rooms for safe patient-centered hospitals. JAMA. 2008;300:954–6.

# 4

# Drug resistant tuberculosis in Saudi Arabia: an analysis of surveillance data 2014–2015

Maha Al Ammari[1], Abdulrahman Al Turaiki[1], Mohammed Al Essa[1,2], Abdulhameed M. Kashkary[3],
Sara A. Eltigani[3] and Anwar E. Ahmed[4*]

## Abstract

**Background:** There is limited data that investigates the national rates of drug-resistant tuberculosis (TB) in Saudi Arabia. This study aimed to estimate the rates of multi-drug-resistant tuberculosis (MDR-TB), rifampicin-resistant tuberculosis (RR-TB), and monoresistance (MR) in Saudi Arabia.

**Methods:** A retrospective cohort study was conducted on all TB cases reported to the National TB Control and Prevention Program (NTCPP) registry at the Saudi Ministry of Health between January 1, 2014 and December 31, 2015. A total of 2098 TB patients with positive TB cultures were included in the study. Subgroup analyses and multivariate binary logistic regression models were performed with IBM SPSS 23.0.

**Results:** Of the total TB cases, 4.4% (95% CI: 3.59%–5.40%) were found to have MDR-TB. The rates of MR were 3.8% (95% CI: 2.99%–4.67%) for ethambutol, 5.4% (95% CI: 4.50%–6.49%) for pyrazinamide, 10.2% (95% CI: 5.89%–11.52%) for isoniazid, 11% (95% CI: 9.70%–12.43%) for streptomycin, and 5.9% (95% CI: 4.90%–6.96%) for rifampicin. The high rates of MDR and RR-TB were found among the younger age group, female gender, and those who had a previous history of TB. We also discovered that renal failure tends to increase the risk of rifampicin resistance.

**Conclusions:** National TB data in Saudi Arabia shows that the rate of MDR-TB was similar to the global rate reported by the World Health Organization (WHO). It is a relatively high rate as compared to Western countries. The proportion of MDR/RR-TB patients tends to be higher in the younger age group, female gender, and in patients with a previous history of TB treatment. Effective strategies for prevention of all multi-drug-resistant TB cases are warranted.

**Keywords:** Mdr-Tb, RR-Tb, Tuberculosis, Anti-TB drugs, Saudi Arabia

## Background

Tuberculosis (TB) is a major public health concern in Saudi Arabia's health system [1]. Despite the implementation of prevention and control measures, TB remains a public health concern in several of the developed world's health systems [2–5]. The World Health Organization (WHO) reported around 10 million newly diagnosed TB cases in 2016 [6].

According to WHO, TB has been ranked Number 11 of the top leading causes of death in Saudi Arabia. A total of 64,345 new TB cases were reported in Saudi Arabia during a period of 20 years (1991 to 2010) [7]. Although TB can be

treated in most cases, patient and health-system challenges exist regarding proper utilization of TB treatment, compliance [8], and direct observation of each TB patient under treatment [9]. Unfortunately, TB bacilli may develop resistance to Anti-TB drugs. [10].

MDR-TB (MDR-TB) is defined as resistance to isoniazid and rifampicin, the two most potent anti-TB drugs [11]. Developing resistance to anti-tuberculosis medications has immense implications on the management of TB by 1) increasing the treatment duration, 2) having to use second-line medications with broader side-effects profiles, 3) the increased cost of therapy, and 4) the lower success rates (82% for drug-susceptible TB, 52% for MDR-TB, 28% for XDR-TB) [6, 12, 13].

* Correspondence: ahmeda5@vcu.edu
[4]College of Public Health and Health Informatics, King Saud bin Abdulaziz University for Health Sciences, Riyadh, Saudi Arabia
Full list of author information is available at the end of the article

Globally, of all TB patients diagnosed in 2015, 4.6% of the new TB cases were found to have MDR-TB, in addition to 21% of the previously treated patients, and it was estimated that there were 480,000 new cases of MDR-TB worldwide [6]. The Saudi region-specific rates of MDR-TB were reported between 1 and 5% [14–16]. A single national study reported an overall MDR-TB rate of 4% [17]. To date, there has been no other national study that investigates the MDR-TB rate in Saudi Arabia. This epidemiological study aimed to estimate the rates of MDR-TB, RR-TB, and monoresistance to anti-TB drugs in Saudi Arabia. We also assessed the association between the demographic and clinical characteristics and the rate of high MDR-TB and RR-TB in the Saudi population.

## Methods

A retrospective cohort study was conducted on all TB cases reported to the National TB Control and Prevention Program (NTCPP) registry at the Saudi Ministry of Health between January 1, 2014 and December 31, 2015. The NTCPP registry is a data registry at the Saudi Ministry of Health, where all suspected and confirmed TB cases are registered from all Saudi Arabian regions, with all related variables that enable researchers and stakeholders to retrieve and analyze any data at any period of time. The authors used a retrospective design because it can be useful in identifying the factors associated with the high rates of drug-resistant TB using large-scale existing data. We assessed the drug-resistant TB over a two-year period (January 1, 2014 through December 31, 2015). The Institutional Review Board (IRB) approval was obtained from King Abdullah International Medical Research Center (KAIMRC) in December 2016. All registered TB cases in the NTCPP registry from January 2014 through December 31, 2015 were reviewed. The eligibility criterion was defined as TB cases with positive TB cultures as culture is considered the gold standard method that provides viable organisms to perform DST. DST is the definite diagnostic tool for confirming resistance of *Mycobacterium tuberculosis* against isoniazid, rifampicin, ethambutol, pyrazinamide, and streptomycin as per program guidelines. No subsample was selected as all TB patients fulfilling the eligibility criteria were included in the study. We extracted demographic data (age, gender, nationality, and place of residence); co-morbidity (renal disease, HIV, diabetes, lung disease, and immunosuppression); type of TB (pulmonary or extra pulmonary); history of previous TB treatment; and the drug susceptibility test for isoniazid, rifampicin, ethambutol, pyrazinamide, and streptomycin.

## Statistical analysis

We analyzed the data using IBM SPSS Statistics for Windows, version 23 (IBM Corp., Armonk, N.Y., USA). Summary statistics were used to describe the sample

characteristics (Table 1). The rates of multi-drug-resistant tuberculosis (MDR-TB), rifampicin-resistant tuberculosis (RR-TB), and monoresistance (MR) were described by percentage and 95% confidence intervals (CI). We estimated the rates of MDR-TB and RR-TB by each of the variables.

### Subgroup analyses

Chi-square/Fisher's Exact were used to test the associations between the sample characteristics across MDR-TB and RIF-resistance (Table 2).

**Table 1** Sample characteristics $N = 2098$

| Characteristics | Levels | Mean | SD |
|---|---|---|---|
| Age/year | | 36.6 | 15.9 |
| | | n | % |
| Gender | Male | 1449 | 69.1 |
| | Female | 649 | 30.9 |
| Occupation | Driver | 147 | 7 |
| | Housemaid | 246 | 11.7 |
| | Housewife | 172 | 8.2 |
| | Handcraft | 48 | 2.3 |
| | Student | 148 | 7.1 |
| | Unemployed | 283 | 13.5 |
| | Prisoner | 123 | 5.9 |
| | Other | 931 | 44.4 |
| Nationality | Saudi | 879 | 41.9 |
| | Non-Saudi | 1219 | 58.1 |
| Region | Center | 557 | 26.5 |
| | West | 796 | 37.9 |
| | East | 340 | 16.2 |
| | South | 290 | 13.8 |
| | North | 115 | 5.5 |
| TB site | Pulmonary | 1901 | 90.6 |
| | EPTB | 197 | 9.4 |
| Diabetes | Yes | 267 | 12.7 |
| | No | 1831 | 87.3 |
| HIV | Yes | 45 | 2.1 |
| | No | 2053 | 97.9 |
| Lung diseases | Yes | 54 | 2.6 |
| | No | 2044 | 97.4 |
| Chronic renal failure | Yes | 19 | 0.9 |
| | No | 2079 | 99.1 |
| Immunosuppressive | Yes | 13 | 0.6 |
| | No | 2085 | 99.4 |
| Previous TB treatment | Yes | 143 | 6.8 |
| | No | 1955 | 93.2 |

*SD* Standard deviation, *HIV* human immunodeficiency virus, *TB* tuberculosis

## Multivariate analyses

We used multivariate logistic models to identify the factors related to MDR-TB and RIF-resistance (Table 3). All variables assessed by the subgroup analyses were included in the multivariate models. The strength of the relation was assessed using unadjusted and adjusted odds ratios OR and aOR)and 95% CI (Table 2 and Table 3, respectively). In all analyses, the significance level was determined at $P \leq 0.05$.

## Results

A total of 6753 patients included in NTCPP registry from January 1, 2014 through December 31, 2015 were

**Table 2** Bivariate factors associated with MDR-TB and RR-TB

| Characteristics | Levels | MDR-TB 93(4.4%) | | | | 95% CI for OR | | RR-TB 123(5.9%) | | | | 95% CI for OR | |
|---|---|---|---|---|---|---|---|---|---|---|---|---|---|
| | | Mean Difference | SE Difference | P | OR | Lower | Upper | Mean Difference | SE Difference | P | OR | Lower | Upper |
| Age/year | | 3.8 | 1.4 | 0.006[a] | .983 | .968 | .998 | 2.547 | 1.5 | .084 | .989 | .977 | 1.001 |
| | | | | | | 95% CI for OR | | | | | | 95% CI for OR | |
| | | n | % | P | OR | Lower | Upper | n | % | P | OR | Lower | Upper |
| Gender | Male | 60 | 4.1 | 0.332 | 1.240 | .803 | 1.916 | 84 | 5.8 | 0.848 | 1.039 | .702 | 1.537 |
| | Female | 33 | 5.1 | | | | | 39 | 6 | | 1 | | |
| Occupation | Driver | 8 | 5.4 | 0.984 | 1.133 | .523 | 2.455 | 10 | 6.8 | 0.918 | 1.060 | .530 | 2.119 |
| | Housemaid | 10 | 4.1 | | | .834 | .414 | 1.680 | 12 | 4.9 | | .744 | .394 | 1.407 |
| | Housewife | 6 | 3.5 | | | .712 | .299 | 1.695 | 7 | 4.1 | | .616 | .277 | 1.371 |
| | Handcraft | 2 | 4.2 | | | .856 | .201 | 3.639 | 3 | 6.3 | | .968 | .292 | 3.205 |
| | Student | 6 | 4.1 | | | .832 | .349 | 1.986 | 7 | 4.7 | | .721 | .323 | 1.608 |
| | Unemployed | 11 | 3.9 | | | .796 | .406 | 1.561 | 17 | 6 | | .928 | .532 | 1.617 |
| | Prisoner | 5 | 4.1 | | | .834 | .325 | 2.144 | 7 | 5.7 | | .876 | .391 | 1.962 |
| | Other | 45 | 4.8 | | | 1 | | | 60 | 6.4 | | 1 | | |
| Nationality | Saudi | 34 | 3.9 | 0.286 | 1.264 | .821 | 1.946 | 51 | 5.8 | 0.920 | 1.019 | .704 | 1.475 |
| | Non-Saudi | 59 | 4.8 | | 1 | | | 72 | 5.9 | | 1 | | |
| Region | West | 43 | 5.4 | 0.014[a] | .937 | .585 | 1.500 | 54 | 6.8 | 0.004[a] | .892 | .587 | 1.356 |
| | East | 5 | 1.5 | | | .245 | .094 | .635 | 6 | 1.8 | | .220 | .093 | .524 |
| | South | 9 | 3.1 | | | .525 | .247 | 1.116 | 17 | 5.9 | | .764 | .427 | 1.367 |
| | North | 4 | 3.5 | | | .591 | .205 | 1.705 | 4 | 3.5 | | .442 | .155 | 1.258 |
| | Center | 32 | 5.7 | | | 1 | | | 42 | 7.5 | | 1 | | |
| TB site | Pulmonary | 87 | 4.6 | 0.320 | 1.527 | .659 | 3.539 | 113 | 5.9 | 0.622 | 1.182 | .608 | 2.296 |
| | EPTB | 6 | 3 | | 1 | | | 10 | 5.1 | | 1 | | |
| Diabetes | Yes | 9 | 3.4 | 0.367 | 1.378 | .685 | 2.775 | 14 | 5.2 | 0.645 | 1.144 | .646 | 2.027 |
| | No | 84 | 4.6 | | 1 | | | 109 | 6 | | 1 | | |
| HIV | Yes | 92 | 4.5 | 1.000 | 2.064 | .281 | 15.148 | 121 | 5.9 | 0.720 | 1.347 | .322 | 5.625 |
| | No | 1 | 2.2 | | 1 | | | 2 | 4.4 | | 1 | | |
| Lung diseases | Yes | 2 | 3.7 | 1.000 | .825 | .198 | 3.442 | 4 | 7.4 | 0.555 | 1.294 | .460 | 3.644 |
| | No | 91 | 4.5 | | 1 | | | 119 | 5.8 | | 1 | | |
| Chronic renal failure | Yes | 2 | 10.5 | 0.205 | 2.570 | .585 | 11.292 | 4 | 21.1 | 0.022[a] | 4.392 | 1.435 | 13.439 |
| | No | 91 | 4.4 | | 1 | | | 119 | 5.7 | | 1 | | |
| Immunosuppressive | Yes | 1 | 7.7 | 0.446 | 1.805 | .232 | 14.032 | 2 | 15.4 | 0.175 | 2.951 | .647 | 13.463 |
| | No | 92 | 4.4 | | 1 | | | 121 | 5.8 | | 1 | | |
| Previous TB treatment | Yes | 36 | 25.2 | 0.001[a] | 11.203 | 7.069 | 17.755 | 41 | 28.7 | 0.001[a] | 9.181 | 6.005 | 14.038 |
| | No | 57 | 2.9 | | 1 | | | 82 | 4.2 | | 1 | | |

[a]Significant at α = 0.05; *OR* odds ratio, *TB* Tuberculosis, *HIV* human immunodeficiency virus, *MDR-TB* multi-drug-resistant tuberculosis, *RR-TB* rifampicin-resistant tuberculosis, *EPTB* extra-pulmonary tuberculosis, *SE* (standard error)

**Table 3** Multivariate factors associated with MDR-TB and RR-TB

| Factor | | MDR-TB | | 95% CI for aOR | | RR-TB | | 95% CI for aOR | |
| --- | --- | --- | --- | --- | --- | --- | --- | --- | --- |
| | | P | aOR | Lower | Upper | P | aOR | Lower | Upper |
| Age | | 0.032[a] | 0.98 | 0.962 | 0.998 | 0.047[a] | 0.98 | 0.970 | 1.000 |
| Female | Male | 0.015[a] | 2.21 | 1.170 | 4.181 | 0.044[a] | 1.78 | 1.015 | 3.120 |
| Occupation: Driver | Other | 0.232 | 1.68 | 0.718 | 3.932 | 0.285 | 1.51 | 0.708 | 3.237 |
| Occupation: Housemaid | Other | 0.116 | 0.49 | 0.200 | 1.193 | 0.147 | 0.55 | 0.246 | 1.234 |
| Occupation: Housewife | Other | 0.036[a] | 0.33 | 0.114 | 0.932 | 0.010[a] | 0.28 | 0.109 | 0.744 |
| Occupation: Hand Craft | Other | 0.390 | 1.93 | 0.430 | 8.654 | 0.241 | 2.11 | 0.606 | 7.342 |
| Occupation: Student | Other | 0.113 | 0.44 | 0.157 | 1.217 | 0.037[a] | 0.37 | 0.144 | 0.940 |
| Occupation:Unemployed | Other | 0.395 | 0.72 | 0.338 | 1.534 | 0.267 | 0.70 | 0.370 | 1.317 |
| Occupation: Prisoner | Other | 0.771 | 0.86 | 0.313 | 2.369 | 0.584 | 0.79 | 0.330 | 1.868 |
| Saudi | Non-Saudi | 0.921 | 0.97 | 0.569 | 1.664 | 0.583 | 1.14 | 0.716 | 1.813 |
| West | Center | 0.624 | 0.88 | 0.522 | 1.477 | 0.371 | 0.81 | 0.514 | 1.282 |
| East | Center | 0.038[a] | 0.35 | 0.131 | 0.942 | 0.005[a] | 0.28 | 0.115 | 0.685 |
| South | Center | 0.181 | 0.57 | 0.254 | 1.296 | 0.552 | 0.82 | 0.437 | 1.556 |
| North | Center | 0.710 | 0.81 | 0.274 | 2.418 | 0.273 | 0.55 | 0.189 | 1.601 |
| TB Type: Pulmonary | EPTB | 0.480 | 1.38 | 0.565 | 3.375 | 0.766 | 1.11 | 0.548 | 2.260 |
| Diabetes | No | 0.835 | 0.92 | 0.411 | 2.052 | 0.874 | 0.95 | 0.486 | 1.847 |
| HIV | No | 0.469 | 2.34 | 0.234 | 23.392 | 0.416 | 2.14 | 0.343 | 13.353 |
| Lung diseases | No | 0.549 | 0.63 | 0.138 | 2.868 | 0.789 | 0.85 | 0.271 | 2.693 |
| Chronic renal failure | No | 0.102 | 4.01 | 0.759 | 21.231 | 0.004[a] | 6.61 | 1.860 | 23.495 |
| Immunosuppressive | No | 0.738 | 1.56 | 0.116 | 21.008 | 0.262 | 3.18 | 0.420 | 24.113 |
| Previous TB treatment | No | 0.001[a] | 12.08 | 7.325 | 19.927 | 0.001[a] | 9.33 | 5.920 | 14.717 |
| (Intercept) | | 0.003 | 0.02 | | | 0.002 | 0.04 | | |

[a]Significant at α = 0.05; *aOR* adjusted odds ratio, *TB* Tuberculosis, *HIV* human immunodeficiency virus, *MDR-TB* multi-drug-resistant tuberculosis, *RR-TB* rifampicin-resistant tuberculosis, *EPTB* extra-pulmonary tuberculosis. The percentages of correct classification were 95.6% for MDR-TB and 94.1% for RR-TB

reviewed. Around 4655 patients were excluded due to non-availability of culture results, or non-availability of rifampicin-susceptibility test results. A total of 2098 patients with positive TB cultures enrolled in the study for the final analysis.

The mean age was 36.6 (SD = 15.9) years. Of the TB cases, 69.1% were male, 11.7% were housemaids, and 41.9% were Saudi. About 38% of these TB cases occurred in the Western region of Saudi Arabia. Pulmonary tuberculosis was common in TB patients (90.6%), while 9.4% had extra-pulmonary tuberculosis (EPTB). More details can be found in Table 1. The rate for MDR-TB in TB patients studied was 4.4% (95% CI: 3.59%–5.40%), while the resistance rate was 3.8% (95% CI: 2.99%–4.67%) for ethambutol, 5.4% (95% CI: 4.50%–6.49%) for pyrazinamide, 5.9% (95% CI: 4.90%–6.96%) for rifampicin, 10.2% (95% CI: 5.89%–11.52%) for isoniazid, and 11% (95% CI: 9.70%–12.43%) for streptomycin.

According to subgroup analyses (Table 2), the resistance rates for MDR/RR-TB were low in the Eastern region. The resistance rates for MDR-TB and RR-TB were high in patients with previous anti-TB treatment, and chronic renal

failure was associated with a higher rate of RR-TB. There was no association regarding gender, age, TB site, nationality, or HIV status. According to multivariate logistic models (Table 3), the female gender is more likely to have MDR-TB and RR-TB (2.21 and 1.78 times) as compared to the male gender, respectively. As age increases by 1 year, MDR-TB and RIF-resistance tend to decrease by 2%.

In comparison to patients with no previous anti-TB treatment, MDR-TB and RR-TB were 12.08 and 9.33, respectively, times more likely to occur in patients with previous TB treatment. Patients from the Eastern region are less likely to develop MDR-TB and RR-TB by 65% and 72% respectively, compared with patients from the Central region. Compared to patients with no renal failure, patients with renal failure were 6.61 times more likely to have RR-TB. Housewives, compared to other occupations, were 67% and 72% less likely to have MDR-TB and RR-TB, respectively.

## Discussion

Our data showed that the rate of MDR-TB in Saudi Arabia is within the global average as per the 2016 WHO report [6]. Similar to a previous Al-Hajoj et al. study, our study revealed that the Western and Central regions showed the highest rates of MDR-TB and Eastern region was the lowest [17]. The high rates in the Western region could be due to the presence of the two biggest holy sites (Mecca and Medina), which are visited by millions of Muslim from all around the world, including from countries where TB is highly endemic. During Hajj season, TB is the most frequent cause of hospitalization [18]. In the Central region we expected the higher rate could be due to the presence of four tertiary care hospitals in addition to the MOH central hospital and the chest hospital, that serve as referral centers from the periphery for all suspected and confirmed TB cases.

Comparing our result with the Al-Hajhoj study, there were slightly higher rates of MDR-TB (4.4% vs. 4.0%) and RR-TB in our study (5.8% vs. 5.3%), respectively. Comparing the rate of MDR-TB in the newly treated patients, the Al-Hajhoj study showed 1.8% of newly treated patients had MDR-TB, while our study showed a higher rate of MDR-TB (2.9%) among the newly diagnosed patients [17]. Our study showed consistent results with several published studies regarding previously treated patients and the risk of MDR-TB [17, 19–24].

Our study also revealed that each one-year increase was associated with a 2% decrease in MDR-TB. This was similar to what was seen in a European meta-analysis, which showed that patients younger than 65 years of age were associated with a higher risk of MDR-TB [19] and in an Ethiopian study, which showed that patients younger than 25 years of age had an increased risk of MDR-TB [20]. This association could be explained by the fact that younger patients have lower compliance to the medication compared with the elderly.

In our study, the female gender was associated with a higher rate of MDR-TB compared with males. This finding contradicted the results of the previously mentioned meta-analysis, which showed that males have a higher chance of developing MDR-TB when compared to females [19].

This study has several limitations: the data were collected retrospectively, and due to the nature of the study, we did not include modifiable factors such as patient compliance and appropriateness of regimen. These factors could be important in developing anti-TB resistance as is shown in a study conducted in Turkey in 2004 [24]. Data were not available for close contact with other MDR-TB patients, alcohol use, and monthly income in our patients, which may be important factors for a high rate of MDR-TB as was shown in the Mulu study [20]. No data on intravenous drug abuse was collected, however it was found to be associated with MDR-TB in a 2014 study conducted in Portugal [23]. Despite these limitations, the study determined the overall MDR-TB rate and TB patients with high risk in Saudi Arabia. The study may be helpful to policymakers wanting to address the rising concern of MDR-TB in Saudi Arabia.

## Conclusion

National TB data in Saudi Arabia shows the rate of MDR-TB is in accordance with global rates, however, it is a relatively high rate when compared to Western countries. The proportion of MDR/RR-TB cases tends to increase in younger age group, female gender, and in patients with previous TB treatment. The rates of MDR/RR-TB varied between regions in Saudi Arabia, with the Eastern region reporting the lowest MDR-TB rate. Further studies are required to understand the association between the suggested high risk and drug-resistant TB. It will help in addressing the early identification of the drug-resistant TB patients and their management.

### Acknowledgements
We would like to thank the National Tuberculosis Control and Prevention Program personnel for providing the data used in this research and for their support. The authors would like to thank King Abdullah International Medical Research Center for approving and funding this study.

### Funding
Funding for publication fees for open access was obtained from King Abdullah International Medical Research Center.

### Authors' contributions
MA, AA, and MAA conceived and designed the study and drafted the manuscript. AEA carried out the data analysis, prepared the results and the abstract sections, and revised the manuscript. AMK and SAE revised the draft of the manuscript. All authors read and approved the final manuscript.

### Competing interests
The authors declare that they have no competing interests.
Open Choice: Yes.

### Author details
[1]King Abdullah International Medical Research Center (KAIMRC)/King Abdulaziz Medical City(KAMC), Ministry of National Guard - Health Affairs, Riyadh, Saudi Arabia. [2]College of Pharmacy, King Saud bin Abdulaziz University for Health Sciences, Riyadh, Saudi Arabia. [3]Ministry of Health Kingdom of Saudi Arabia, Riyadh, Saudi Arabia. [4]College of Public Health and Health Informatics, King Saud bin Abdulaziz University for Health Sciences, Riyadh, Saudi Arabia.

### References
1. Abouzeid MS, Zumla AI, Felemban S, Alotaibi B, O'Grady J, Memish ZA. Tuberculosis trends in Saudis and non-Saudis in the Kingdom of Saudi Arabia–a 10 year retrospective study (2000–2009). PLoS One. 2012;7(6):e39478.
2. Main CL, Ying E, Wang EE. How much does it cost to manage paediatric tuberculosis? One-year experience from the Hospital for Sick Children. Can J Infect Dis Med Microbiol. 1998;9(6):354–8.
3. McGowan JE, Blumberg HM. Inner-city tuberculosis in the USA. J Hosp Infect. 1995;30:282–95.
4. Fiebig L, Kollan C, Hauer B, Gunsenheimer-Bartmeyer B, an der Heiden M, Hamouda O, Haas W. HIV-prevalence in tuberculosis patients in Germany, 2002–2009: an estimation based on HIV and tuberculosis surveillance data. PLoS One. 7(11):e49111.

5. Allen AR, Minozzi G, Glass EJ, et al. Bovine tuberculosis: the genetic basis of host susceptibility. Proceedings of the Royal Society B: Biological Sciences. 2010;277(1695):2737—45. https://doi.org/10.1098/rspb.2010.0830.

6. World Health Organization. Global tuberculosis report 2016.

7. Al-Orainey I, Alhedaithy MA, Alanazi AR, Barry MA, Almajid FM. Tuberculosis incidence trends in Saudi Arabia over 20 years: 1991-2010. Annals Thoracic Med. 2013;8(3):148.

8. Cambau E, Viveiros M, Machado D, Raskine L, Ritter C, Tortoli E, Matthys V, Hoffner S, Richter E, Del Molino MP, Cirillo DM. Revisiting susceptibility testing in MDR-TB by a standardized quantitative phenotypic assessment in a European multicentre study. J Antimicrob Chemother. 2015;70(3):686–96.

9. Jain A, Dixit P. Multidrug resistant to extensively drug resistant tuberculosis: what is next? J Biosci. 2008;33(4):605.

10. Villarino ME, Geiter LJ, Simone PM. The multidrug-resistant tuberculosis challenge to public health efforts to control tuberculosis. Public Health Rep. 1992;107(6):616.

11. Laserson KF, Thorpe LE, Leimane V, Weyer K, Mitnick CD, Riekstina V, Zarovska E, Rich ML, Fraser HS, Alarcón E, Cegielski JP. Speaking the same language: treatment outcome definitions for multidrug-resistant tuberculosis. Int J Tuberc Lung Dis. 2005;9(6):640–5.

12. World Health Organization (WHO). Treatment of tuberculosis: guidelines for national programmes. Geneva: WHO; 2003. WHO/CDS/TB/2003.313.

13. Cegielski JP. Extensively drug-resistant tuberculosis:"there must be some kind of way out of here". Clin Infect Dis. 2010;50(Supplement 3):S195–200.

14. Chaudhry LA, Rambhala N, Al-Shammri AS, Al-Tawfiq JA. Patterns of antituberculous drug resistance in eastern Saudi Arabia: a 7-year surveillance study from 1/2003 to 6/2010. J Epidemiol Global Health. 2012;2(1):57–60.

15. Asaad AM, Alqahtani JM. Primary anti-tuberculous drugs resistance of pulmonary tuberculosis in southwestern Saudi Arabia. J Infect Public Health. 2012;5(4):281–5.

16. Elhassan M, Hemeg HA, Elmekki MA, Turkistani KA, Abdul-Aziz AA. Burden of Multidrug Resistant Mycobacterium tuberculosis Among New Cases in Al-Madinah Al-Monawarah, Saudi Arabia. Infect Disord Drug Targets (Formerly Current Drug Targets-Infectious Disorders). 2017;17(1):14—23.

17. Al-Hajoj S, Varghese B, Shoukri MM, Al-Omari R, Al-Herbwai M, AlRabiah F, Alrajhi AA, Abuljadayel N, Al-Thawadi S, Zumla A, Zignol M. Epidemiology of antituberculosis drug resistance in Saudi Arabia: findings of the first national survey. Antimicrob Agents Chemother. 2013;57(5):2161–6.

18. Alzeer A, Mashlah A, Fakim N, Al-Sugair N, Al-Hedaithy M, Al-Majed S, Jamjoom G. Tuberculosis is the commonest cause of pneumonia requiring hospitalization during hajj (pilgrimage to Makkah). J Infect. 1998;36(3):303–6.

19. Faustini A, Hall AJ, Perucci CA. Risk factors for multidrug resistant tuberculosis in Europe: a systematic review. Thorax. 2006;61(2):158–63.

20. Mulu W, Mekkonnen D, Yimer M, Admassu A, Abera B. Risk factors for multidrug resistant tuberculosis patients in Amhara National Regional State. Afr Health Sci. 2015;15(2):368–77.

21. Barroso EC, Mota RM, Santos RO, Sousa AL, Barroso JB, Rodrigues JL. Risk factors for acquired multidrug-resistant tuberculosis. J Pneumol 2003;29(2):89-97.

22. Gomes M, Correia A, Mendonça D, Duarte R. Risk factors for drug-resistant tuberculosis. J Tuberc Res. 2014;3:2014.

23. Ruddy M, Balabanova Y, Graham C, Fedorin I, Malomanova N, Elisarova E, Kuznetznov S, Gusarova G, Zakharova S, Melentyev A, Krukova E. Rates of drug resistance and risk factor analysis in civilian and prison patients with tuberculosis in Samara region, Russia. Thorax. 2005;60(2):130–5.

24. Karabay O, Otkum M, Akata F, Karlikaya C, Tugrul M, Dundar V. Antituberculosis drug resistance and associated risk factors in the European section of Turkey. Indian J Chest Dis Allied Sci. 2004;46:171–8.

# 5

# Superbugs in the supermarket? Assessing the rate of contamination with third-generation cephalosporin-resistant gram-negative bacteria in fresh Australian pork and chicken

Jade E. McLellan[1†], Joshua I. Pitcher[1†], Susan A. Ballard[2], Elizabeth A. Grabsch[2], Jan M. Bell[3], Mary Barton[4] and M. Lindsay Grayson[1,2,5*] [iD]

## Abstract

**Background:** Antibiotic misuse in food-producing animals is potentially associated with human acquisition of multidrug-resistant (MDR; resistance to ≥ 3 drug classes) bacteria via the food chain. We aimed to determine if MDR Gram-negative (GNB) organisms are present in fresh Australian chicken and pork products.

**Methods:** We sampled raw, chicken drumsticks (CD) and pork ribs (PR) from 30 local supermarkets/butchers across Melbourne on two occasions. Specimens were sub-cultured onto selective media for third-generation cephalosporin-resistant (3GCR) GNBs, with species identification and antibiotic susceptibility determined for all unique colonies. Isolates were assessed by PCR for SHV, TEM, CTX-M, AmpC and carbapenemase genes (encoding IMP, VIM, KPC, OXA-48, NDM).

**Results:** From 120 specimens (60 CD, 60 PR), 112 (93%) grew a 3GCR-GNB ($n = 164$ isolates; 86 CD, 78 PR); common species were *Acinetobacter baumannii* (37%), *Pseudomonas aeruginosa* (13%) and *Serratia fonticola* (12%), but only one *E. coli* isolate. Fifty-nine (36%) had evidence of 3GCR alone, 93/163 (57%) displayed 3GCR plus resistance to one additional antibiotic class, and 9/163 (6%) were 3GCR plus resistance to two additional classes. Of 158 DNA specimens, all were negative for ESBL/carbapenemase genes, except 23 (15%) which were positive for AmpC, with 22/23 considered to be inherently chromosomal, but the sole *E. coli* isolate contained a plasmid-mediated CMY-2 AmpC.

**Conclusions:** We found low rates of MDR-GNBs in Australian chicken and pork meat, but potential 3GCR-GNBs are common (93% specimens). Testing programs that only assess for *E. coli* are likely to severely underestimate the diversity of 3GCR organisms in fresh meat.

**Keywords:** Infection, Antibiotic resistance, Foodborne

* Correspondence: Lindsay.Grayson@austin.org.au
†Equal contributors
[1]Department of Medicine, Austin Health, University of Melbourne, Melbourne, VIC, Australia
[2]Infectious Diseases & Microbiology Departments, Austin Health, Melbourne, VIC, Australia
Full list of author information is available at the end of the article

## Background

The emergence of multi-drug resistant (MDR) bacteria is a major health problem that has been likened in its global future impact on human health to that of terrorism [1, 2]. Widespread inappropriate use of antimicrobials in food production (especially meat/seafood, some fruit) has been linked to environmental contamination with MDR pathogens and outbreaks of MDR infections in humans, but direct cause-and-effect has often been difficult to confirm, despite the strength of the observed associations [3–8]. Most food testing programs for antimicrobial resistance (AMR) have focused on specific organisms (e.g. *E. coli*, Salmonella *spp.*, Listeria *spp.*), assuming direct food-to-human pathogen transfer, rather than considering resistant gene transfer between bacterial species [6, 8, 9]. Furthermore, the optimum site of specimen collection (e.g. on-farm animal, manure, abattoir, point-of-sale supermarket products) has been debated [9–13]. Although Australia has reasonably strict regulations regarding antimicrobial use in agriculture [13, 14], use of some agents for prophylaxis and treatment (e.g. trimethoprim-sulfamethoxazole, some beta-lactams and macrolides) is common in some food sectors [2, 13, 15, 16], such that this may have some implications for acquisition by consumers of multi-resistant pathogens via food consumption [6, 7].

Hence, we aimed to assess the rates of contamination with potential extended-spectrum beta-lactamase (ESBL)-producing Gram-negative organisms (without restricting to specific species) in Australian-produced chicken and pork meat. To best identify any potential risk to the consumer and to be certain that the meat was produced in Australia, we purchased chicken drumsticks and pork ribs at local fresh food outlets, since national legislation requires that bone-containing meat products must be Australian-produced (by conventional or organic production), whereas de-boned meats (e.g. bacon) can be imported into Australia [17].

## Methods

### Study design

This was a prospective cross-sectional survey undertaken during a four-month period from March to June 2014 in the eastern suburbs of Melbourne, Australia. We identified ten regions within the medical catchment area of the Austin Hospital and sampled from 2 to 4 retailers within each region (see Additional file 1: Figure S1 for locations). We tested raw, skin-covered chicken drumsticks (CD) and pork spare ribs (PR), each weighing approximately 150 g, from a total of 30 meat retailers (26 supermarkets, 4 butchers shops). Samples were purchased from each site on two occasions (approximately one month between each sample). Each sample from a supermarket was derived from a pre-packaged container with multiple CD or PR specimens, while each sample from a butcher was selected for purchase individually and was not pre-packaged.

### Specimen handling, culture and susceptibility

Similar to methods previously described [18, 19], each specimen was placed individually into separate zip lock bags (22 × 22 cm, Hercules, Australia), to which 100 mL of buffered peptone water (Thermofisher Scientific, Australia) was added and the specimen was massaged manually for 2 min. Of the subsequent rinsate, 50 mL was added in a sterile manner to 50 mL of double-strength tryptone soya broth (TSB; Thermofisher Scientific, Australia) which was incubated for 24 h at 37 °C. From this broth, 100 μL was inoculated into 10 mL of TSB containing ceftriaxone (0.25 mg/L) and vancomycin (8 mg/L), and incubated (37 °C, 24 h) before 10 μL was inoculated and spread onto ChromID ESBL agar (BioMérieux, France) and incubated for 48 h at 37 °C [18, 19]. All unique colonial morphologies on this selective medium were purity-plated onto Columbia horse blood agar/MacConkey agar (HBA/MAC; Thermofisher Scientific, Australia) and then subcultured onto Columbia HBA (Thermo Scientific, Australia) and incubated (37 °C, 24 h) before being identified using MALDI-TOF MS (BioMérieux, France) and tested for antibiotic susceptibility by Vitek2® (BioMérieux, France) using CLSI clinical breakpoint criteria. For those species and antibiotics where there were no defined criteria (e.g. *Pseudomonas* spp., *Stenotrophomonas* spp.), the Vitek-derived MIC value was compared to the relevant EUCAST distribution to categorise (for the purpose of this study) the presence of resistance (either intrinsic or acquired) [20–23]. If MALDI-TOF MS was unable to confidently identify (< 90% match) the organism after three attempts, Vitek2® was used for identification.

Isolates which grew on ChromID ESBL agar and displayed phenotypic resistance by Vitek2 to third-generation cephalosporins (ceftriaxone; 3GCR) were considered to be potential ESBL-producers or intrinsically 3GCR [24–26] and were classified according to the number of antibiotic classes to which they were resistant – including third-generation cephalosporins, carbapenems (meropenem), aminoglycosides (gentamicin), fluoroquinolones (ciprofloxacin) and anti-folates (trimethoprim-sulfamethoxazole). Similar to previously, multi-drug-resistance (MDR) was defined as resistance to ≥3 classes of antibiotics [27].

### Molecular assessment for beta-lactamase genes

DNA was extracted from all potential ESBL-producing isolates using previously described methods (DNeasy Blood and Tissue kit, Qiagen, USA), then screened for the presence of the bla$_{TEM}$, and bla$_{SHV}$ genes using a real-time polymerase chain reaction (PCR) platform (LC-480) and published primers [28, 29]. A multiplex real-time TaqMan PCR was used to detect CTX-M-type genes (groups 1, 2, 9, 8, 25) [30]. Strains were probed for plasmid-borne AmpC enzymes using the method described by Pérez-Pérez and Hanson (including blaACC-like, blaDHA-like, blaCIT/CMY-like, blaMOX-like, blaFOX-like, blaMIR/ACT-like; [31]) and subjected to molecular tests for MBL (bla$_{VIM}$, bla$_{IMP}$ and bla$_{NDM}$), bla$_{KPC}$, and blaOXA-48-like genes using real-time PCR [32, 33]. Isolates suspected of containing transferable ESBL or MBL genes underwent whole genome sequencing whereby unique dual indexed libraries were prepared from genomic DNA using the Nextera XT DNA sample preparation kit (Illumina). Libraries were sequenced on the Illumina NextSeq 500 with 150-cycle paired end chemistry as described by the manufacturer's protocols and sequences were accessed for known resistance genes using KmerResistance 2.2 [34].

### Data analysis and statistics

The rates of contamination with potential ESBL-producing Gram-negative organisms were assessed according to specimen type (CD, PR), the geographic site of specimen purchase and the type of meat outlet (supermarket vs butcher). Similar rates were reported for PCR-confirmed ESBL isolates and those where the ESBL was likely to be plasmid-mediated. Comparisons between rates for CD and PR were undertaken using Chi-square.

### Results

Of a total of 120 meat specimens (60 CD, mean ± SD weight: 155.4 ± 26.5 [range 78.5–223.9] grams; 60 PR, 160.5 ± 48.9 [range: 91.5–355.1] grams) that were assessed from 30 retailers (see locations in Additional file 1: Figure S1), 112 (56 CD, 93%; 56 PR; 93%) were contaminated with a total of 164 (86 CD; 78 PR) 3GCR (i.e. potential ESBL-producing) isolates (Table 1). Among these isolates, 59 (36%; 26 CD, 33 PR) displayed phenotypic evidence of 3GCR alone, 96 (59%; 54 CD, 42 PR) were 3GCR plus were also resistant to either anti-folates, aminoglycosides or carbapenems and 9 isolates (5.5%; 6 CD, 3 PR; 9 specimens; 5 Pseudomonas aeruginosa, 2 Pseudomonas spp., 1 Bordetella trematum, 1 Chryseobacterium gleum) were MDR with evidence of being 3GCR plus resistance to two other antibiotic classes. Resistance to anti-folates was most common (n = 91 [55%] isolates, 49 CD, 42 PR, Table 1; 82 [68.3%] specimens). The four most common 3GCR species identified were Acinetobacter baumannii complex (n = 59), Pseudomonas aeruginosa (n = 22), Serratia fonticola (n = 19) and Hafnia alvei (n = 15). Only one E. coli isolate was identified – this was in a CD specimen.

Among the 164 isolates, 158 had DNA available for PCR analysis. Beta-lactamase genes were identified in 23 (15%) isolates (7CD, 14PR [2 PR each had two isolates], p = 0.15; 17.5% specimens). All were AmpC, with 22/23 considered to be inherently chromosomally located (ACC, n = 12 [H. alvei, 10; S. fonticola, 2]; CMY-like n = 7 [C. freundii, 6; C. youngae/freundii, 1]; FOX, n = 1 [A. sobria]; MIR-like/ACT-like, n = 2; [E. cloacae complex]), while the sole E. coli isolate contained a CMY-like AmpC gene that was likely to be plasmid-mediated and was subsequently shown on whole genome sequencing to be a CMY-2 (see Table 1). All DNA samples were PCR-negative for other ESBL genes (including SHV, TEM, CTX-M) and all carbapenemase encoding gene families (including IMP, VIM, KPC, OXA-48-like and NDM).

Among the 30 food outlets, there were four supermarket chains (two large [n = 10 and 11 stores sampled]; two smaller [n = 2 and 3 stores] and 4 separate (unlinked) butcher shops. Overall, there were no differences in rates of contamination between supermarkets and unlinked butchers shops. All supermarkets and butcher shops had at least one CD or PR specimen that grew a potential ESBL-producing isolate, at some time. Only 8 specimens were culture-negative (4 CD, 4 PR; one supermarket site had both its PR specimens culture-negative). The numbers of 3GCR isolates per specimen were as follows: single isolate in 63 specimens; two isolates in 44 specimens; 3 isolates in 3 specimens, and one specimen contained 4 potential ESBL-producing isolates. Interestingly, it was this latter specimen (which was collected from a butcher's shop) that grew the CMY-2-containing E. coli, along with an A. baumannii, S. fonticola and an E. cloacae complex isolate – although none of these latter 3 isolates contained any definable ESBL genes (Table 1).

### Discussion

This study of Australian chicken and pork is notable for a number of reasons. Firstly, we assessed for a broad range of Gram-negative organisms, not simply the traditional species of E. coli or Salmonella spp. [6, 8–10]. Taking this approach, we identified that 93% of specimens appeared to be contaminated with a wide variety of 3GCR species, including particularly Acinetobacter baumannii complex, Pseudomonas aeruginosa, Serratia fonticola and Hafnia alvei. We were surprised by the relatively high rates of these potential pathogens and initially speculated that perhaps they were due to a point-source within certain supermarkets or butcher shops, such as has been reported in one outbreak of multidrug-resistant K. pneumoniae [35]. However, they were identified from both CD and PR products purchased from a wide variety of food outlets which had no common supply chain. Notably, only one E. coli isolate was identified – so testing programs which only assess for this species

**Table 1** Summary of isolates grown from fresh retail chicken and pork

| Isolate | Overall total n=164 | Chicken (n=86) | | | | | | | Pork (n=78) | | | | | | | |
|---|---|---|---|---|---|---|---|---|---|---|---|---|---|---|---|---|
| | | Total | 3GCR alone | AF | Mero | AF+Mero | AF+FQ | Mero+AMG | Total | 3GCR alone | AF | Mero | AMG | AF+Mero | AF+FQ | Mero+AMG |
| Acinetobacter baumannii complex | 59 | 34 | – | 34 | – | – | – | – | 25 | – | 25 | – | – | – | – | – |
| Acinetobacter ursingii | 2 | – | – | – | – | – | – | – | 2 | – | 2 | – | – | – | – | – |
| Aeromonas sobria | 1[f] | – | – | – | – | – | – | – | 1 | – | – | 1 | – | – | – | – |
| Bordetella trematum | 1 | – | – | – | – | – | – | – | 1 | – | – | – | – | – | 1 | – |
| Chryseobacterium gleum | 1 | – | – | – | – | – | – | – | 1 | – | – | – | – | – | – | 1 |
| Citrobacter braakii | 7 | – | – | – | – | – | – | – | 7[b] | 7[b] | – | – | – | – | – | – |
| Citrobacter freundii | 6[e] | – | – | – | – | – | – | – | 6 | 6 | – | – | – | – | – | – |
| Citrobacter youngae | 1[e] | 1 | 1 | – | – | – | – | – | – | – | – | – | – | – | – | – |
| Enterobacter cloacae complex | 9[g] | 1 | 1 | – | – | – | – | – | 8 | 8 | – | – | – | – | – | – |
| Escherichia coli | 1[a] | 1[a] | 1[a] | – | – | – | – | – | – | – | – | – | – | – | – | – |
| Hafnia alvei | 15[c] | 6 | 6 | – | – | – | – | – | 9 | 9 | – | – | – | – | – | – |
| Pseudomonas aeruginosa | 22 | 11 | – | 7 | – | 4 | – | – | 11 | – | 10 | – | – | 1 | – | – |
| Pseudomonas alcaligenes | 1 | 1 | – | – | 1 | – | – | – | – | – | – | – | – | – | – | – |
| Pseudomonas oleovorans | 3 | 1 | – | 1 | – | – | – | – | 2 | – | 2 | – | – | – | – | – |
| Pseudomonas putida | 11 | 10 | – | 1 | 8 | – | – | – | 1 | – | 1 | – | – | – | – | – |
| Pseudomonas spp. | 3 | 3 | – | – | – | – | 2 | – | – | – | – | – | – | – | – | – |
| Serratia fonticola | 19[d] | 16 | 15 | 1 | – | – | – | – | 3 | 3 | – | – | – | – | – | – |
| Stenotrophomonas maltophilia | 1 | – | – | – | – | – | – | – | 1 | – | – | – | 1 | – | – | – |
| Yokenella regensburgei | 1 | 1 | – | – | 1 | – | – | – | – | – | – | – | – | – | – | – |

3GCR Third-generation cephalosporin resistance, AF Anti-folates, FQ Fluoroquinolones, Mero Meropenem, AMG Aminoglycosides

[a] E. coli was an ST 349 isolate and contained a plasmid-mediated CMY-2 AmpC ESBL

[b] Includes 4× C. braakii/freundii and 1× C. braakii/werkmanii isolates

[c] 10 H. alvei isolates contained ACC AmpC ESBLs - 4 were from chicken and 6 from pork

[d] Two S. fonticola isolates contained ACC AmpC ESBLs – 1 was from chicken and 1 from pork

[e] All isolates contained CMY-like AmpC ESBL

[f] Isolate contained a FOX AmpC ESBL

[g] Two isolates contained an EBC AmpC ESBL – both from pork

would have reported a much lower rate of potential contamination.

Secondly, our results highlight the importance of not relying solely on selective media such as ChromID ESBL agar in such programs, but instead confirming the presence of ESBL genes by PCR. Phenotypic detection methods alone may identify intrinsically 3GCR isolates or those that falsely suggest ESBL production [24–26]. AmpC genes were identified in 15% isolates assessed (17.5% specimens), with most (22/23) being inherently chromosomal in location [26]. Notably, however, the sole *E. coli* isolate identified contained a plasmid-mediated CMY-2 which was potentially transferable.

The fact that resistance to anti-folate agents was the most common resistance phenotype identified among potential ESBL-producing strains and was noted in 68.3% of all CD/PR specimens is important, given that trimethoprim-sulfamethoxazole is widely used in pork production and some chicken farms [15, 16]. Hence these results may be no surprise, but at least serve as a potential "wake up call" to farmers who are concerned about the consequences of frequent antibiotic use. Importantly, 9 isolates (7.5% CD/PR specimens) displayed an MDR phenotype, with only one strain (*Bordetella trematum*) being resistant to fluoroquinolones – consistent with Australia's strict controls on fluoroquinolone use in agriculture and similar to previous studies on this issue [14].

*Acinetobacter, Serratia, Hafnia* and *Pseudomonas* spp. are all known to be common in the environment and to be present on some fruit and vegetables [36, 37], but their presence may be a potential source of resistance genes [38].

Given the uncertainty about which testing regimen would be ideally suited for a large national food safety screening program for MDR contamination [9–13], we believe our methodology was a practical approach that is potentially relevant and meaningful to retail consumers and which could be up-scaled without the need for major infrastructure or specialised training. In comparison, all previous published Australian studies have assessed non-meat items such as animal faeces or eggs [39–42].

Our findings differ from those by other authors. Overdevest et al. [8] reported that 79.8% of retail chicken meat samples in the Netherlands had organisms with ESBL genes present, while only 1.8% of pork samples grew an ESBL-producing organism. However, this study focused particularly on *E. coli* and *K. pneumoniae* without commenting on other organisms isolated. Stewardson et al. [7] reported 86% contamination of chicken meat products delivered to a tertiary hospital in Switzerland with ESBL-producing *Enterobacteriaceae* species. Similar to our results, MDR strains were uncommon.

This study has some limitations. Firstly, the sample size of 120 specimens, while consistent with similar studies, is relatively small in the context of overall Australian supply [2, 7, 8, 43–47]. Secondly, we were not able to track the original farm source of the CD and PR products, although one might expect larger supermarket chains to have a limited number of defined contracted suppliers. Further research to investigate the rates of contamination at each step of the meat production process, including samples from animals in farms, carcasses and meat products in slaughterhouses and of meat products distributed to third party organisations for packaging and distribution, may be helpful to identify if there is a common source of contamination. Thirdly, our sample preparation (including initial 24 h culture in non-selective media), the subsequent selective culturing techniques provided enhanced sensitivity for 3GCR-GNBs but did not allow us to accurately quantify the burden of contamination in each CD/PR sample. Importantly, we did not assess for phenotypic colistin resistance since laboratory methods are evolving [48, 49], nor did we assess for *mcr* genes since this resistance mechanism was only first reported in 2016 [50]. Notably, colistin resistance appears to be currently rare in Australia [51, 52] and colistin is infrequently used in Australian agriculture [2, 53]. Finally, Australia does not import fresh chicken meat, nor any fresh bone-containing pork products [13, 17], which means that all of our specimens came from animals born and grown in Australia. As such we cannot comment on any possible difference in contamination between these Australian products and similar, but boned, imported chicken and pork processed meat products.

We believe our findings raise important questions regarding future food testing programs and potentially highlight the importance of routine public health measures related to safe food preparation such as appropriate hand hygiene before/after handling uncooked meat products, adequate washing of kitchen utensils and surfaces that have contact with uncooked meat and appropriate cooking methods to ensure destruction of any contaminating bacteria. These public health messages may be of particular importance to patient groups where immunosuppression is likely, such as those with haematological malignancy or transplant recipients. Further research into the potential source(s) of retail meat contamination is warranted.

## Conclusion

Overall, we found low rates of MDR-GNBs in Australian chicken and pork meat, but potential 3GCR-GNBs are common (93% specimens), as is resistance to trimethoprim-sulfamethoxazole. Food testing programs that only assess for *E. coli* are likely to severely underestimate the diversity of 3GCR organisms in fresh meat.

**Acknowledgements**
We are grateful to John Bourke for his assistance with education regarding the Australian pork industry and Ms. Trudi Bannam for technical laboratory assistance.

**Funding**
No specific funding was received for this project – it was supported internally by the Infectious Diseases Department, Austin Health.

**Authors' contributions**
JEM, JIP, MB and MLG designed the study, including approach to specimen sampling, handling and laboratory methods used. JEM, JIP, SAB, EAG and JMB undertook the laboratory testing. JEM, JIP and MLG undertook any necessary statistical analyses and prepared the manuscript with feedback/input from all other authors. All authors read and approved the final manuscript.

**Competing interests**
The authors declare that they have no competing interests.

**Author details**
[1]Department of Medicine, Austin Health, University of Melbourne, Melbourne, VIC, Australia. [2]Infectious Diseases & Microbiology Departments, Austin Health, Melbourne, VIC, Australia. [3]Infectious Diseases and Microbiology, SA Pathology, Adelaide, South Australia, Australia. [4]School of Pharmacy and Medical Sciences, University of South Australia, Adelaide, South Australia, Australia. [5]Department of Epidemiology and Preventive Medicine, Monash University, Melbourne, VIC, Australia.

**References**
1. Davies S. (2013). Annual report of the chief medical officer, 2011 – volume 2. https://www.gov.uk/government/publications/chief-medical-officer-annual-report-volume-2 Accessed 16th July 2016.
2. Australian Government. Department of Health, Department of Agriculture (2015). Responding to the Threat of Antimicrobial Resistance. https://www.health.gov.au/internet/main/publishing.nsf/.../amr-strategy-2015-2019.pdf. Accessed 8th Nov 2016.
3. O'Neill J. Tackling drug-resistant infections globally: final report and recommendations. London: H M Government/Wellcome Trust; 2016. p. 2016.
4. WHO – World Health Organization (2012).The evolving threat of antimicrobial resistance – Options for action. http://www.who.int/patientsafety/implementation/amr/publication/en/ Accessed 8th Nov 2016.
5. WHO (2015). Global action plan on antimicrobial resistance. Geneva: World Health Organization, 2015. http://www.who.int/drugresistance/global_action_plan/en/ Accessed 8th Nov 2016.
6. Kluytmans JA, Overdevest IT, Willemsen I, et al. Extended-spectrum β-lactamase-producing Escherichia Coli from retail chicken meat and humans: comparison of strains, plasmids, resistance genes, and virulence factors. Clin Infect Dis. 2013;56(4): 478–87.
7. Stewardson AJ, Renzi G, Maury N, et al. Extended-spectrum β-lactamase-producing Enterobacteriaceae in hospital food: a risk assessment. Infect Control Hosp Epidemiol. 2014;35(4):375–83.
8. Overdevest I, Willemsen I, Rijnsburger M, Eustace A, Xu L, Hawkey P, Heck M, Savelkoul P, Vandenbroucke-Grauls C, van der Zwaluw K, Huijsdens X, Kluytmans J. Extended-Spectrum ß-lactamase genes of Escherichia coli in chicken meat and humans, the Netherlands. Emerg Infect Dis. 2011;17(7):1216–22.
9. EFSA (European Food Safety Authority) and ECDC (European Centre for Disease Prevention and Control) (2015). EU Summary Report on antimicrobial resistance in zoonotic and indicator bacteria from humans, animals and food in 2013. EFSA Journal 2015;13:4036. http://ecdc.europa.eu/en/publications/Publications/antimicrobial-resistance-zoonotic-bacteria-humans-animals-food-EU-summary-report-2013.pdf. Accessed 8th Nov 2016.
10. DANMAP (2014). DANMAP 2013 - use of antimicrobial agents and occurrence of antimicrobial resistance in bacteria from food animals, food and humans in Denmark. September 2015. Copenhagen. http://www.danmap.org/~/media/Projekt%20sites/Danmap/DANMAP%20reports/DANMAP%202014/Danmap_2014.ashx. Accessed 8th Nov 2016.
11. ECDC (European Centre for Disease Prevention and Control), EFSA (European Food Safety Authority) and EMA (European Medicines Agency) (2015). ECDC/EFSA/EMA first joint report on the integrated analysis of the consumption of antimicrobial agents and occurrence of antimicrobial resistance in bacteria from humans and food-producing animals. Stockholm/Parma/London: ECDC/EFSA/EMA, 2015. EFSA Journal 13: 4006. https://www.efsa.europa.eu/en/efsajournal/pub/4006 Accessed 8th Nov 2016.
12. Guerra B, Fischer J, Helmuth R. An emerging public health problem: acquired carbapenemase-producing microorganisms are present in food-producing animals, their environment, companion animals and wild birds. Vet Microbiol. 2014;171:290.
13. JETACAR (Joint Expert Advisory Committee on Antibiotic Resistance [JETACAR]). The use of antibiotic in food producing animals: antibiotic-resistant bacteria in animals and humans. 1999. Commonwealth of Australia. http://www.health.gov.au/internet/main/publishing.nsf/Content/health-pubs-jetacar-cnt.htm/$FILE/jetacar.pdf. Accessed 6th Mar 2015.
14. Cheng AC, Turnidge J, Collignon P, Looke D, Barton M, Gottlieb T. Control of fluoroquinolone resistance through successful regulation, Australia. Emerg Infect Dis. 2012;18(9):1453–60.
15. APVMA - Australian Pesticides and Veterinary Medicines Authority (2014). Quantity of antimicrobial products sold for veterinary use in Australia. Australian Pesticides and Veterinary Medicines Authority. Kingston. Australia. https://apvma.gov.au/node/11816. Accessed 8th Nov 2016.
16. Jordan D, Chin JJ, Fahy VA, Barton MD, Smith MG, Trott DJ. Antimicrobial use in the Australian pig industry: results of a national survey. Aust Vet J. 2009;87(6):222–9.
17. Australia - Pork meat import restrictions (PRRS/PMWS). European Commission Trade, Market Access Database. Agriculture and Fisheries Sector. 2012 May 2.
18. Government of Canada. Sample Collection, Preparation & Laboratory Methodologies. January 2010. National Integrated Enteric Disease Surveillance Program. http://www.phac-aspc.gc.ca/foodnetcanada/niedsp10-pnisme10/s02-eng.php Accessed 8th Nov 2016.
19. Kanki M, Sakata J, Taguchi M, Kumeda Y, Ishibashi M, Kawai T, Kawatsu K, Yamasaki W, Inoue K, Miyahara M. Effect of sample preparation and bacterial concentration on Salmonella enterica detection in poultry meat using culture methods and PCR assaying of preenrichment broths. Food Microbiol. 2009;26:1–3.
20. Clinical and Laboratory Standards Institute (CLSI). M100-S25 Performance Standards for Antimicrobial Susceptibility Testing; Twenty-fifth informational supplement. January 2015. Vol 35, No. 3.
21. European Committee on Antimicrobial Susceptibility Testing (EUCAST). EUCAST Expert Rules Version 3.1. Intrinsic Resistance and Exceptional Phenotypes Tables. http://www.eucast.org/expert_rules_and_intrinsic_resistance/ (Accessed 30th Jan 2018).
22. European Committee on Antimicrobial Susceptibility Testing (EUCAST). Antimicrobial wild type distributions of microorganisms. https://mic.eucast.org/Eucast2/SearchController/search.jsp?action=performSearch&BeginIndex=0&Micdif=mic&NumberIndex=50&Antib=-1&Specium=430. (Accessed 29th Jan 2018).
23. European Committee on Antimicrobial Susceptibility Testing (EUCAST). Antimicrobial wild type distributions of microorganisms. https://mic.eucast.org/Eucast2/SearchController/search.jsp?action=performSearch&BeginIndex=0&Micdif=mic&NumberIndex=50&Antib=-1&Specium=218. (Accessed 29th Jan 2018).
24. Jiang X, Zhang Z, Li M, et al. Detection of extended-Spectrum -lactamases in clinical isolates of Pseudomonas aeruginosa. Antimicrob Agents Chemother. 2006;50:2990–5.
25. Beceiro A, Fernández-Cuenca F, Ribera A, et al. False extended-spectrum beta-lactamase detection in Acinetobacter spp. due to intrinsic susceptibility to clavulanic acid. J Antimicrob Chemother. 2008;61:301–8.
26. Thomson KS. Extended-Spectrum-β-lactamase, AmpC, and Carbapenemase issues. J Clin Microbiol. 2010;48:1019–25.
27. Magiorakos AP, Srinivasan A, Carey RB, Carmeli Y, Falagas ME, Giske CG, et al. Multidrug-resistant, extensively drug-resistant and pandrug-resistant bacteria: an international expert proposal for interim standard definitions for acquired resistance. Clin Microbiol Infect. 2012;18(3):268–81.
28. Hanson ND, Thomson KS, Moland ES, Sanders CC, Berthold G, Penn RG. Molecular characterization of a multiply resistant Klebsiella pneumoniae encoding ESBLs and a plasmid-mediated AmpC. J Antimicrob Chemother. 1999;44:377–80.
29. Chia JH, Chu C, Su LH, Chiu CH, Kuo AJ, Sun CF, et al. Development of a multiplex PCR and SHV melting-curve mutation detection system for detection

of some SHV and CTX-M β-lactamases of *Escherichia coli, Klebsiella pneumoniae,* and *Enterobacter cloacae* in Taiwan. J Clin Microbiol. 2005;43:4486–91.

30. Birkett CI, Ludlam HA, Woodford N, Brown DFJ, Brown NM, Roberts MTM, et al. Real-time TaqMan PCR for rapid detection and typing of genes encoding CTX-M extended-spectrum β-lactamases. J Med Microbiol. 2007;56(Pt 1):52–5.

31. Perez-Perez FJ, Hanson ND. Detection of plasmid-mediated AmpC beta-lactamase genes in clinical isolates by using multiplex PCR. J Clin Microbiol. 2002;40:2153–62.

32. Poirel L, Héritier C, Tolün V, Nordmann P. Emergence of oxacillinase-mediated resistance to imipenem in *Klebsiella pneumoniae.* Antimicrob Agents Chemother. 2004;48:15–22.

33. Mendes RE, Kiyota KA, Monteiro J, Castanheira M, Andrade SS, Gales AC, et al. Rapid detection and identification of metallo-β-lactamase-encoding genes by multiplex real-time PCR assay and melt curve analysis. J Clin Microbiol. 2007;45:544–7.

34. Clausen PT, Zankari E, Aarestrup FM, Lund O. Benchmarking of methods for identification of antimicrobial resistance genes in bacterial whole genome data. J Antimicrob Chemother. 2016;71(9):2484–8.

35. Calbo E, Freixas N, Xercavins M, et al. Foodborne nosocomial outbreak of SHV1 and CTX-M-15-producing Klebsiella Pneumoniae: epidemiology and control. Clin Infect Dis. 2011;52(6):743–9.

36. Doughari HJ, Ndakidemi PA, Human IS, Benade S. The ecology, biology and pathogenesis of Acinetobacter spp.:an overview. Microbes Environ. 2011;26: 101–12.

37. Janda JM, Abbott SL. The genus hafnia: from soup to nuts. Clin Microbiol Rev. 2006;19:12–8.

38. Argudín MA, Deplano A, Meghraoui A, et al. Bacteria from animals as a pool of antimicrobial resistance genes. Antibiotics (Basel). 2017;6(2):E12.

39. van Breda LK, Dhungyel OP, Ward MP. Antibiotic resistant *Escherichia coli* in southeastern Australian pig herds and implications for surveillance. Zoonoses Public Health. 2018;65(1):e1–7.

40. Obeng AS, Rickard H, Ndi O, Sexton M, Barton M. Antibiotic resistance, phylogenetic grouping and virulence potential of Escherichia Coli isolated from the faeces of intensively farmed and free range poultry. Vet Microbiol. 2012;54(3–4):305–15.

41. Pande VV, Gole VC, McWhorter AR, Abraham S, Chousalkar KK. Antimicrobial resistance of non-typhoidal salmonella isolates from egg layer flocks and egg shells. Int J Food Microbiol. 2015;203:23–6.

42. Smith MG, Jordan D, Gibson JS, Cobbold RN, Chapman TA, Abraham S, Trott DJ. Phenotypic and genotypic profiling of antimicrobial resistance in enteric Escherichia Coli communities isolated from finisher pigs in Australia. Aust Vet J. 2016;94(10):371–6.

43. Folster JP, Pecic G, Singh A, Dvual B, Rickert R, Ayers S, Abbott J, McGlinchey B, Bauer-Turpin J, Haro J, Hise K, Zhao S, Fedorka-Cray PJ, Whichard J, McDermott PF. Characterization of extended-Spectrum cephalosporin-resistant *Salmonella enterica* Serovar Heidelberg isolated from food animals, retail meat, and humans in the United States 2009. Foodborne Pathog Dis. 2012;9(7):638–45.

44. Mihaiu L, Lapusan A, Tanasuica R, Sobolu R, Mihaiu R, Oniga O, Mihaiu M. First study of *Salmonella* in meat in Romania. J Infect Dev Ctries. 2014;8(1):50–8.

45. Ojer-Usoz E, Gonzalez D, Vitas AI, et al. Prevalence of extended-spectrum beta-lactamase-producing Enterobacteriaceae in meat products sold in Navarra, Spain. Meat Sci. 2013;93(2):316–21.

46. Silva N, Costa L, Goncalves A, Sousa M, Radhouani H, Brito F, et al. Genetic characterisation of extended-spectrum beta-lactamases in Escherichia Coli isolated from retail chicken products including CTX-M-9 containing isolates: a food safety risk factor. Br Poult Sci. 2012;53(6):747–55.

47. Egea P, Lopez-Cerero L, Navarro MD, Rodriguez-Bano J, Pascual A. Assessment of the presence of extended-spectrum beta-lactamase-producing Escherichia Coli in eggshells and ready-to-eat products. Eur J Clin Microbiol Infect Dis. 2011;30(9):1045–7.

48. Matuschek E, Åhman J, Webster C, Kahlmeter G. Antimicrobial susceptibility testing of colistin - evaluation of seven commercial MIC products against standard broth microdilution for Escherichia coli, Klebsiella pneumoniae, Pseudomonas aeruginosa, and Acinetobacter spp. Clin Microbiol Infect. 2017;17:30667–5.

49. Carretto E, Brovarone F, Russello G, et al. Clinical validation of the SensiTest™ Colistin, a broth microdilution based method to evaluate colistin MICs.

J Clin Microbiol. 2018:01523–17. https://doi.org/10.1128/JCM.01523-17. [Epub ahead of print]

50. Liu YY, Wang Y, Walsh TR, et al. Emergence of plasmid-mediated colistin resistance mechanism MCR-1 in animals and human beings in China: a microbiological and molecular biological study. Lancet Infect Dis. 2016;16:161–8.

51. Hadjadj L, Riziki T, Zhu Y, Li J, Diene SM, Rolain JM. Study of mcr-1 gene-mediated colistin resistance in Enterobacteriaceae isolated from humans and animals in different countries. Genes (Basel). 2017;8(12):E394.

52. Ellem JA, Ginn AN, Chen SC, et al. Locally Acquired mcr-1 in *Escherichia coli,* Australia, 2011 and 2013. Emerg Infect Dis. 2017;23(7):1160–3.

53. Australian Commission on Safety and Quality in Health Care. AURA 2016: first Australian report on antimicrobial use and resistance in human health. Commonwealth of Australia, 2016. https://www.safetyandquality.gov.au/publications/aura-2016-first-australian-report-on-antimicroibal-use-and-resistance-in-human-health/ (Accessed 29th Jan 2018).

# 6

# Duration of colonization with and risk factors for prolonged carriage of multidrug resistant organisms among residents in long-term care facilities

I-Wen Lin[1], Chiao-Yu Huang[2,3], Sung-Ching Pan[4], Yng-Chyi Chen[5] and Chia-Ming Li[6*]

## Abstract

**Background:** Residents of long-term care facilities (LTCFs) colonized with multidrug resistant organisms (MDROs) are often placed under contact isolation to ensure appropriate infection control. This isolation may reduce opportunities for rehabilitation and social stimuli and may also increase medical costs. However, the number of previous studies investigating the duration of colonization in LTCFs is limited. This study was conducted to determine the duration of colonization and risk factors for prolonged carriage of MDROs among residents of a LTCF.

**Methods:** This retrospective study was conducted in a hospital-affiliated nursing home with 59 beds. Fifty-four residents in the nursing home were isolated for MDROs between January 1, 2013 and December 31, 2015. Clinical data were collected from the charts of these 54 residents, including catheter use, colonizing MDRO species and site, underlying diseases, Charlson Comorbidity Index (CCI) scores, and Barthel index scores before and after isolation. Forty-seven residents were included into the statistic analysis. Multivariate Cox regression analyses were performed using duration of colonization as the dependent variable.

**Results:** The most frequently isolated MDROs were vancomycin-resistant enterococci (VRE) (44.7%), and the median duration of colonization was 72 (4–407) days. An increased CCI score significantly increased the risk of prolonged colonization (HR: 0.86, 95% CI: 0.76–0.98, $p$ value 0.02).

**Conclusion:** Among residents of the LTCF, the average duration of MDRO colonization was approximately 3 months. CCI scores were positively associated with the duration of the MDRO colonization of the LTCF residents. Further studies should be conducted to determine whether implementing isolation protocols for MDRO-colonized LTCF residents is associated with a decline in ADL.

**Keywords:** Colonization, Long-term care facilities, Multidrug-resistant organisms

* Correspondence: jeremyli2005@gmail.com
[6]Department of Family Medicine, National Taiwan University Hospital, Bei-Hu Branch, No.87, Neijiang Street, Taipei City 10845, Taiwan
Full list of author information is available at the end of the article

## Background

The number of residents living in long-term care facilities (LTCFs) has increased due to changes in societal age structures. Residents of LTCFs may be at increased risk of infection as a result of sharing common living areas and participating in group activities. Additionally, due to the frequent hospitalization of LTCF residents, pathogens may be transmitted between LTCFs and hospitals [1–6]. Serious infections may increase medical costs and mortality rates. Residents colonized with multidrug resistant organisms (MDROs) are often placed under contact isolation and prohibited from group activities to ensure infection control. When LTCF staff come into direct contact with a colonized patient or potentially contaminated areas in the resident's environment, frequently employed contact precautions include wearing a gown and using gloves [1, 7–9]. However, isolation may reduce the opportunity for rehabilitation and social stimuli, potentially resulting in functional decline [1]. Thus, LTCFs perform repeated cultures for MDRO pathogens to determine whether isolation may be discontinued.

Risk factors previously identified as potentially associated with an increased probability of microorganism colonization include age, immobility, incontinence, nutrition, functional status, underlying chronic diseases, medication usage (e.g., drugs that affect consciousness, immune functions, gastric acid secretions, and normal flora, including antimicrobial therapy), invasive catheter use, frequency of hospitalization [10–13] and Charlson Comorbidity Index (CCI) score [1].

Several previous studies have investigated the factors that may be associated with the duration of MDRO colonization. For instance, persistent carriage of Klebsiella pneumoniae carbapenemase (KPC)-producing Klebsiella pneumoniae has been found to be associated with catheter use and a low functional status [14], and the risk factors for prolonged carriage of vancomycin-resistant enterococci (VRE) that have been previously identified include surgery, antibiotic use at admission, dialysis, and discharge to a nursing home or other health care institution [15]. One study found persistent methicillin-resistant Staphylococcus aureus (MRSA) carriage to be associated with admission at another health care institution and disruption of the skin barrier [16]. However, prior studies have predominantly focused on patients admitted to hospitals.

Several previous studies have investigated risk factors for MDRO colonization in LTCFs. A cross-sectional study of 84 nursing home residents in an LTCF in Boston, Massachusetts found that having a diagnosis of advanced dementia was a major risk factor for harboring MDRGN (multidrug-resistant gram-negative bacteria) [17]. Another nested case-control study was conducted in four co-located LTCFs in Australia. Of the 115 residents included in this study, 41 carried MDROs. This study reported that wound management, medical device use and pressure ulcers were independent risk factors for MDRO colonization [18].

Previous studies investigating the duration of MDRO colonization have been predominantly conducted in hospitals [2, 3, 6, 8, 14–16]. No prior studies have investigated the factors that affect the duration of MDRO colonization in the LTCF setting. However, the implementation of MDRO isolation protocols to control infection may lead to the limitation of resident activities, thereby shortening the golden time for functional recovery after hospitalization. The consequences of contact isolation may also include increased medical costs and increased health care worker (HCW) and caregiver workloads. Information regarding the length of time required for MDRO clearance would be of benefit to both HCWs and families. To answer these questions, we conducted a retrospective observational study to determine the duration of MDRO colonization and risk factors associated with colonization duration in LTCF residents.

## Methods
### Setting
The setting for this study was a hospital-affiliated nursing home with 59 beds. In this facility, infection control protocols are strictly enforced under the supervision of the hospital infection control center. Urine, sputum, and anal swab samples were collected for bacterial culture from every new resident and from all residents who were readmitted after hospitalization on the date of LTCF admission. If the culture results indicate the presence of MDROs, residents were placed under contact isolation. If the resident had been isolated during hospitalization, the LTCF maintained contact isolation after the resident was transferred back to the LTCF and performed monthly follow-up bacterial cultures to determine whether isolation could safely be discontinued.

The residents with MDRO colonization in this facility were arranged in a single-patient room as a priority. If a single-patient room was not available, residents with the same MDROs would be placed together or lived with residents with a low risk of contracting an infection. In multi-patient rooms, at least 1 m of spatial separation was provided, and curtains would be used. The caregivers were required to ensure contact precautions, such as wearing a gown and gloves for all interactions that may involve contact with the patient or potentially contaminated areas in the patient's environment.

MDROs are defined as Methicillin-resistant Staphylococcus aureus, Vancomycin-resistant Enterococcus spp., Carbapenem-resistant Enterobacteriaceae spp., or other multi-drug resistant pathogens with non-susceptibility to at least one agent in at least 3 antimicrobial classes of the following 6 classes: ampicillin/sulbactam, cephalosporins, β-lactam/β-lactamase inhibitor combination, carbapenems, fluoroquinolones, and aminoglycosides [19]. VRE was initially identified by CHROMagar VRE.

The following criteria were used to determine MDRO resolution: (1) absence of infectious symptoms at the site of original infection/colonization; (2) discontinuation of antibiotics; (3) removal of related catheters; (4) one negative nasal swab culture for MRSA and one negative throat swab culture for multidrug-resistant *Acinetobacter baumannii* (MDRAB); and (5) three negative anal swab cultures for VRE, and one negative anal swab

culture for carbapenem-resistant gram-negative bacteria (CRGNB). MDRO resolution needed to meet 1 to 3, plus 4 or 5, depending on the species of MDRO.

### Enrollment

We identified the residents of a single LTCF localized in Taipei City, Taiwan from whom a MDRO was isolated from Jan 1, 2013 to Dec 31, 2015. We reviewed the charts of identified patients and extracted clinical and demographic data, including age, sex, catheter use (including nasogastric tube, indwelling urinary catheter,

**Table 1** Baseline characteristics of study subjects ($N = 47$)

| Variable | N (%) | Duration of colonization, (Mean ± SD), days | Duration of colonization, (Median(Range)), days |
|---|---|---|---|
| Total | 47(100) | 94.6 ± 75.6 | 72(4–407) |
| Subjects who died before decolonization | 8(17.0) | | |
| Age, y | 83.9 ± 7.8 | | |
| Gender, N(%) | | | |
| Men | 27(57.4) | 92.7 ± 85.9 | 63(14–107) |
| Women | 20(42.6) | 97.2 ± 61.2 | 75(4–263) |
| Origin of case, N(%) | | | |
| Hospital | 37(78.7) | 96.0 ± 62.8 | 72(32–314) |
| Long term care facility | 10(21.3) | 89.6 ± 115.9 | 59.5(4–407) |
| Type of indwelling devices, N(%) | | | |
| Nasogastric tube | 32(68.1) | 97.7 ± 86.5 | 72(14–107) |
| Foley catheter | 22(46.8) | 71.1 ± 44.6 | 62(4–158) |
| Tracheostomy | 8(17.0) | 116.8 ± 121.2 | 70.5(32–407) |
| Type of MDROs, N(%) | | | |
| VRE | 21(44.7) | 108.1 ± 72.7 | 80(35–314) |
| MRSA | 6(12.8) | 100.0 ± 61.5 | 111(4–158) |
| MDRAB | 7(14.9) | 111.1 ± 137.6 | 48(14–107) |
| CRGNB | 13(27.7) | 61.4 ± 19.5 | 60(31–111) |
| Barthel index score before isolation | 6.4 ± 20.2 | | |
| Barthel index score after isolation | 5.1 ± 17.3 | | |
| Charlson comorbidity index score | 5.8 ± 2.5 | | |
| Underlying comorbidity, N(%) | | | |
| Dementia | 43(91.5) | 96.8 ± 77.5 | 72(14–107) |
| Cerebrovascular disease | 33(70.2) | 85.9 ± 67.7 | 62(4–314) |
| Cardiovascular diseases | 25(53.2) | 103.6 ± 72.2 | 74(4–314) |
| Chronic lung disease | 21(44.7) | 82.0 ± 80.9 | 61(14–407) |
| Moderate or severe renal disease | 21(44.7) | 85.9 ± 67.7 | 72(4–407) |
| Diabetes mellitus | 21(44.7) | 99.8 ± 62.5 | 78(4–314) |
| Peptic ulcer disease | 18(38.3) | 93.7 ± 99.3 | 59(14–407) |
| Cancer | 7(14.9) | 148.1 ± 118.4 | 128(72–407) |
| Moderate or severe liver disease | 4(8.5) | 88.3 ± 30.6 | 77(66–133) |

*MDROs* multiple drug resistant organisms; *VRE* vancomycin-resistant enterococci; *MRSA* methicillin-resistant *Staphylococcus aureus*; *MDRAB* multidrug-resistant *Acinetobacter baumannii*; *CRGNB* Carbapenem-resistant gram-negative bacilli

and tracheostomy tube), colonizing MDRO species, site of colonization (including sputum, urine, anus, blood, or wound colonization), antibiotics used most recently prior to MDRO detection, chronic illnesses, CCI scores, and Barthel index scores before and after isolation.

The Charlson comorbidity index (CCI) was developed to predict the one-year mortality of patients based on comorbidity information. The CCI included 19 items: myocardial infarction, congestive heart failure, peripheral vascular disease, cerebrovascular disease without sequelae, hemiplegia, dementia, chronic pulmonary disease, connective tissue disease, peptic ulcer disease, mild liver disease, moderate or severe liver disease, moderate or severe renal disease, diabetes without end-organ damage, diabetes with end-organ damage, tumor without metastasis, leukemia, lymphoma, metastatic solid tumor, and acquired immunodeficiency syndrome (AIDS). CCI has been used to predict the outcome and risk of death from many comorbid diseases [20, 21].

The Barthel index is a widely used instrument to evaluate the functional status of and the dependency of daily life and includes 10 items: feeding, moving from wheelchair to bed and returning, personal care, getting on and off the toilet, bathing oneself, walking on a level surface, ascending and descending stairs, dressing, controlling bowels, and controlling the bladder [22].

The dates of isolation and resolution were defined by the dates on which positive and negative bacterial cultures were obtained, respectively.

### Statistical analysis

The data were summarized as frequencies or percentages for categorical variables and as median and range (inter-quartile range) for continuous variables. Study subjects were censored at the time of death or loss to follow-up. A time-to-event analysis of the weeks between the date of readmission or admission to the LTCF

**Table 2** Cox regression analysis for the probability of MDRO decolonization

| Variable | Univariate regression analysis | | | Multivariate regression analysis | | |
|---|---|---|---|---|---|---|
| | Raw HR | 95%CI | P value | Adjusted HR | 95%CI | P value |
| Age[c] | 1.00 | 0.96–1.04 | 0.831 | 1.01 | 0.97–1.06 | 0.532 |
| Gender[a, c] | 1.36[a] | 0.71–2.58[a] | 0.352[a] | 1.92[a] | 0.90–4.09[a] | 0.093[a] |
| Origin of case[b] | 1.26[b] | 0.57–2.74[b] | 0.569[b] | | | |
| Type of indwelling devices, N(%) | | | | | | |
| Nasogastric tube | 0.97 | 0.50–1.91 | 0.939 | | | |
| Foley catheter[c] | 1.69 | 0.88–3.22 | 0.114 | | | |
| Tracheostomy | 0.82 | 0.34–1.96 | 0.649 | | | |
| Type of MDROs, N(%) | | | | | | |
| VRE | 0.66 | 0.35–1.26 | 0.209 | | | |
| MRSA | 0.90 | 0.37–2.18 | 0.818 | | | |
| MDRAB | 0.88 | 0.34–2.27 | 0.792 | | | |
| CRGNB[c] | 2.46 | 1.13–5.33 | 0.023 | | | |
| Charlson comorbidity index score[c] | 0.89 | 0.79–1.01 | 0.064 | 0.86 | 0.76–0.98 | 0.02 |
| Underlying comorbidity | | | | | | |
| Dementia | 0.62 | 0.22–1.77 | 0.367 | | | |
| Cerebrovascular disease | 1.35 | 0.68–2.67 | 0.389 | | | |
| Cardiovascular diseases | 0.77 | 0.41–1.47 | 0.434 | | | |
| Chronic lung disease | 1.52 | 0.80–2.90 | 0.203 | | | |
| Moderate or severe renal disease | 0.82 | 0.43–1.59 | 0.562 | | | |
| Diabetes mellitus | 0.81 | 0.43–1.52 | 0.504 | | | |
| Peptic ulcer disease[c] | 1.57 | 0.82–3.00 | 0.176 | | | |
| Cancer[c] | 0.51 | 0.20–1.30 | 0.156 | | | |
| Moderate or severe liver disease | 1.28 | 0.45–3.68 | 0.644 | | | |

*MRSA* Methicillin-resistant *Staphylococcus aureus*; *MDRAB* Multidrug-resistant *Acinetobacter baumannii*; *CRGNB* Carbapenem-resistant gram-negative bacilli
[a]Comparison between male and female subjects (reference)
[b]Comparison of cases originating from the long-term care facility and cases originating from hospitals (reference)
[c]age, gender and variables with a *p* value less than 0.2 in the univariate model were included in the multivariate model

and the date of the resolution of MDRO colonization was performed using the Kaplan-Meier method. We performed univariate and multivariate Cox proportional hazard regression analyses in which the duration of colonization was used as the dependent variable. Age, sex and variables with a *p* value less than 0.2 in the univariate model were included in the multivariate model. A backward stepwise regression analysis was performed. The SPSS version 11.0 statistical package (SPSS Inc., Chicago, IL) was used for analysis. A *p* value <0.05 was considered statistically significant.

## Results

In total, MDROs were isolated from 54 patients during the study period. Seven patients were excluded due to missing data; thus, 47 patients were included in the final analysis, and 8 patients died before MDRO clearance. The mean age of the patients was 83.9 ± 7.8 years; 27 patients were male, and 20 were female. The mean Barthel index score was 6.4 ± 20.2 before isolation and 5.1 ± 17.3 after isolation. Of the 47 included patients, 37 (78.7%) were colonized with MDROs during hospitalization, whereas the remaining patients were colonized with MDROs at the LTCF. Overall, 89.4% of the patients had at least one indwelling device. The most frequently isolated MDROs were VRE (44.7%). The mean CCI score was 5.8 ± 2.5. The most prevalent underlying disease among the patients was dementia (91.5%). The mean duration of colonization was 94.6 ± 75.6 days, and the median duration of colonization was 72 (4–407) days. The median

durations of colonization for each pathogen were 80 (35–314) days for VRE, 111 (4–158) days for MRSA, 48 (14–107) days for MDRAB, and 60 (31–111) days for CRGNB. Detailed descriptive statistics are shown in Table 1.

Age, sex, Foley catheter use, CCI score, and CRGNB colonization were included in the model. Multivariate analysis revealed that only an increased CCI score was associated with increased risk of prolonged colonization after accounting for age and sex (HR: 0.86, 95% CI: 0.76–0.98, *p* value 0.02). The origin of MDRO colonization, type of indwelling device, and species of MDRO did not affect the duration of colonization (Table 2). The Kaplan–Meier estimate for the duration of MDRO colonization is shown in Fig. 1.

## Discussion

The median colonization days of MDROs were more than 2 months in this study. In addition, 8 patients died before MDRO clearance. The results of this study suggest that the duration of colonization for MDRO-colonized LTCR residents may be longer than expected. Sohn KM, et al. found the median duration of VRE colonization to be 5.57 weeks after hospital discharge [15], and Scanvic A, et al. reported an estimated median time of MRSA clearance of 8.5 months [16]. Overall, large variations are observed in different study settings.

Patients with a higher CCI score had a significantly longer duration of colonization. In these residents, MDRO colonization may be prolonged due to the presence of a greater number of comorbidities. This

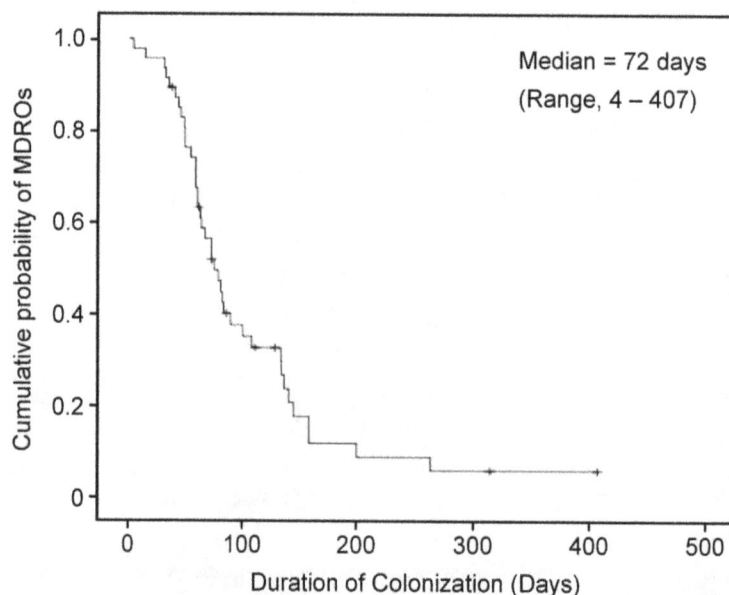

**Fig. 1** The Kaplan–Meier estimate for the duration of MDRO colonization

hypothesis is reasonable because comorbidities may contribute to a more complex disease course or more frail condition, thereby leading to a decrease capacity for MDRO clearance. The risk factors identified in this study were consistent with those of studies conducted in the hospital setting [2, 3, 6, 8, 14–16].

We attempted to determine the manner in which the implementation of isolation protocols for MDRO-colonized patients affected their activities of daily living (ADL, measured by the Barthel index). However, the ADL scores of the residents included in our study were mostly low, which made a direct evaluation of the correlation between ADL score and isolation duration difficult and limited our ability to assess this issue, as a result. This important issue should be investigated further in multicenter studies that are conducted in LTCFs, that include a large number of patients, and that enroll residents with a wider spectrum of ADL scores.

The risk factors identified in this study are not currently modifiable. However, the findings of this study may influence the isolation protocols implemented for MDRO-colonized patients. As we noticed that MDRO colonization was longer than 2–3 months for those with increased CCI scores, rehabilitation should be maintained even during the isolation period to prevent further functional decline. For example, isolating colonized residents in the same location, sharing the same environment or rehabilitation modality, may retain their rehabilitation program and at the same time prevent further transmission of MDROs to uncolonized residents. Furthermore, identification of the modifiable risk factors that influence the duration of colonization may reduce or even avoid the costs of isolation.

There are some limitations to our study. First, we only included a small number of patients from whom MDROs were isolated. Second, this study was conducted only in a single LTCF, but this single LTCF regularly performed follow-up cultures for MDROs to determine if isolation could be discontinued. Moreover, we simultaneously evaluated multiple types of MDROs, but different MDROs may be associated with different risk factors that affect the duration of patient isolation.

## Conclusion

The average duration of colonization among MDRO-colonized LTCF residents was approximately 3 months. Among LTCF residents, CCI scores were positively associated with the duration of colonization. Further studies should be conducted to determine whether implementing the isolation protocols for MDRO-colonized LTCF residents is associated with a decline in ADL.

## Abbreviations

ADL: activities of daily living; CCI: Charlson Comorbidity Index; CRGNB: carbapenem-resistant gram-negative bacteria; HCW: health care worker; KPC: *Klebsiella pneumoniae* carbapenemase; LTCFs: long-term care facilities; MDRAB: multidrug-resistant *Acinetobacter baumannii*; MDRGN: multidrug-resistant gram-negative bacteria; MDROs: multidrug-resistant organisms; MRSA: methicillin-resistant *Staphylococcus aureus*; VRE: Vancomycin-resistant enterococci

## Acknowledgements

The authors would like to thank registered nurse Haiyen Chou and all colleagues of the Nursing home, National Taiwan University Hospital Beihu Branch for data collection.

## Funding

The English editing fee of this paper was supported by a grant from the National Taiwan University Hospital, Beihu Branch, No.10504.

## Authors' contributions

IWL mainly contributed to chart reviewing and primary article writing. CYH mainly contributed to statistical analyses. YCC mainly contributed to case enrollment. SCP and CML supervised the study. All authors read and approved the final manuscript.

## Competing interests

The authors declare that they have no competing interests.

## Author details

[1]Department of Family Medicine, National Taiwan University Hospital, Bei-Hu Branch, No.87, Neijiang Street, Taipei City 10845, Taiwan. [2]Department of Family Medicine, Renai Branch, No.10, Sec. 4, Ren'ai Rd., Da'an Dist, Taipei City 106, Taiwan, Republic of China. [3]Institute of Health Policy and Management, National Taiwan University, No. 1, Sec. 4, Roosevelt Rd, Taipei 10617, Taiwan, Republic of China. [4]Department of Internal Medicine, National Taiwan University Hospital, No.7, Zhongshan S. Rd., Zhongzheng Dist, Taipei City 100, Taiwan, Republic of China. [5]Department of Nursing, National Taiwan University Hospital, Bei-Hu Branch, No.87, Neijiang Street, Taipei City 10845, Taiwan. [6]Department of Family Medicine, National Taiwan University Hospital, Bei-Hu Branch, No.87, Neijiang Street, Taipei City 10845, Taiwan.

## References

1.  Healthcare Infection Control Practices Advisory Committee (HICPAC). Guideline for isolation precautions. http://www.cdc.gov/hicpac/2007IP/2007ip_part1.html#3; 2007. Accessed Jan 25, 2016.
2.  Evans RS, Lloyd JF, Abouzelof RH, Taylor CW, Anderson VR, Samore MH. System-wide surveillance for clinical encounters by patients previously identified with MRSA and VRE. Stud Health Technol Inform. 2004;107:212–6.
3.  Mylotte JM, Goodnough S, Tayara A. Antibiotic-resistant organisms among long-term care facility residents on admission to an inpatient geriatrics unit: retrospective and prospective surveillance. Am J Infect Control. 2001;29:139–44.
4.  Strausbaugh LJ, Jacobson C, Yost T. Methicillin-resistant Staphylococcus Aureus in a nursing home and affiliated hospital: a four-year perspective. Infect Control Hosp Epidemiol. 1993;14:331–6.
5.  Wiener J, Quinn JP, Bradford PA, Goering RV, Nathan C, Bush K, et al. Multiple antibiotic-resistant Klebsiella and Escherichia Coli in nursing homes. JAMA. 1999;281:517–23.
6.  Pop-Vicas AE, D'Agata EM. The rising influx of multidrug-resistant gram-negative bacilli into a tertiary care hospital. Clin Infect Dis. 2005;40:1792–8.
7.  Donskey CJ. The role of the intestinal tract as a reservoir and source for transmission of nosocomial pathogens. Clin Infect Dis. 2004;39:219–26.
8.  Bhalla A, Pultz NJ, Gries DM, Ray AJ, Eckstein EC, Aron DC, et al. Acquisition of nosocomial pathogens on hands after contact with environmental surfaces near hospitalized patients. Infect Control Hosp Epidemiol. 2004;25:164–7.
9.  Duckro AN, Blom DW, Lyle EA, Weinstein RA, Hayden MK. Transfer of vancomycin-resistant enterococci via health care worker hands. Arch Intern Med. 2005;165:302–7.
10. High KP, Bradley S, Loeb M, Palmer R, Quagliarello V, Yoshikawa T. A new

paradigm for clinical investigation of infectious syndromes in older adults: assessment of functional status as a risk factor and outcome measure. Clin Infect Dis. 2005;40:114–22.

11. Loeb MB, Craven S, McGeer AJ, Simor AE, Bradley SF, Low DE, et al. Risk factors for resistance to antimicrobial agents among nursing home residents. Am J Epidemiol. 2003;157:40–7.

12. Nicolle LE. The chronic indwelling catheter and urinary infection in long-term-care facility residents. Infect Control Hosp Epidemiol. 2001;22:316–21.

13. Gomes GF, Pisani JC, Macedo ED, Campos AC. The nasogastric feeding tube as a risk factor for aspiration and aspiration pneumonia. Curr Opin Clin Nutr Metab Care. 2003;6:327–33.

14. Feldman N, Adler A, Molshatzki N, Navon-Venezia S, Khabra E, Cohen D, et al. Gastrointestinal colonization by KPC-producing Klebsiella Pneumoniae following hospital discharge: duration of carriage and risk factors for persistent carriage. Clin Microbiol Infect. 2013;19:E190–6.

15. Sohn KM, Peck KR, Joo EJ, Ha YE, Kang CI, Chung DR, et al. Duration of colonization and risk factors for prolonged carriage of vancomycin-resistant enterococci after discharge from the hospital. Int J Infect Dis. 2013;17:e240–6.

16. Scanvic A, Denic L, Gaillon S, Giry P, Andremont A, Lucet JC. Duration of colonization by methicillin-resistant Staphylococcus Aureus after hospital discharge and risk factors for prolonged carriage. Clin Infect Dis. 2001;32:1393–8.

17. Pop-Vicas A, Mitchell SL, Kandel R, Schreiber R, D'Agata EM. Multidrug-resistant gram-negative bacteria in a long-term care facility: prevalence and risk factors. J Am Geriatr Soc. 2008;56:1276–80.

18. Lim CJ, Cheng AC, Kennon J, Spelman D, Hale D, Melican G, et al. Prevalence of multidrug-resistant organisms and risk factors for carriage in long-term care facilities: a nested case-control study. J Antimicrob Chemother. 2014;69:1972–80.

19. Centers for Disease Control and Prevention. Multidrug-resistant organism & Clostridium difficile infection (MDRO/CDI) module; 2017. https://www.cdc.gov/nhsn/PDFs/pscManual/12pscMDRO_CDADcurrent.pdf. Accessed July 10, 2017.

20. Charlson ME, Pompei P, Ales KL, MacKenzie CR. A new method of classifying prognostic comorbidity in longitudinal studies: development and validation. J Chronic Dis. 1987;40:373–83.

21. Huang YQ, Gou R, Diao YS, Yin QH, Fan WX, Liang YP, et al. Charlson comorbidity index helps predict the risk of mortality for patients with type 2 diabetic nephropathy. J Zhejiang Univ Sci B. 2014;15:58–66.

22. Mahoney FI, Barthel DW. Functional evaluation: the Barthel index. Md State Med J. 1965;14:61–5.

# 7

# Multiple drug resistance and biocide resistance in *Escherichia coli* environmental isolates from hospital and household settings

Bothyna Ghanem and Randa Nayef Haddadin[*]

## Abstract

**Background:** Antibiotic resistance of environmental *Escherichia coli* in hospitals could be increased due to extensive use of biocides resulting in serious infections. In this study, the prevalence of antibiotic resistance of environmental isolates of *E. coli* from hospitals and household settings were evaluated and compared. In addition, the association between biocide minimum inhibitory concentration (MIC) and multiple drug resistance (MDR) was investigated.

**Methods:** Environmental samples were collected from different homes and hospitals in Amman, Jordan. The isolates were identified phenotypically and by PCR. Antibiotic susceptibility tests and MIC of selected biocides were performed on the isolates. Screening for *bla*CTX-M group 1 was also performed.

**Results:** Of 21 *E. coli* strains isolated, 47.6% were MDR and 67.9% were phenotypically identified as extended spectrum beta-lactamase (ESBL) producers. The occurrence of these ESBL isolates was comparable between household and hospital settings ($P > 0.05$). The MIC values of the biocides tested against all isolates were well below the in-use concentration of biocides. Moreover, the MICs of biocides were comparable between isolates from households and those from hospitals ($P > 0.05$). No association was found between MDR and biocide MIC ($P > 0.05$). Most of ESBL isolates harboured *bla*CTX-M 1.

**Conclusions:** The extensive use of biocides in hospitals is not associated with MDR nor does it affect the MIC of biocides against *E.coli*.

**Keywords:** *Escherichia coli*, Biocide, Environment, ESBL, Hospital, Multiple drug resistance

## Background

Health care associated infections (HAIs) are known to contribute to morbidity and mortality among patients affected by them. In addition, they cause significant medical and financial consequences accompanied by emotional devastation [1]. Among the factors contributing to increased risk of HAIS are poor facilities cleaning and inadequate disinfection of health care settings [1]. These issues have led to the extensive use of biocides (including antiseptics and disinfectants) in hospitals. Since biocides have some common properties with antibiotics regarding their activity, mechanism of action and

development of resistance [2], there is a possibility that resistance to biocides can contribute to resistance to antibiotics [3]. However, the contribution of biocide use to antibiotic resistance is still controversial and, despite some evidence, remains largely unproven. Several studies have shown that certain disinfectants have increased the expression of specific multiple drug resistant (MDR) efflux pumps which eventually resulted in resistance to some antibiotics [4]. Other studies have shown that over-exposure of bacteria to disinfectants results in reduced susceptibility towards some antibiotics [2, 5]. On the other hand, other studies have failed to show any cross-resistance between biocides and antibiotics [6, 7].

*E. coli* is a highly diverse species with respect to its virulence and pathogenicity. It is widely distributed in

* Correspondence: r_haddadin@ju.edu.jo
Department of Pharmaceutics and Pharmaceutical Technology, School of Pharmacy, The University of Jordan, Amman 11942, Jordan

open systems and can easily spread in the environment causing risks to human health [8]. *E. coli* is one of the most common bacteria causing nosocomial infections. Its presence on inanimate surfaces in hospitals is one of the major infection control challenges facing hospitals [9]. In fact, contaminated surfaces and inanimate objects (fomites) are considered reservoirs for pathogen transmission to the patients. Therefore, the use of biocides in hospitals is of a paramount importance to control infections and transmission of pathogens.

In this study the biocides were selected to represent different chemical classes that are used extensively in Jordan in hospital and/ or household settings. Ethanol is an alcohol, which is used as antiseptic in hospitals and community settings. 4-Chloro-3,5-xylenol (known as chloroxylenol) is a phenolic compound that is used as a general antiseptic and disinfectant in the community. Iodine is a halogen, which is used in the form of povidone-iodine as a preoperative antiseptic in hospitals and for wound disinfection in household and hospital settings. Cetrimide is a member of the quaternary ammonium compounds that are incorporated in many biocidal preparations in combination with other biocides that are used in hospitals as antiseptics or disinfectants.

The aim of this research is to evaluate and compare the prevalence of antibiotic resistance in *E. coli* isolated from two distinct environments; hospital settings, where biocides are extensively used, and household settings, where biocide use is limited. *E. coli* was selected since it is recognized as an indicator for the presence of other Enterobacteriaceae and is a common cause of nosocomial infections. The collected isolates were assessed for the presence of potential association between antibiotic resistance and resistance to biocides, which was measured by an increase in their minimum inhibitory concentration (MIC).

## Materials and methods
### Sample collection
The environmental samples included in the study were collected from two hospitals, Prince Hamzeh (PH) Hospital and Jordan University (JU) Hospital and ten resident homes located in Amman-Jordan. Sample collection was performed from March to October 2016. The samples were collected using sterile swabs (Amies Transport media, Max Protect, China) that were pre-moistened with Amies medium present in the tube. The swab was rolled and moved over the surface to be sampled. After sampling, the swabs were transferred to the laboratory within one to two hours to be processed. In the laboratory, the swabs were cut off aseptically and placed in Lauryl sulphate tryptose broth (LSB) for enrichment and incubated overnight at $35° \pm 2°Ċ$.

The two hospitals included in the study are among the largest in Amman. Each hospital treats on average more than 500,000 patients annually. Ethical permission to undertake sampling was obtained from both hospitals. Biocides used within the hospitals were recorded. The two hospitals use ethanol based gels and solutions as antiseptic for healthcare personnel, pre-injection disinfection and for visitor use. Different quaternary ammonium compounds based products are used for general disinfection and antisepsis within the two hospitals. Iodine in the form of povidone-iodine is used for wound disinfection and preoperative skin treatment. The hospitals apply strict disinfection policies that are monitored by infection control teams. Samples from hospital environments were collected from the floors, elevators, curtains, patient beds, windows, door knobs, nursing cabinets, bathroom sinks, drains, pressure devices, magnetic resonance device, operation equipment, dialysis device, trolleys, and any device that is transferrable among patients and medical staff. The samples were collected from different hospital wards. In total 344 swab samples were collected from both hospitals.

The homes included in the study apply routine cleaning to the premises using detergents. These homes occasionally use hypochlorite (a halogen) or chloroxylenol (e.g. Dettol®) based preparations for general disinfection. Povidone iodine and ethanol (70%) were the most common antiseptics used in these homes to treat bruises or cuts if occurred. Samples from household environment were collected from the floors, door knobs, bathroom sinks and kitchen sinks. The number of samples collected from the 10 homes was 86.

### E. coli Isolation and identification
A loopful of LSB culture was streaked on MacConkey agar medium and incubated overnight at $35° \pm 2°Ċ$. Morphologically distinctive pink colonies were isolated and identified biochemically for oxidase production, Kligler's iron agar, urease, gas, indole production and then identified using API 20 E kit (Biomerieux, France). The potential *E. coli* isolates were confirmed genetically using PCR method.

### Antibiotic susceptibility test
Antibiotic susceptibility test was performed using disc diffusion test according to Clinical and Laboratory Standard Institute (CLSI, 2016) guideline [10] using the following antibiotics: Amoxicillin, Amoxicillin-clavulanic acid, Cefaclor, Cefixime, Nitrofurantoin, Cefuroxime, Amikacin, Ciprofloxacin, Imipenem, Trimethoprim-Sulfamethoxazole, Doxycycline. These antibiotics represent the major antibiotic classes which have known activity against *E. coli* and are used clinically. *E. coli* ATCC 25922 was used as a quality control strain to validate the method [10].

The isolates were further tested to phenotypically detect extended spectrum beta lactamase (ESBL) producing bacteria using double disc diffusion test [10]. In this test, cefotaxime and ceftazidime discs alone and in combination of clavulanate were used. The isolate is considered ESBL producing if there is ≥5-mm increase in the zone diameter for antibiotic tested in combination with clavulanate vs the zone diameter of the antibiotic when tested alone [10].

## MIC determination of biocides

Minimum inhibitory concentrations of ethanol, chloroxylenol, cetrimide and iodine were determined using a broth microdilution method according to CLSI, but with slight modification. Stock solutions of ethanol, cetrimide and chloroxylenol were prepared in Mueller Hinton broth (MHB) to get final concentration of 200 mg/ml, 400 µg/ml and 300 µg/ml respectively. In order to enhance the solubility of chloroxylenol in MHB, it was dissolved first in dimethylsulfoxide (DMSO) and the final volume completed by the addition of MHB. The lowest concentration of DMSO needed to ensure complete solubility of chloroxyleneol in MHB was 5%. To ensure that DMSO at 5% concentration has no inhibitory effect on the isolates, positive control containing 5% DMSO in MHB was prepared for each isolate. Since MHB medium contains starch as an ingredient, TSB was used for MIC determination of iodine. Iodine was solubilized with potassium iodide at 1:2 ratio ($I_2$: KI) in TSB to get a stock solution of iodine (1300 µg/ml). Aliquots (200 µl) of each stock solution were dispensed into the wells of a microtitre plate. Double serial dilutions were performed using broth. Each trial was performed in five replicates. Aliquots (20 µl) of each bacterial culture adjusted to $5 \times 10^6$ CFU/ ml were used to inoculate the microtitre plate wells to yield a final concentration of ca $5 \times 10^5$ CFU/ ml. The microtitre plate was incubated for 20 h at $35° \pm 2°C$. MIC was determined by visual inspection. For ethanol, since the difference between consecutive concentrations is large, linear serial dilutions were performed after determining its MIC by double serial dilutions. E. coli Nissle 1917 was used as a control for MIC testing. This strain is a kind gift from Ardeypharm GmbH, Germany. It is a probiotic non-pathogenic microorganism utilized clinically to treat many gastrointestinal disorders including diarrhoea, ulcerative colitis and uncomplicated diverticular disease [11].

## DNA extraction

The Wizard® Genomic DNA Purification Kit (Promega, England) was used to isolate DNA from the isolated E. coli strains. The kit was used according to manufacturer's instructions.

## PCR primers and conditions

blaCTX-M group 1 gene and E. coli16s rRNA gene: PCR reaction was performed using 3 µl of the extracted DNA (2 µl for E. coli 16S rRNA gene), and 0.4 µM of each of the blaCTX-M group 1 gene forward and reverse primer and the (16 E1, 16 E2 and 16 E3) primers of E. coli 16S rRNA gene (Table 1). The gene was amplified using 12.5 µl of PCR Master Mix 2× (GoTaq® Green Master Mix, Promega, USA). The volume was made up to 25 µl using nuclease free water. Cycling conditions for E. coli 16S rRNA gene were applied according to Tsen et al., [12]. Cycling conditions for blaCTX-M 1 gene were applied according to Mirzaee et al., [13]. The amplified gene products were analyzed using 2% agarose gel electrophoresis and visualized by (UVP) system (Alpha Imager®, Japan) using Redsafe™ (Intron biotechnology, Korea).

## Statistical analysis

The results were statistically analysed using the nonparametric Mann Whitney U test and the Chi square test as relevant. Analyses at 95% confidence level were performed. The analysis was performed using IBM SPSS Statistics version 23.

## Results

The total number of samples collected was 430; 175 samples were taken from PH hospital, 169 samples from JU hospital and 86 samples from household settings. The potential number of E. coli isolates identified by API kit was 21. These isolates were confirmed to be E. coli by PCR followed by agarose gel electrophoresis. Accordingly, the prevalence rate of E. coli in all the settings was 4.9%; seven isolates from PH hospital, four isolates from JU hospital and 10 isolates from households (Table 2).

**Table 1** The targeted genes, primer sequence and product size

| Target | Detection primer | Primer (sequence 5' to 3') | Product size (bp) | Reference |
|---|---|---|---|---|
| E. coli 16S rRNA | 16 E1 (F) | GGGAGTAAAGTTAATACCTTTGCTC | 584 | 12 |
| | 16 E2 (R) | TTCCCGAAGGCACATTCT | | |
| | 16 E3 (R) | TTCCCGAAGGCACCAATC | | |
| blaCTX-M group 1 | CTX-M-7 (F) | GCGTGATACCACTTAACCTC | 260 | 13 |
| | CTX-M-8 (R) | TGAAGTAAGTGACCAGAATC | | |

**Table 2** The antibiogram of *E coli* isolates from the environment of the two hospitals and 10 homes

| Facility | Isolate | Amx | Amc | Cfc | Cfu | Cfx | Ctz | Ctx | Imp | Nit | Amk | Cip | Tms | Dox | MDR |
|---|---|---|---|---|---|---|---|---|---|---|---|---|---|---|---|
| Household settings | A126 | R | S | R | R | R | R | R | S | S | S | S | S | S | No |
| | A409-c | I | I | R | R | R | R | R | S | S | S | S | R | I | No |
| | A410-a | R | R | S | S | S | R | R | S | S | S | S | R | S | Yes |
| | A410-b | R | R | R | R | R | R | R | S | I | R | S | R | S | Yes |
| | A411 | R | S | R | R | R | R | R | S | S | S | S | R | I | Yes |
| | A413 | R | R | R | R | R | R | R | S | S | S | S | R | S | Yes |
| | A414 | R | S | R | R | R | S | S | S | S | S | R | R | S | Yes |
| | A801 | R | I | S | I | S | S | S | S | S | S | S | R | I | No |
| | A814-a | I | S | S | I | S | S | S | S | S | S | S | S | S | No |
| | A824-a | S | S | S | S | S | S | S | S | S | S | S | S | S | No |
| PH Hospital | B107-a | R | S | R | R | R | S | S | S | R | S | R | R | R | Yes |
| | B425-a | S | S | R | R | R | R | R | S | S | S | S | R | I | No |
| | B425-b | S | S | R | R | R | S | R | S | S | S | S | R | S | No |
| | B426-a | R | R | R | R | R | R | I | S | S | S | R | R | R | Yes |
| | B475-a | R | I | R | R | R | R | R | S | S | S | R | R | R | Yes |
| | B506-a | S | S | S | S | S | S | S | S | S | S | S | R | R | No |
| | B705-b | R | S | R | R | R | R | R | S | S | S | S | R | S | Yes |
| JU Hospital | C604 | R | S | S | I | S | S | S | S | S | S | S | R | I | No |
| | C705 | S | S | R | I | S | R | R | S | S | S | S | S | S | No |
| | C715-b | I | S | S | I | S | S | S | S | S | S | S | S | S | No |
| | C906 | R | S | R | R | R | R | R | S | S | S | R | S | I | Yes |
| | E. coli ATCC | S | S | S | S | S | S | S | S | S | S | S | S | S | No |

Amx: amoxicillin, Amc: amoxicillin-clavulanate, Cfc: cefaclor, Cfu: cefuroxime, Cfx: cefixime, Ctz: ceftazidime, Ctx: cefotaxime, Imp: imipenem, Nit: nitrofurantoin, Amk: amikacin, Cip: ciprofloxacin, Tms: trimethoprim-sulfamethoxazole, Dox: doxycycline. MDR: multiple drug resistant

Antibiotic susceptibility tests have shown that the majority of the isolates (71.4%) exhibited resistance to Trimethoprim-sulfamethoxazole (Fig. 1). Resistance to amoxicillin was seen in 61.9% of the isolates. When clavulanic acid was combined with amoxicillin (amoxicillin-clavulanic acid), the resistance was seen in only 19% of the isolates. Resistance to cephalosporins (second and third generation) was considerable and ranged from 57% to 66.7% of the isolates. However, no resistance was detected against imipenem. Multiple drug resistance (MDR), that is resistance to three antibiotics or more from different classes, was observed in 10 isolates from the 21 *E. coli* strains (47.6%, Table 2). MDR *E. coli* isolates were found to comprise 50% (5 isolates), 57.1% (4 isolates) and 25% (1 isolate) of the isolated *E. coli* strains from households, PH hospital and JU hospital respectively (Table 2). The prevalence of MDR *E. coli* in the household environment was comparable to that in hospitals ($p = 0.59$). Moreover, 13 strains out of 21 were phenotypically identified as ESBL-producers (61.9%). The prevalence of the phenotypically identified ESBL *E. coli* in households was 60% and in hospital settings were 71.4% and 50% for PH & JU Hospital respectively.

*bla*CTXM group 1 was found in 11 strains (52%) out of the 21 strains.

The results of biocides MIC against *E. coli* isolates are given in Table 3. All MIC values measured are well below the in-use concentrations of these biocides (Table 3). It is noteworthy that the quality control strain (ATCC 25922) and the probiotic strain (Nissle 1917) have MIC values that overlap with MIC values of hospital and household isolates. Moreover, the MIC values of the isolates collected from hospitals were found to be comparable to those collected from households ($p = 0.23$).

## Discussion

The pattern of antibiotic resistance detected in the studied isolates is in line with the resistance encountered in different strains of *E. coli* isolated from various clinical or environmental sources worldwide [14, 15]. In the last few years it has been observed that *E. coli* is exhibiting resistance to more antibiotic classes, hence rendering these drugs ineffective in treating its infections. On the other hand, the high prevalence of *bla*CTXM 1 gene is expected since this gene was found to be the most prevalent ESBL enzyme producing genes in Jordan, particularly in *E. coli* [16, 17].

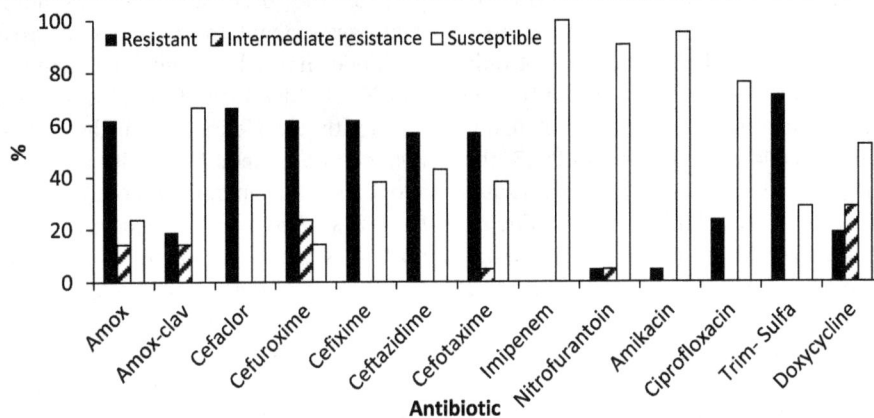

**Fig. 1** Percentage of resistant, intermediate resistant and susceptible *E. coli* strains versus the antibiotics tested

**Table 3** MIC values of the biocides tested (mg/ ml) against different isolates compared to the in-use concentration (mg/ ml). Each result is the average of five replicates ± SD

| Environment | Strain NO. | Cetrimide MIC±SD | Chloroxylenol MIC±SD | Ethanol MIC±SD | Iodine MIC±SD |
|---|---|---|---|---|---|
| Household settings | A126 | 0.2 ± 0 | 0.1 ± 0 | 55 ± 12 | 0.4 ± 0.2 |
| | A409-c | 0.2 ± 0 | 0.2 ± 0 | 75 ± 0 | 0.4 ± 0.1 |
| | A410-a | 0.4 ± 0.1 | 0.2 ± 0 | 55 ± 12 | 0.4 ± 0.2 |
| | A410-b | 0.4 ± 0.1 | 0.1 ± 0 | 55 ± 12 | 0.4 ± 0.1 |
| | A411 | 0.2 ± 0 | 0.1 ± 0 | 65 ± 14 | 0.4 ± 0.1 |
| | A413 | 0.2 ± 0 | 0.1 ± 0 | 75 ± 0 | 0.4 ± 0.1 |
| | A414 | 0.2 ± 0 | 0.1 ± 0 | 55 ± 12 | 0.2 ± 0.2 |
| | A801 | 0.2 ± 0 | 0.2 ± 0.1 | 85 ± 14 | 0.2 ± 0.2 |
| | A814-a | 0.2 ± 0 | 0.2 ± 0 | 50 ± 0 | 0.4 ± 0.2 |
| | A824-a | 0.2 ± 0 | 0.1 ± 0 | 55 ± 12 | 0.4 ± 0.2 |
| PH Hospital | B107-a | 0.4 ± 0.1 | 0.2 ± 0.1 | 50 ± 0 | 0.4 ± 0.2 |
| | B425-a | 0.4 ± 0.1 | 0.2 ± 0.1 | 65 ± 14 | 0.4 ± 0.1 |
| | B425-b | 0.4 ± 0.1 | 0.1 ± 0 | 50 ± 0 | 0.4 ± 0.1 |
| | B426-a | 0.2 ± 0.1 | 0.1 ± 0 | 50 ± 0 | 0.4 ± 0.2 |
| | B475-a | 0.4 ± 0.1 | 0.2 ± 0 | 65 ± 14 | 0.4 ± 0.1 |
| | B506-a | 0.2 ± 0 | 0.2 ± 0 | 55 ± 12 | 0.2 ± 0.1 |
| | B705-b | 0.2 ± 0 | 0.2 ± 0 | 60 ± 14 | 0.2 ± 0.1 |
| JU Hospital | C604 | 0.2 ± 0 | 0.2 ± 0 | 55 ± 12 | 0.4 ± 0.1 |
| | C705 | 0.4 ± 0.1 | 0.1 ± 0 | 50 ± 0 | 0.4 ± 0.1 |
| | C715-b | 0.2 ± 0 | 0.2 ± 0 | 75 ± 0 | 0.4 ± 0.1 |
| | C906 | 0.2 ± 0 | 0.1 ± 0 | 55 ± 12 | 0.2 ± 0.1 |
| | *E. coli* ATCC | 0.2 ± 0 | 0.1 ± 0 | 25 ± 0 | 0.4 ± 0.1 |
| | *E. coli* Nissle | 0.2 ± 0.1 | 0.2 ± 0.1 | 50 ± 0 | 0.4 ± 0.1 |
| In- use concentration of the biocides | | 6[22] | 4–4.8* | 390–710[22] | 2.5–5[22] |

*Calculated from manufacturer's instructions for use

The results showing the prevalence of MDR and ESBL producing *E. coli* in the environment are alarming since they reveal the dissemination of ESBL bacteria not only in hospital environment, but also in the community. The spread of ESBL-producing microorganisms is of major concern to health organizations worldwide. In 2013, the CDC published a report listing the top 18 drug resistant threats to the United States [18]. ESBL-producing *Enterobacteriaceae* were within the group categorized as *"serious threat"*. Moreover, the spread of MDR organisms has caused the WHO to issue a recent report classifying ESBL-producing *Enterobacteriaceae* as a *"critical priority"*, where effective treatment is urgently required [19]. Infections with ESBL-producing bacteria leave limited choices in antibiotic treatment, where carbapenems are the only approved drugs of choice. This effectiveness was observed in this study where all isolates were susceptible to imipenem (Fig. 1).

The biocides investigated in this study were chosen from different classes; alcohols (ethanol), quaternary ammonium compounds (cetrimide), phenolics (chloroxylenol: 4-Chloro-3,5-xylenol,) and halogens (iodine). These classes are used extensively by health care sectors and /or household settings.

A large difference between the MIC and the in-use concentrations of the studied biocides was seen. This suggests that these biocides are effective against the isolated *E. coli* strains, whether MDR or non-MDR. Moreover, the MICs of household isolates and hospital isolates were comparable for all the biocides tested. They were also comparable to the quality control strain and the non pathogenic strain. These findings indicate that the extensive use of biocides in hospitals didn't increase the MIC values of biocides, i.e. they didn't have an impact on the resistance of *E. coli* isolates. Furthermore, we investigated the possible association of MDR with the MIC values of the isolates. No significant difference or association was found ($p > 0.05$).

The occurrence of potential cross-resistance between antimicrobial agents and antibiotics is still not well understood. Some reports have shown a relationship between biocide resistance and antibiotic resistance whilst others have failed to do so [2, 20, 21]. Cole et al. [20], performed a study on 1238 (Gram-positive and Gram-negative) bacterial isolates taken from different surfaces and locations from 60 houses. They didn't observe any cross resistance between antibiotics and biocides. On the contrary, Moken et al. [21] reported cross-resistance between pine oil disinfectant and MDR. In their study, the cross resistance was thought to be through over-expression of multiple antibiotic resistance (*marA*) gene. Other studies have reported the induction of some resistant mechanisms, such as over-expression of efflux pumps or a decrease in growth rates and alteration in gene expression [2]. These are believed to be part of the bacterial stress response. The scientific controversy about the presence of cross-resistance with antibiotics has led the Scientific Committee on Emerging and Newly Identified Health Risks / Directorate General for Health and Consumers in the European Commission (Directorate General for Health and Consumers, 2009) to adopt and issue an opinion about *"Assessment of the Antibiotic Resistance Effects of Biocides"* in 2009 [2]. In this report, they state that *"there is convincing evidence that common mechanisms that confer resistance to biocides and antibiotics are present in bacteria"*. However, due to the limitations in identifying and characterizing cross-resistance in the targeted environment (in situ), the report concluded that more research is needed in this field.

## Conclusion

*E. coli* isolates from household and hospital environments showed high resistance rates to different classes of antibiotics without any significant differences between the two environments. For both groups, many *E. coli* isolates showed antibiotic multiple resistant patterns. ESBL-producing isolates were detected in both environments. *E. coli* isolates from both environments showed comparable MIC values of four of the widely used biocides, although the use of biocides in hospitals is more extensive than in households. Data generated from this study failed to show an association between antibiotic resistance and biocide resistance in *E. coli* isolates.

### Acknowledgements

The authors would like to thank Dr. Phillip Collier for revising the manuscript and providing valuable comments.

### Funding

This research was funded by the Deanship of Academic Research and Quality Assurance, The University of Jordan.

### Authors' contributions

RH supervised the work, directed the research, interpreted the results and wrote the manuscript. BG performed the work and the literature survey. Both authors read and approved the final manuscript.

### Competing interests

The authors declare that they have no competing interests.

### References

1. Health Care-Associated Infections. Office of disease prevention and health promotion. U.S. Department of health and human services. 2017 https://health.gov/hcq/prevent-hai.asp. Accessed 16 Sep 2017.
2. Assessment of the antibiotic resistance effects of biocides. Scientific Committee on Emerging and Newly Identified Health Risks (SCENIHR). Directorate general for health and consumers. European commission. 2009.
3. D'Costa M, King C, Kalan L, Morar M, Sung W, Schwarz C, Froese D, Zazula, G, Calmels F, Debruyne R, Golding G, Poinar H, Wright G. Antibiotic resistance is ancient. Nature 2011; 477,457–461.

4.  Hansen L, Sorensen S, Jorgensen H, Jensen L. The prevalence of the OqxAB multidrug efflux pump amongst olaquindox-resistant *Escherichia coli* in pigs. Microb Drug Resist. 2005;11:378–82.

5.  Karatzas K, Webber M, Jorgensen F, Woodward M, Piddock L, Humphrey T. Prolonged treatment of *Salmonella enteric serovar* typhimurium with commercial disinfectants selects for multiple antibiotic resistance, increased efflux and reduced invasiveness. J Antimicrob Chemother. 2007;60:947–55.

6.  McBain A, Ledder R, Sreenivasan P, Gilbert P. Selection for high-level resistance by chronic triclosan exposure is not universal. J Antimicrob Chemother. 2004;53:772–7.

7.  Ledder R, Gilbert P, Willis C, McBain A. Effects of chronic triclosan exposure upon the antimicrobial susceptibility of 40 ex-situ environmental and human isolates. J Appl Microbiol. 2006;100:1132–40.

8.  Tenaillon O, Skurnik D, Picard B, Denamur E. The population genetics of commensal Escherichia coli. Nature Rev Microbiol. 2010;8(3):207–17.

9.  Ekrami A, Kayedani A, Jahangir M, Kalantar E, Jalali M. Isolation of common aerobic bacterial pathogens from the environment of seven hospitals, Ahvaz, Iran. Jundishapur J Microbiol. 2011;4(2):75–82.

10. Clinical and Laboratory Standard Institute (CLSI). 2016. M 100S performance standards for antimicrobial susceptibility testing, 26th edition.

11. Scaldaferri F, Gerardi V, Mangiola F, Lopetuso L, Pizzoferrato M, Petito V, et al. Role and mechanisms of action of Escherichia coli Nissle 1917 in the maintenance of remission in ulcerative colitis patients: an update. World J Gastroenterol. 2016;22(24):5505–11.

12. Tsen H, Lin C, Chi W. Development and use of 16S rRNA gene targeted PCR primersfor the identification of Escherichia coli cells in water. J Appl Microbiol. 1998;85:554–60.

13. Mirzaee M, Owlia P, Mansouri S. Distribution of CTX-M β-lactamase genes among *Escherichia coli* strains isolated from patients in Iran. Lab Medicine. 2009;40(12):724–7.

14. van der Donk CF, van de Bovenkamp JH, De Brauwer E, De Mol P, Feldhoff K, Kalka-Moll W, et al. Antimicrobial resistance and spread of multi drug resistant Escherichia coli isolates collected from nine urology services in the Euregion Meuse-Rhine. PLoS One. 2012; https://doi.org/10.1371/journal.pone.0047707.

15. Poonia S, Singh T, Tsering D. Antibiotic susceptibility profile of bacteria isolated from natural sources of water from rural areas of East Sikkim. Indian J Community Med. 2014;39(3):156–60.

16. Abu Salah M, Badran E, Shehabi A. High incidence of multidrug resistant *Escherichia coli* producing CTX-M-type ESBLs colonizing the intestine of Jordanian infants. Int Arab J Antimicrob Agents. 2013;3(4:3)

17. Badran EF, Qamer Din RA, Shehabi AA. Low intestinal colonization of Escherichia coli clone ST131 producing CTX-M-15 in Jordanian infants. J Med Microbiol. 2016;65(2):137–41. https://doi.org/10.1099/jmm.0.000210.

18. Biggest Threats, Antibiotic / Antimicrobial Resistance. Centers for Disease Control and Prevention (CDC- USA). 2017; https://www.cdc.gov/drugresistance/biggest_threats.html (access date1/9/2017).

19. Lawe-Davies O, Bennett S. WHO publishes list of bacteria for which new antibiotics are urgently needed, World Health Organization, Geneva. 2017; http://www.who.int/mediacentre/news/releases/2017/bacteria-antibiotics-needed/en/ (access date, 1/9/2017).

20. Cole E, Addison R, Rubino J, Lese K, Dulaney P, Newell M, et al. Investigation of antibiotic and antibacterial agent cross-resistance in target bacteria from homes of antibacterial product users and nonusers. J Appl Microbiol. 2003; 95:664–76.

21. Moken M, McMurry L, Levy S. Selection of multiple-antibiotic-resistant (mar) mutants of *Escherichia coli* by using the disinfectant pine oil: roles of the mar and acrAB loci. Antimicrob Agents Chemother. 1997;41(12):2770–2.

22. Al Adham I, Haddadin R, Collier P. Types of microbicidal and microbistatic agents. In: Fraise AP, Maillard J, Satter SA, editors. *Russell, Hugo & Ayliffe's Principles and practice of disinfection, preservation and sterilization* 5th edition UK: Wiley Blackwell; 2013. p. 5–57.

# 8

# Successful treatment of extensively drug-resistant *Acinetobacter baumannii* ventriculitis with polymyxin B and tigecycline

Wei Guo, Shao-Chun Guo, Min Li, Li-Hong Li and Yan Qu[*]

## Abstract

**Background:** *Acinetobacter baumannii* nosocomial ventriculitis/meningitis, especially those due to drug-resistant strains, has substantially increased over recent years. However, limited therapeutic options exist for the *Acinetobacter baumannii* ventriculitis/meningitis because of the poor penetration rate of most antibiotics through the blood-brain barrier.

**Case presentation:** A 57-year-old male patient developed ventriculitis from an extensively drug-resistant strain of *Acinetobacter baumannii* after the decompressive craniectomy for severe traumatic brain injury. The patient was successfully treated with intraventricular and intravenous polymyxin B together with intravenous tigecycline.

**Conclusions:** The case illustrates intraventricular polymyxin B can be a therapeutic option against extensively drug-resistant *Acinetobacter baumannii* ventriculitis.

**Keywords:** *Acinetobacter Baumannii*, Multidrug resistance, Polymyxin B, Ventriculitis, Intraventricular therapy

## Background

*Acinetobacter baumannii* has emerged as a major nosocomial central nervous system infection, with mortality rates ranging from 15% to 71% for acinetobacter meningitis [1]. Successful treatments with intraventricular/intrathecal polymyxins have been reported; however, the incidence of potential toxicity was not negligible [2]. Here, we report a successful microbiological cure for extensively drug-resistant *A. baumannii* ventriculitis using intravenous and intraventricular polymyxin B together with intravenous tigecycline.

## Case presentation

A 57-year-old male patient was transferred from another hospital to the neurosurgical intensive care unit of the Tangdu hospital. The patient had experienced a falling accident at work and then was diagnosed as having a severe traumatic brain injury. The patient underwent a decompressive craniectomy and an external ventricular drain (EVD) insertion. Eight days after the operation, the patient presented with remittent fever (peak at 39.0 °C) associated with meningeal signs and altered mental status. Empirical antimicrobial therapy was initiated with meropenem and vancomycin. Twelve days after the operation, the patient was transferred to our intensive care unit. A right frontal EVD was inserted because of bilateral hydrocephalus. Cerebrospinal fluid (CSF) analysis revealed a WBC count of $5550 \times 10E6/L$, with 70% polymorphonuclear leukocytes, a glucose concentration of 1.11 mmol/L, and protein levels of 3662.1 mg/L. CSF sample was cultured on columbia agar with 5% sheep blood at 35 °C in aerobic conditions for 48 h. The bacteria were identified by an automated mass spectrometry microbial identification system (VITEK MS, bioMérieux). On day 5 of the hospitalization, the patient's CSF culture showed that the *A. baumannii* was susceptible only to polymyxin (MIC = 1 μg/mL) and tigecycline (MIC ≤1 μg/mL). According to the Clinical and Laboratory Standards Institute criteria, polymyxin breakpoints are susceptible (≤2 μg/ml)

* Correspondence: Yanqu0123@icloud.com
Department of Neurosurgery, Tangdu Hospital, Fourth Military Medical University, Xi'an, Shaanxi 710038, China

and resistant (≥4 µg/ml). For tigecycline, the U.S. Food Drug Administration proposed breakpoints are susceptible (≤2 µg/ml), intermediate (4 µg/ml) and resistant (8 µg/ml). A chest computed tomography scan showed lung infiltrates, which were suggestive of pneumonia. Sputum sample was cultured on Columbia agar with 5% sheep blood and MacConkey at 35 °C in aerobic conditions for 48 h. The same strain of A. baumannii was isolated from the sputum (polymyxin susceptibility was not tested). The antimicrobial therapy was changed to intraventricular (IVT) polymyxin B (50,000 U q24h), intravenous polymyxin B (450,000 U q12h), and tigecycline (50 mg q12h). The patient became afebrile 5 days after the polymyxin B and tigecycline therapy, with negative CSF cultures thereafter. However, in the treatment process, decreased CSF drainage and a contractible right ventricle were observed gradually. Ten days after the right frontal EVD placement, the right EVD was removed, and another EVD was inserted into the left lateral ventricle. Antimicrobial treatment was switched to IVT polymyxin B (25,000 U q12h), intravenous polymyxin B (475,000 U q12h), and tigecycline (50 mg q12h). A contractible left ventricle was also observed after the IVT polymyxin B administration. Next, the antimicrobial regimen was changed by stopping the IVT polymyxin B administration and continuing the intravenous polymyxin B (500,000 U q12h) and tigecycline (50 mg q12h) administration for another 14 days until the patient's clinical conditions were stable. On day 31 of the hospitalization, the patient was discharged.

## Discussion and conclusion

Over the years, Acinetobacter baumannii, which is associated with post-neurosurgical meningitis and ventriculitis, has increasingly been regarded as an important nosocomially acquired pathogen [1, 3]. Statistical data showed that 3.6–11.2% of post-neurosurgical meningitis cases are caused by A. baumannii [2, 4]. Antimicrobial-resistant A. baumannii are divided into three categories: multidrug-resistant (MDR), extensively drug-resistant (XDR) and pandrug-resistant (PDR). XDR is defined as non-susceptibility to all penicillins and cephalosporins (including inhibitor combinations), fluroquinolones, aminoglycosides, and carbapenems. [5]. In the present case, XDR A. baumannii that was susceptible only to polymyxin and tigecycline was cultured from the cerebral spinal fluid (CSF) and sputum. As a result of the poor blood-brain barrier penetration, intraventricular (IVT) therapy polymyxin B was used through the external ventricular derivation (EVD).

Emerging evidence has indicated that intrathecal (IT) or IVT colistin administration is a safe and effective treatment for XDR A. baumannii meningitis [6]. Karaiskos et al. [2]. summarized 36 studies and a total of 81 patients who were diagnosed with meningitis secondary to neurosurgical procedures. A total of 89% (72/81) of the cases treated with IVT/ITH colistin were eventually cured, and the median time to achieve sterilization of the CSF was 4 days. De Bonis et al. [3]. compared the outcomes of the XDR A. baumannii ventriculomeningitis patients treated with intravenous (IV) colistin or IV plus IVT colistin. Compared with 33.3% of the cases in the IV alone group, 100% of the cases achieved CSF sterilization (a negative CSF culture result) in the IV + IVT group. The results showed that IVT colistin administration is significantly more effective than IV colistin alone [3]. To the best of our knowledge, polymyxin B and colistin (polymyxin E) were regarded as equivalent because of their similar chemical structures and their activity spectra [7]. However, compared to colistin, there is limited clinical data for the use of polymyxin B in ventriculitis treatment. Piparsania et al [8]. showed successful treatment of multidrug-resistant A. baumannii neonatal meningo-ventriculitis with IVT polymyxin B in combination with IV netilmicin and polymyxin B. IVT polymyxin B (40,000 units per dose) was given alternate day for four weeks. In the present case, sterilization of CSF was detected 5 days after the IVT polymyxin B administration. Hence, we speculate that IVT polymyxin B administration could be as effective as IVT colistin administration.

In the present case, tigecycline was used intravenously. Tigecycline, which belongs to a new class of antibiotics known as the glycylcyclines [9], has demonstrated excellent activity against Acinetobacter strains [10]. Pallotto et al. [11] showed the weak penetration of tigecycline to the CSF in a patient with ventriculo-atrial shunt infection. The average CSF concentration of tigecycline equals to 7.9% of the serum concentration. That is the reason why tigecycline is not currently recommended for Acinetobacter ventriculitis. Recently, Lauretti et al. reported a successful case of the IVT tigecycline use to treat PDR A. baumannii meningitis [12].

Potential toxicity is a concern associated with local administration of polymyxins. Chemical ventriculitis and meningitis which usually cause fever and altered mental state, are the most severe adverse effects reported with IVT/ITH polymyxin treatment. Karaiskos reviewed the literature and found that out of 81 patients with IVT/ITH colistin administration, chemical meningitis and chemical ventriculitis were diagnosed in 3 (3.7%) and 2 (2.4%) cases, respectively [2]. A recent retrospective study showed that out of 9 patients with IVT colistin administration, no cases of chemical meningitis were encountered [3]. However, to the best of our knowledge, limited reports on the adverse effects of IVT/ITH polymyxin B were published.

In the treatment process, two observations were noted. First, the transient ventricular adhesion due to the IVT polymyxin B administration was observed from the CT scan (Fig. 1). Initially, the IVT polymyxin B was

Therefore, we conclude that IVT and intravenous polymyxin B combined with intravenous tigecycline could be an effective therapeutic option in the treatment of XDR *A. baumannii* ventriculitis. Currently, IVT administration of antibiotics with favorable outcomes is widely reported. However, multicenter randomized studies are still needed to demonstrate the efficacy and safety of intraventricular administration on these patients.

### Abbreviations

CSF: Cerebrospinal fluid; EVD: External ventricular drain; IT: Intrathecal; IV: Intravenous; IVT: Intraventricular; MDR: Multidrug-resistant; PDR: Pandrug-resistant; XDR: Extensively drug-resistant

### Acknowledgements

Not applicable

### Funding

Not applicable

### Authors' contributions

YQ was in charge of case reviewing and preparation of the manuscript. WG and LHL collected clinic opinions regarding on this case and drafted the manuscript. SCG and ML participated in its coordination and revised the manuscript. All authors read and approved the final manuscript.

### Competing interests

The authors declared no potential conflicts of interest with respect to the research, authorship, and/or publication of this article.

### References

1. Kim BN, Peleg AY, Lodise TP, Lipman J, Li J, Nation R, Paterson DL. Management of meningitis due to antibiotic-resistant Acinetobacter species. Lancet Infect Dis. 2009;9(4):245–55.
2. Karaiskos I, Galani L, Baziaka F, Giamarellou H. Intraventricular and intrathecal colistin as the last therapeutic resort for the treatment of multidrug-resistant and extensively drug-resistant Acinetobacter baumannii ventriculitis and meningitis: a literature review. Int J Antimicrob Agents. 41(6):499–508.
3. De Bonis P, Lofrese G, Scoppettuolo G, Spanu T, Cultrera R, Labonia M, Cavallo MA, Mangiola A, Anile C, Pompucci A. Intraventricular versus intravenous colistin for the treatment of extensively drug resistant Acinetobacter Baumannii meningitis. Eur J Neurol. 23(1):68–75.
4. Wang KW, Chang WN, Huang CR, Tsai NW, Tsui HW, Wang HC, Su TM, Rau CS, Cheng BC, Chang CS. Post-neurosurgical nosocomial bacterial meningitis in adults: microbiology, clinical features, and outcomes. J Clin Neurosci. 2005;12(6):647–50.
5. Magiorakos AP, Srinivasan A, Carey RB, Carmeli Y, Falagas ME, Giske CG, Harbarth S, Hindler JF, Kahlmeter G, Olsson-Liljequist B. Multidrug-resistant, extensively drug-resistant and pandrug-resistant bacteria: an international expert proposal for interim standard definitions for acquired resistance. Clin Microbiol Infect. 18(3):268–81.
6. Hoenigl M, Drescher M, Feierl G, Valentin T, Zarfel G, Seeber K, Krause R, Grisold A. Successful management of nosocomial ventriculitis and meningitis caused by extensively drug-resistant Acinetobacter baumannii in Austria. Can J Infect Dis Med Microbiol. 24(3):e88–90.
7. Cai Y, Lee W, Kwa AL. Polymyxin B versus colistin: an update. Expert Rev Anti-Infect Ther. 13(12):1481–97.
8. Piparsania S, Rajput N, Bhatambare G. Intraventricular polymyxin B for the treatment of neonatal meningo-ventriculitis caused by multi-resistant Acinetobacter Baumannii– case report and review of literature. Turk J Pediatr. 2012;54:548–54.
9. Pankey GA. Tigecycline. J Antimicrob Chemother. 2005;56(3):470–80.
10. Karageorgopoulos DE, Falagas ME. Current control and treatment of multidrug-resistant Acinetobacter Baumannii infections. Lancet Infect Dis. 2008;8(12):751–62.

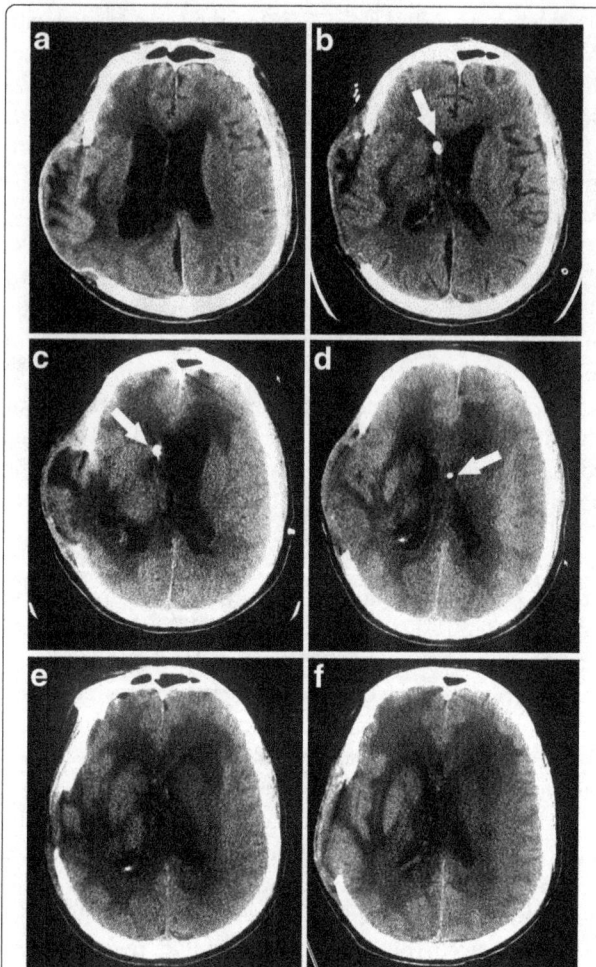

**Fig. 1** Transient ventricular adhesion due to intraventricular (IVT) polymyxin B administration observed from CT scan. **a** CT scan obtained on day 1 of the hospitalization, showing bilateral hydrocephalus. **b** On day 6 of the hospitalization, CT scan showing the contractible right ventricle and enlarged left ventricle after IVT polymyxin B administration through right EVD (arrows). **c** On day 11 of the hospitalization, CT scan showing the contractible right ventricle and enlarged left ventricle after IVT polymyxin B administration through right EVD (arrows). **d** On day 18 of the hospitalization, CT scan showing the contractible left ventricle after IVT polymyxin B administration through left EVD (arrows). **e** CT scan obtained on day 20 of the hospitalization. **f** CT scan obtained on day 23 of the hospitalization

administered through the right EVD. However, decreased CSF drainage and a contractible right ventricle were detected after the IVT polymyxin B administration. Six days later, when the left EVD were used for the polymyxin B administration, left ventricle shrinkage was observed. These phenomena indicate that there is a direct correlation between polymyxin B usage and ventricular adhesion. Second, at the 6-month follow-up, the neurological conditions of the patients had not improved, and the patient was still in a comatose status.

# 9

# Prevalence and patterns of drug resistance among pulmonary tuberculosis patients in Hangzhou, China

Qingchun Li[1†], Gang Zhao[1†], Limin Wu[1], Min Lu[1], Wei Liu[1], Yifei Wu[1], Le Wang[1], Ke Wang[1], Han-Zhu Qian[2] and Li Xie[1*] (iD)

## Abstract

**Background:** To evaluate prevalence and patterns of drug resistance among pulmonary tuberculosis (TB) patients in Hangzhou City, China.

**Methods:** Sputum samples of smear positive TB patients enrolled in 2011 and 2015 were collected and tested for drug susceptibility, and demographic and medical record data were extracted from the electronic database of China Information System for Disease Control and Prevention. Chi-square test was used to compare drug resistance prevalence between new and treated patients and between male and female patients, and Chi-square test for trend was used to compare the prevalence over calendar years 2011 and 2015.

**Results:** Of 1326 patients enrolled in 2015, 22.3% had resistance to any first-line anti-TB drugs and 8.0% had multi-drug resistance (MDR); drug resistance rates among previously treated cases were significantly higher than among new cases. Significant declines of resistance to isoniazid, rifampin, ethambutol and streptomycin, and MDR from 2011 to 2015 were observed among previously treated patients, while a significant decline of resistance to rifampin was observed among new cases.

**Conclusions:** While the prevalence of acquired drug resistance decreased due to due to implementation of DOTS-Plus program, the prevalence of primary drug resistance due to transmission remained high. Greater efforts should be made to screen drug resistance for case finding and to reduce transmission through improving the treatment and management of drug-resistant patients.

**Keywords:** Tuberculosis, Drug sensitivity testing, Drug resistance, China

## Background

China is one of the countries with the highest burden of tuberculosis (TB) disease in the world. Although its ranking in total TB cases dropped in 2015 from second to third behind India and Indonesia [1], the epidemic of drug-resistant TB (DR-TB) and multi-drug resistant TB (MDR-TB) is still a severe public health issue in China. A national survey published in 2012 showed 5.7% of new cases and 25.6% of previously treated cases had MDR-TB, both higher than the global averages [2]. The prevalence of DR-TB and MDR-TB varied geographically, and 57% TB patients were resistant to any first-line drugs and 24.1% were resistant to multiple drugs in high-burden regions [3, 4]. Studies have been conducted to investigate the prevalence of TB drug resistance across the country in recent years [3, 5], but few have evaluated the temporal trend. A study in Shanghai City in the middle of China's east coast found the drug resistance rates increased significantly from 2000 to 2003, and then stabilized during 2004–2006 [6]. A study among TB patients in Hangzhou City in east China showed DR-TB and MDR-TB prevalence was 31.3% and 11.6%, respectively [7]. Little is known about the patterns of drug resistance and recent trend of the epidemic in Hangzhou City. This study reports drug resistance patterns and the

* Correspondence: jiefangsuo@sina.com
†Equal contributors
[1]Hangzhou Center for Disease Control and Prevention, Mingshi Road, Hangzhou City 310021, Zhejiang Province, China
Full list of author information is available at the end of the article

epidemic trend from 2011 to 2015 in Hangzhou City in eastern China.

## Methods
### Study population
Hangzhou City is located in eastern China, about a hundred miles away from Shanghai. It comprises 13 districts, one county-level city, and two counties, and has 7.2 million local residents and over 2 million migrant populations.

All smear-positive pulmonary TB patients who lived in Hangzhou in years 2011 and 2015 were included in this study. The highest value was used for analysis if patients had multiple drug susceptibility testing (DST) results in the study years.

### Data collection and bacteriologic examinations
TB is a notifiable disease in China. Over 68,000 health facilities report notifiable diseases to the national, real-time, internet-based disease reporting system, known as the China Information System for Disease Control and Prevention (CIS-DCP). Hangzhou City Center for Disease Control and Prevention (CDC) is authorized for access to the sociodemographic information and medical records of TB patients who live in Hangzhou in this system.

TB cases were diagnosed following Chinese clinical guideline for TB diagnosis and treatment. Three sputum samples were collected from each participant at different time points (clinic visit, early morning, and night) prior to initiation of treatment, and were examined for acid-fast bacilli (AFB). Two specimens with the highest bacterial counts were used for culture. TB culture was performed as follows: First, decontaminating and digesting the sputum with equal volume of 4% sodium hydroxide for 15 min; Then, inoculating 0.1 ml specimen into the Lowenstein–Jensen medium, and culturing it in incubator at 37 °C; After that, observing the colony growth, which was confirmed by microscopic examination for AFB through Ziehl-Neelsen staining.

Species identification of mycobacteria was performed by conventional biochemical tests. Drug sensitivity test was performed using the proportion method on Löwenstein-Jensen medium, with the following concentrations: 0.2 micrograms per milliliter (μg/ml) for isoniazid, 2.0 μg/ml for ethambutol, 2.0 μg/ml for ofloxacin, 4.0 μg/ml for streptomycin, 30 μg/ml for kanamycin, and 40 μg/ml for rifampin. The critical growth proportion for drug resistance was 1% for all drugs. All drugs were obtained from Sigma Life Science Company (USA). The standard sensitive strain H37Rv was tested in each set of the tests and again within each set if the batch of medium was changed. The drug sensitivity test result or the H37Rv should be sensitive. All drug sensitivity tests in years 2011 and 2015 were performed by the same staff in the TB reference laboratory at Hangzhou CDC, a part

of World Health Organization/International Union against Tuberculosis and Lung Disease Global Project on Anti-Tuberculosis Drug Resistance Surveillance.

### Statistical analysis
Statistical analysis was conducted with SPSS 12.0 software. Chi-square tests or Fisher's exact tests were used comparing drug resistance rates between new and treated patients and between male and female patients. Chi-square tests for trend were used for comparing the difference of drug resistance rates from 2011 to 2015. $P$ value $< 0.05$ was considered statistically significant.

## Results
### Demographic characteristics of TB patients
The general characteristics and drug resistance rates of 1184 participants in 2011 were reported elsewhere [7]; of these participants, 903 (76.3%) were new TB patients and 281 (23.7%) were previously treated patients. In 2015, a total of 1888 smear-positive pulmonary TB patients who lived in Hangzhou were diagnosed, of whom 1583 (83.8%) had positive sputum culture results and 1332 (70.6%) were positive for *M. tuberculosis*. Six patients were excluded due to lack of drug sensitivity test results for first-line anti-TB drugs; therefore, 1326 (70.2%) patients were included in the analysis.

Of 1326 patients, 961 (72.5%) were male and 365 (27.5%) were female; 1305 (98.42%) were Han Chinese and 21 (1.58%) were other ethnic minorities; age ranged from 12 to 94 years (mean 54); 289 (21.8%) were migrants; 1020 (76.9%) were new cases and 306 (23.1%) were previously treated cases; 874 (65.9%) had a drug sensitivity test result for ofloxacin and 875 (66.0%) for kanamycin.

### TB drug resistance patterns in 2015
In 2015, about 18% (184/1020) new TB patients were resistant to at least one first-line drug, while the prevalence of drug resistance among previously treated patients was double (36.6%, 112/306) (Table 1). The majority of drug resistance cases had resistance to a single drug, such as streptomycin, isoniazid, rifampin, ofloxacin, ethambutol and kanamycin. Eight percent of TB patients had multi-drug resistance (MDR), 3.8% among new patients and 22.2% among previously treated patients; the common combinations of MDR were isoniazid with rifampin or streptomycin. One new patient and two previously treated patients had extensive drug resistance (XDR) (Table 1).

The difference in the prevalence of resistance to any single drug or to multiple drugs between new and treated patients was statistically significant (Table 2). This difference was same for both male and female patients, separately (not shown in tables). There was no statistically significant difference of drug resistance prevalence between male and

**Table 1** Drug resistance patterns among 1326 tuberculosis patients in Hangzhou, China, 2015

| Type of TB resistance | New cases (N = 1020) | | Treated cases (N = 306) | |
|---|---|---|---|---|
| | n | % | n | % |
| Resistance to any first-line drugs | 184 | 18.0 | 112 | 36.6 |
| Resistance to individual drugs in any tests | | | | |
| Isoniazid | 102 | 10.0 | 89 | 29.1 |
| Rifampin | 57 | 5.6 | 78 | 25.5 |
| Ethambutol | 15 | 1.5 | 23 | 7.5 |
| Streptomycin | 119 | 11.7 | 58 | 19.0 |
| Ofloxacin | 20 | 2.0 | 15 | 4.9 |
| Kanamycin | 7 | 0.7 | 4 | 1.3 |
| Resistance to single drug only | | | | |
| Isoniazid | 33 | 3.2 | 15 | 4.9 |
| Rifampin | 15 | 1.5 | 8 | 2.6 |
| Ethambutol | 2 | 0.2 | 0 | 0 |
| Streptomycin | 57 | 5.6 | 10 | 3.3 |
| Ofloxacin | 14 | 1.4 | 3 | 1.0 |
| Kanamycin | 2 | 0.2 | 0 | 0 |
| Resistance to two drugs | | | | |
| Isoniazid+ethambutol | 1 | 0.1 | 1 | 0.3 |
| Isoniazid+streptomycin | 27 | 2.7 | 3 | 1.0 |
| Rifampin+ethambutol | 1 | 0.1 | 0 | 0 |
| Rifampin+streptomycin | 3 | 0.3 | 1 | 0.3 |
| Ethambutol+streptomycin | 1 | 0.1 | 1 | 0.3 |
| Rifampin+ofloxacin | 0 | 0 | 1 | 0.3 |
| Streptomycin+ofloxacin | 2 | 0.2 | 1 | 0.3 |
| Isoniazid+ofloxacin | 1 | 0.1 | 1 | 0.3 |
| Streptomycin+ kanamycin | 1 | 0.1 | 0 | 0 |
| Isoniazid+rifampin | 9 | 0.9 | 19 | 6.2 |
| Resistance to three drugs | | | | |
| Isoniazid+rifampin+ethambutol | 0 | 0 | 6 | 2.0 |
| Isoniazid+rifampin+Streptomycin | 16 | 1.6 | 24 | 7.8 |
| Ethambutol+streptomycin+ofloxacin | 0 | 0 | 1 | 0.3 |
| Isoniazid+rifampin+ofloxacin | 1 | 0.1 | 1 | 0.3 |
| Isoniazid+rifampin+kanamycin | 1 | 0.1 | 0 | 0 |
| Isoniazid+ethambutol+ofloxacin | 0 | 0 | 1 | 0.3 |
| Resistance to four drugs | | | | |
| Isoniazid+rifampin+ethambutol +streptomycin | 8 | 0.8 | 10 | 3.3 |
| Isoniazid+rifampin+ethambutol +ofloxacin | 0 | 0 | 2 | 0.7 |
| Isoniazid+rifampin+streptomycin +ofloxacin | 1 | 0.1 | 1 | 0.3 |
| Isoniazid+rifampin+streptomycin +kanamycin | 0 | 0 | 2 | 0.7 |

**Table 1** Drug resistance patterns among 1326 tuberculosis patients in Hangzhou, China, 2015 (Continued)

| Type of TB resistance | New cases (N = 1020) | | Treated cases (N = 306) | |
|---|---|---|---|---|
| | n | % | n | % |
| Resistance to five drugs | | | | |
| Isoniazid+rifampin+ethambutol +streptomycin+ofloxacin | 0 | 0 | 2 | 0.7 |
| Isoniazid+rifampin+ethambutol +streptomycin+kanamycin | 1 | 0.1 | 0 | 0 |
| Multi-drug resistance (MDR) | 38 | 3.7 | 68 | 22.2 |
| Extensive drug resistance (XDR) | | | | |
| Isoniazid+rifampin+ofloxacin +kanamycin (or cycloserine)[a] | 1 | 0.1 | 2 | 0.7 |

[a]Of these 3XDR patients, two were resistant to kanamycin, and one to cycloserine

female participants, and no difference by age group (not shown in tables).

### Time trend of drug resistance from 2011 to 2015

A significant decline of resistance to any first-line drugs from 2011 to 2015 was observed: from 31.3% to 22.3% among all TB patients, and from 23.4% to 18% in new and 57% to 36.6% in previously treated patients ($P < 0.01$). There were significant declines in resistance to isoniazid, rifampin, ethambutol, streptomycin, and multi-drugs among previously treated patients, while among new patients there was a significant decline for rifampin only (Table 3).

### Discussion

Our study showed that 22.3% of TB patients in Hangzhou City in 2015 were resistant to at least one first-line anti-TB drugs and 8.0% were MDR, and the prevalence of MDR was lower among new cases (3.7%) than among treated cases (22.2%). The MDR prevalence is comparable to the global average, e.g., 3.3% among new cases and 20% among previously treated cases [1]. Among TB patients in Zhejiang province where Hangzhou City is located, 23.6% were resistant to any first-line drugs and 5.0% were MDR [8]. The prevalence rates of any first-line drug resistance and MDR in six Chinese provinces were 23.4% and 13.5%, respectively [9], whereas in other areas, the rate of resistance to any first-line drugs ranged from 16.6% and 57%, and MDR from 4.0% to 24.1% [5, 6, 10–13]. In summary, the drug resistance prevalence in Hangzhou City was in the lower range of the epidemics in China.

Studies have shown that there is increasing or persistently high prevalence of drug resistance among TB patients in Mainland China [3, 5, 6, 14], a review showed that primary MDR-TB prevalence in China was below 4.0% before 1995, and reached 10% by 2005; The acquired MDR-TB prevalence increased from 5% in 1995 to 32.

**Table 2** Comparison of drug resistance among 1326 new and treated tuberculosis cases in Hangzhou, China, 2015

| Type of TB resistance | All (N = 1326) n, % | New cases (N = 1020) n, % | Treated cases (N = 306) n, % | $\chi^2$ | P |
|---|---|---|---|---|---|
| Resistance to any first-line drugs | 296 (22.3) | 184 (18.0) | 112 (36.6) | 46.8 | < 0.01 |
| Isoniazid | 191(14.40) | 102 (10.00) | 89 (29.08) | 69.5 | < 0.01 |
| Rifampin | 135 (10.2%) | 57 (5.6) | 78 (25.5) | 102.0 | < 0.01 |
| Ethambutol | 38 (2.9) | 15 (1.5) | 23 (7.5) | 30.9 | < 0.01 |
| Streptomycin | 177(13.4) | 119 (11.7) | 58 (19.0) | 10.8 | < 0.01 |
| Multi-drug resistance (MDR) | 106 (8.0) | 38 (3.8) | 68 (22.2) | 109.5 | < 0.01 |

4% in 1990 and then stayed around 30% until 2005 [15]. We observed significant decline of TB drug resistance in Hangzhou City, particularly among previous diagnosed TB patients, and the findings have significant implications. First, primary drug resistance among treatment-naïve TB patients is caused by transmission; while drug resistance among treated patients can also be acquired due to inappropriate treatment. The decline of resistance to most first-line drugs among treated patients, but only to rifampin among new patients during 2011–2015 suggests that the prevalence of acquired drug resistance (ADR) mutations in treated patients declined, but the prevalence of transmitted drug resistance (TDR) mutations remained high. This decline may be due to the improvement of TB treatment and management in Hangzhou City, as it has implemented the DOTS Plus program—a DOTS program with components for MDR TB diagnosis, management, and treatment. A recent study in Shanghai showed the primary resistance due to exogenous reinfection was the major cause of drug resistance among treated TB patients [16], and this observation was also confirmed in other parts of China [17]. Another study found that 60% MRD patients had primary drug resistance attributable to transmission [18]. It is suggested that more efforts are needed to enhance detection, treatment and management of drug resistant patients, and more effective strategies are needed to prevent and interrupt transmission of drug resistant tuberculosis.

Second, the widely used regimens for both new and treated TB patients in China are two months of isoniazid, rifampicin, pyrazinamide and ethambutol followed by four months of isoniazid and rifampicin (2HRZE/4HR) or two months of isoniazid, rifampicin, pyrazinamide, ethambutol and streptomycin followed by six months of isoniazid and rifampicin (2HRZES/6HR) [19].Previous studies showed that about 90% TB patients with resistance to rifampin

**Table 3** Prevalence trend of drug resistance among tuberculosis patients in Hangzhou, China, from 2011 to 2015

| Type of TB resistance | Treatment history | 2011 (N = 1184) | 2015 (N = 1326) | $\chi^2$ | P |
|---|---|---|---|---|---|
| Resistance to any first-line drugs | All | 371 (31.3) | 296 (22.3) | 26.0 | < 0.01 |
| | New cases | 211 (23.4) | 184 (18.0) | 8.3 | < 0.01 |
| | Treated cases | 160 (57.0) | 112 (36.6) | 24.4 | < 0.01 |
| Isoniazid | All | 231 (19.5) | 191 (14.4) | 11.7 | < 0.01 |
| | New cases | 103 (11.4) | 102 (10.0) | 1.0 | 0.32 |
| | Treated cases | 128 (45.6) | 89 (29.1) | 17.1 | < 0.01 |
| Rifampin | All | 201 (17.0) | 135 (10.2) | 24.9 | < 0.01 |
| | New cases | 82 (9.1) | 57 (5.6) | 8.7 | < 0.01 |
| | Treated cases | 119 (42.4) | 78 (25.5) | 18.7 | < 0.01 |
| Ethambutol | All | 60 (5.1) | 38 (2.9) | 8.1 | < 0.01 |
| | New cases | 13 (1.4) | 15 (1.5) | 0.0 | 0.95 |
| | Treated cases | 47 (16.7) | 23 (7.5) | 11.8 | < 0.01 |
| Streptomycin | All | 203 (17.2) | 177 (13.4) | 7.0 | < 0.01 |
| | New cases | 110 (12.2) | 119 (11.7) | 0.1 | 0.73 |
| | Treated cases | 93 (33.1) | 58 (19.0) | 15.3 | < 0.01 |
| Multi-drug resistance (MDR) | All | 137 (11.6) | 106 (8.0) | 9.2 | < 0.01 |
| | New cases | 37 (4.1) | 38 (3.7) | 0.2 | 0.67 |
| | Treated cases | 100 (35.6) | 68 (22.2) | 12.8 | < 0.01 |

were also resistant to isoniazid, so drug sensitivity test of rifampin could serve as an index for screening MDR [14]. In our study, 78% patients with resistance to rifampin were MDR. Rifampin resistance is associated with poorer clinical outcomes and requires an increase in duration of therapy. Although the drug resistance was relatively low among the new cases, 37% of MDR patients and 62% of patients with resistance to any first-line anti-TB drugs were from the new cases [20]. Therefore, newly diagnosed patients in economically developed areas should be screened for drug resistance prior to initiate TB treatment [20]. The findings are similar to those from a study in Taiwan, which showed that the acquired MDR-TB prevalence was significantly lower after the implementation of the DOTS and DOTS-plus programmes, while the primary MDR-TB prevalence remained stable [21]. The time trends of drug resistance prevalence varied geographically. A meta-analysis published in 2017 revealed that the MDR TB prevalence among newly diagnosed in Ethiopia in East Africa was 1.7% (95% confidence interval [CI], 1.2–2.3%) and among previously treated TB patients, 14.1% (95% CI, 10.9–17.2%); The overall MDR-TB prevalence showed a stable time trend over the past 10 years [22]. Another meta analysis of the studies conducted in India revealed a worsening trend in DR-TB between the two study decades (decade 1 from 1995 to 2005: 37.7% [95% CI, 29.0–46.4%] vs decade 2 from 2006 to 2015: 46.1% [95% CI, 39.0–53.2%]); The pooled estimate of MDR-TB resistance was higher in previously treated patients (decade 1: 29.8% [95% CI, 20.7–39.0%]; decade 2: 35.8% [95% CI, 29.2–42.4%]) as compared with the newly diagnosed cases (decade 1: 4.1% [95% CI, 2.7–5.6%]; decade 2: 5.6% [95% CI, 3.8–7.4%]) [23].

Our study has limitations. First, our study sample only included sputum smear-positive TB patients, but other study showed 17% of drug-resistant and 20% of MDR cases were linked to sputum smear-negative sources [24]. Therefore, the prevalence of drug resistance in our study may be overestimated, and our study findings may not be extrapolated to sputum smear-negative TB cases. Second, we did not do genotyping of TB infections, so we were unable to ascertain the sources of drug-resistant strains among previously treated cases. Third, we did not perform drug sensitivity testing for second-line anti-TB drugs for all MDR patients, the estimations of resistance to second-line anti-TB drugs and extensive drug resistance might be biased.

## Conclusions

In summary, our study found higher prevalence of drug resistance and MDR among treated TB patients than among new patients in Hangzhou City, and showed a decreasing trend from years 2011–2015. DOTS-Plus program should be expanded, and greater efforts should be made to screen drug resistance for case finding and to reduce transmission through improving the treatment and management of drug-resistant patients.

## Abbreviations
AFB: acid-fast bacilli; CDC: Center for Disease Control and Prevention; CIS-DCP: System for Disease Control and Prevention; DR-TB: drug-resistant TB; DST: drug susceptibility testing; MDR: multi-drug resistance; TB: tuberculosis; XDR: extensive drug resistance

## Funding
This study was supported by a grant from Zhejiang Medical and Health Science and Technology Program (2015KYA189).

## Authors' contributions
LQC and ZG equality contributed in study design, data collection, analysis and manuscript writing. WLM, LM, WL, WK participated in study design and data collection; LW and WYF conducted laboratory testing; HZQ revised the manuscript; XL and HZQ participated in study design, data analysis and funding support. All the authors have read the manuscript and have approved it.

## Competing interests
All authors declare that they have no competing interests.

## Author details
[1]Hangzhou Center for Disease Control and Prevention, Mingshi Road, Hangzhou City 310021, Zhejiang Province, China. [2]Department of Biostatistics, Yale School of Public Health, New Haven, Connecticut, USA.

## References
1. World Health Organization. Global Tuberculosis Report 2016. Available at http://www.who.int/tb/publications/global_report/en/. Accessed 3 Nov 2017.
2. Zhao YL, Xu SF, Wang LX, et al. National survey of drug-resistant tuberculosis in China. New Engl J Med. 2012;366:2161–70.
3. Li D, Wang JL, Ji BY, et al. Persistently high prevalence of primary resistance and multidrug resistance of tuberculosis in Heilongjiang Province, China. BMC Infect Dis. 2016;16:516.
4. Liu BB, Hu PL, Gong DF, et al. Profile and influencing factors of drug resistance of Mycobacterium tuberculosis in smear-positive pulmonary tuberculosis patients in Hunan province. Chin J. Infect Control. 2016; 15(2):73–8.
5. He XC, Zhang XX, Zhao JN, et al. Epidemiological trends of drug-resistant tuberculosis in China from 2007 to 2014. Medicine. 2016;95(15):1–7.
6. Shen X, DeRiemer K, Yuan ZA, et al. Drug resistant tuberculosis in shanghai, China, 2000-2006: prevalence, trends, and risk factors. Int J Tuberc Lung Dis. 2009;13(2):253–9.
7. Li QC, Wu LM, Lu M, et al. Surveillance for tuberculosis drug resistance in Hangzhou, Zhejiang. Disease Surveillance. 2014;29(3):210–4.
8. Chen SH, Wu BB, Liu ZW, et al. An analysis on the epidemic characteristics of tuberculosis drug resistance in Zhejiang province. Pre Med. 2016;28(8): 757–65.
9. Song Y, Wan L, Chen SS, et al. Analysis on drug resistance of Mycobacterium tuberculosis and influencing factors in six provinces of China. Chinese Chin J Epidemio. 2016;37(7):945–8.
10. Xi XY, Dai MJ, Yan XB. Drug resistance analysis on Mycobacterium tuberculosis of 2695 sputum smear-positive patients with tuberculosis in Xuzhou area. Chin J Exp Clin Infect Dis (Electronic Edition). 2015;9(3):347–51.
11. Wang ZD, Zhang HQ, Ren ZS, et al. Analysis of tuberculosis drug resistance in Qingdao. Chin J Antituberc. 2015;37(6):637–40.
12. Wang XL, Wang XP, Xiao HX, et al. Survey of drug-resistant Mycobacterium tuberculosis in Ningxia. Chin J Tuberc Respir Dis. 2015;38(10):738–40.
13. Wang JJ, Hu Y, Jiang WL, et al. Population-based molecular epidemiologic study of rifampicin-resistant tuberculosis in rural area of eastern China. Chin. J Epidemiol. 2009;30(11):1189–93.
14. Yin QQ, Jiao WW, Li QJ, et al. Prevalence and molecular characteristics of drug-resistant Mycobacterium tuberculosis in Beijing, China: 2006 versus 2012. BMC Microbiol. 2016;16:85.

15. Yang XY, Li YP, Mei YW, Yu Y, Xiao J, Luo J, Yang Y, Wu SM. Time and spatial distribution of multidrug-resistant tuberculosis among Chinese people, 1981-2006: a systematic review. Int J Infect Dis. 2010;14(10):e828–37.

16. Nsofor CA, Jiang Q, Wu J, et al. Transmission is a noticeable cause of resistance among treated tuberculosis patients in shanghai, China. Sci Rep. 2017;7:7691.

17. Gao Q, Mei J. Transmission is the main cause of high rate of drug-resistant tuberculosis in China. Chin J Antituberc. 2015;37:1091–6.

18. Huai P, Huang X, Cheng J, et al. Proportions and risk factors of developing multidrug resistance among patients with tuberculosis in China: a population-based case-control study. Microb Drug Resist. 2016;22(8):717–26.

19. National Health and Family Planning Commission of the People's Republic of China. Guideline of tuberculosis control program in China. Beijing. 2008: 57–9.

20. Wang Y. Program of MDR TB control and prevention. Beijing: Military Medicine Science Press; 2012.

21. Chien JY, Lai CC, Tan CK, et al. Decline in rates of acquired multidrug-resistant tuberculosis after implementation of the directly observed therapy, short course (DOTS) and DOTS-plus programmes in Taiwan. J Antimicrob Chemoth. 2013;68(8):1910–6.

22. Eshetie S, Gizachew M, Dagnew M, Kumera G, Woldie H, Ambaw F, Tessema B, Moges F. Multidrug resistant tuberculosis in Ethiopian settings and its association with previous history of anti-tuberculosis treatment: a systematic review and meta-analysis. BMC Infect Dis. 2017;17(1):219.

23. Goyal V, Kadam V, Narang P, Singh V. Prevalence of drug-resistant pulmonary tuberculosis in India: systematic review and meta-analysis. BMC Public Health. 2017;17(1):817.

24. Yang CG, Shen X, Peng P, et al. Transmission of Mycobacterium tuberculosis in China: a population-based molecular epidemiologic study. Clin Infect Dis. 2015;61:219–27.

# 10

# Multi-drug resistant Acinetobacter species: a seven-year experience from a tertiary care center in Lebanon

Zeina A. Kanafani[1,2†], Nada Zahreddine[2†], Ralph Tayyar[1], Jad Sfeir[1], George F. Araj[3], Ghassan M. Matar[4] and Souha S. Kanj[1,2*]

## Abstract

**Background:** *Acinetobacter* species have become increasingly common in the intensive care units (ICU) over the past two decades, causing serious infections. At the American University of Beirut Medical Center, the incidence of multi-drug resistant *Acinetobacter baumannii* (MDR-Ab) infections in the ICU increased sharply in 2007 by around 120%, and these infections have continued to cause a serious problem to this day.

**Methods:** We conducted a seven-year prospective cohort study between 2007 and 2014 in the ICU. Early in the epidemic, a case-control study was performed that included MDR-Ab cases diagnosed between 2007 and 2008 and uninfected controls admitted to the ICU during the same time.

**Results:** The total number of patients with MDR-Ab infections diagnosed between 2007 and 2014 was 128. There were also 99 patients with MDR-Ab colonization without evidence of active infection between 2011 and 2014. The incidence of MDR-Ab transmission was 315.4 cases/1000 ICU patient-days. The majority of infections were considered hospital-acquired (84%) and most consisted of respiratory infections (53.1%). The mortality rate of patients with MDR-Ab ranged from 52% to 66%.

**Conclusion:** MDR-Ab infections mostly consisted of ventilator-associated pneumonia and were associated with a very high mortality rate. Infection control measures should be reinforced to control the transmission of these organisms in the ICU.

**Keywords:** Acinetobacter, Intensive care unit, Ventilator-associated pneumonia, Multi-drug resistance, Lebanon

## Background

Multidrug-resistant organisms (MDRO) have significant infection control implications and are currently affecting the clinical course of patients in tertiary care centers. *Acinetobacter baumannii* is of particular importance. The organism is widely distributed in nature and survives on moist and dry surfaces [1, 2]. Worldwide, multidrug-resistant *A. baumannii* (MDR-Ab) has become a significant cause of hospital-acquired infections (HAI) and hospital-acquired colonizations (HAC) resulting in high morbidity and mortality [3] in patients admitted to the intensive care units (ICU) over the past two decades [4]. Strict adherence to infection control

practices and environmental disinfection have been effective in controlling outbreaks [5]. Appropriate strategies and practices must therefore be implemented to prevent the growing transmission of MDR-Ab.

In line with the worldwide emergence of MDR-Ab, similar trends have been observed at various centers in Lebanon. Although national studies are lacking, the available evidence suggests rapidly falling susceptibility rates to carbapenems (from 49.2% in 2011 to 15.1% in 2013 at 16 selected hospitals) [6], and a predominance of OXA-23 and GES-11 with upstream insertion sequence ISAba1 (90% of isolates in a study from 11 centers) [7]. At the American University of Beirut Medical Center (AUBMC), HAI and HAC caused by MDR-Ab initially increased in the ICU in 2007 from 2-3 cases to 5-6 per month. These infections were mostly associated with invasive devices such as ventilators, central venous catheters, and urinary catheters. Investigations carried by the Infection Control and Prevention Program (ICPP)

* Correspondence: sk11@aub.edu.lb
†Equal contributors
[1]Department of Internal Medicine, Division of Infectious Diseases, American University of Beirut, Cairo Street PO Box 11-0236/11D, Riad El Solh, Beirut 1107 2020, Lebanon
[2]Infection Control and Prevention Program, American University of Beirut, Cairo Street PO Box 11-0236/11D, Riad El Solh, Beirut 1107 2020, Lebanon
Full list of author information is available at the end of the article

identified multiple factors that contributed to the transmission of MDR-Ab. We herein describe our experience at the AUBMC with MDR-Ab over a 7-year period and the infection control measures that were implemented to control the spread of this organism in the ICU.

## Methods

### General description and settings

AUBMC is a 386-bed teaching tertiary care center functioning as a referral center at the national and regional levels. The ICU consists of a medical and surgical unit with a nine-bed capacity. Three single- and three double-bed rooms are spread around a central nursing station. The ICU population consists of high-risk patients with multiple comorbidities, as well as patients following major surgical procedures. The beds in the double rooms are maintained at a distance of 3 m and separated by textile curtains.

### Study design

A 7-year prospective cohort study was conducted in the ICU with systematic attempts to assess present practices and to introduce new interventions to contain the transmissions of MDR-Ab in the unit. All ICU patients were evaluated examining the risk factors attributed to the transmission of MDR-Ab HAI or HAC. The ICU team routinely collected specimens from newly admitted patients for baseline bacteriological studies and all patients were placed under contact isolation. A standardized screening method was adopted, where cultures were obtained from deep tracheal aspirates (DTA), urine, oropharyngeal, axillary, umbilical, perianal, and rectal areas. The ICPP team reviewed the culture results on daily basis to advise on the isolation status of patients through daily surveillance rounds. Patients identified with MDR-Ab were kept on contact isolation. Cultures were repeated on weekly basis until discharge. All MDR-Ab HAI and HAC were periodically discussed with the ICU staff for feedback and interventions. Furthermore, environmental cultures were obtained following the identification of clusters or outbreaks from the direct environment of the patient and from the medical equipment used inside the ICU cubicle. Repeated cleaning and disinfection was performed for all surfaces or equipment identified to be contaminated with MDR-Ab. A nested retrospective case-control study from January 2007 till June 2008 was performed in the ICU and the Respiratory Care Unit (RCU) to analyze patient related risk factors leading to MDR-Ab transmissions. Controls were randomly selected from patients admitted to the ICU and the RCU during the same study period but who did not have a positive screening culture for MDR-Ab. Moreover, cases consisted of patients with one or more cultures growing MDR-Ab (either colonized or infected). For patients with multiple MDR-Ab culture results, only the first positive culture was considered. The data were entered into a database using IBM® SPSS® Statistics version 21.

### Definitions

According to the Centers for Disease Control and Prevention (CDC), a multidrug-resistant pathogen is defined as one that is resistant to one or more classes of antimicrobial agents, including carbapenems [5]. In this study, MDR-Ab was defined as an isolate that is resistant to all tested antimicrobial agents except colistin and tigecycline [8]. A culture positive for MDR-Ab was considered to represent colonization when patients showed no evidence of infection. As for the case definition, patients with at least one clinical/surveillance specimen positive for MDR-Ab were defined as cases of transmission of MDR-Ab colonization or infection that was not present on admission. Such patients were considered to have acquired MDR-Ab during their ICU stay. For device-associated infections, the definitions were subject to considerable variation since 2005 based on the updates issued by the CDC and when the reports published by the National Nosocomial Infections Surveillance (NNIS) system were updated and replaced by the National Healthcare Safety Network (NHSN). All infections were classified using the CDC definitions of the corresponding year using laboratory and clinical criteria. Infection control staff collected data on central line-associated primary bloodstream infections (CLABSI), ventilator-associated pneumonias (VAP), and urinary catheter associated urinary tract infections (CAUTI) in patients admitted to the adult ICU. Corresponding ICU denominator data consisting of patient-days and device-days were also collected by infection control staff for the same calendar month [9, 10].

### Description of clusters and outbreaks

A cluster was defined as an aggregation of MDR-Ab cases (more than 2 cases), closely grouped in time and place. When the number of cases in the cluster exceeded 4 transmissions, it was considered an outbreak.

### Organism identification and susceptibility testing

*Acinetobacter* isolates were identified using the MALDI-TOF platform for identification. All isolates were tested using the disk diffusion method based on the Clinical and Laboratory Standards Institute (CLSI) breakpoints. The colistin sensitivity testing was made based on VITEC-2 Bio System and disk diffusion according to the method reported by Galani et al. in 2008 study [11, 12].

### Ethical considerations

A written informed consent was not needed for our study as the information was obtained from the daily surveillance rounds of the ICPP team. The medical records of patients were routinely reviewed as part of the ongoing ICPP work. Patients were not contacted and medical records were not retrieved a second time to write the manuscript. Over the years, statistics were collected and stored for statistical analysis and periodic reports within the institution. All figures included in the manuscript were retrieved from the preexisting ICPP files without having to perform a review of patient records. Furthermore, the available statistics did not include any identifiable information to maintain patient confidentiality.

## Results

### Results of the case-control study of Acinetobacter infections 2007–2008

A total of 73 cases infected with *Acinetobacter spp.* (carbapenem-sensitive and resistant Acinetobacter isolates) and 73 controls (uninfected patients) were included. The mean age of the infected patients was $61.7 \pm 17.7$ years with a male predominance (male:female ratio of 2:1). Culture specimens consist mostly of respiratory secretions (58%), followed by wound (22%), blood (12%), and urine (8%). Moreover, the microbiological distribution of the isolates was predominated by one species, namely *Acinetobacter baumannii* complex (70 isolates, 96%) with the other 4% distributed between *A. junii* (2 isolates, 2.7%) and *A. lwoffi* (1 isolate, 1.3%). In addition, 40 patients (55%) had carbapenem-resistant isolates, 26 of which were tested against colistin and found to be susceptible. Most infections were deemed to be hospital-acquired (84%) with only 16% being community-acquired. Furthermore, underlying comorbidities such as diabetes mellitus, renal insufficiency, chronic obstructive pulmonary disease (COPD), and malignancy were significant risk factors for developing an Acinetobacter infection. In addition, patients who had undergone surgical interventions and those who received antibiotics within 30 days prior to admission were at significant risk for developing an Acinetobacter infection ($p < 0.05$) (Table 1).

All complications due to Acinetobacter infections, except for acute respiratory distress syndrome (ARDS), were encountered more with resistant strains as compared to sensitive ones, but none of these complications was of statistical significance (Table 2).

### Results of the prospective study of MDR-Ab transmissions in ICU 2007–2014

The total number of patients with Acinetobacter infections diagnosed between 2007 and 2014 was 128 (Table 3). There were also 99 patients with MDR-Ab colonization without evidence of active infection between 2011 and 2014. Prior to 2011, screening of patients on admission to the ICU was not performed.

The mean age of the 128 patients was 58.3 years (range 19–96) with a male predominance (60.2%). The mean length of ICU stay was 3.6 days (range 1–14 days). Outliers for patients staying for more than 30 days (maximum recorded length of stay was 5 months) were documented but were not included in the calculation of the mean length of stay (3 patients). The most common site of infection among the isolates was the respiratory tract (53.1%), followed by surgical wound (18.8%), blood (15.6%), urine (10.2%) and others (2.3%) (Table 4). The most common colonization site among the 99 cases was the respiratory tract (80.8%) followed by skin colonization (12.4%). The mortality rate (22%) in the ICU was associated with old age, trauma, cancer, multiple comorbidities, and invasive device use.

During the outbreak period from December 2012 to December 2014, 130 patients out of 1267 (10.3%) admitted to the ICU became colonized or infected with MDR-Ab, with patients from the surgical ICU having slightly less risk than those from the medical ICU. The overall colonization pressure (number of MDR-Ab patient-days $\times$ 1000/total number of patient-days) of MDR-Ab between 2012 and 2014 was 315.4 cases per 1000 ICU patient-days (range

**Table 1** Bivariable analysis of patient characteristics in the case-control study

| Variable | Cases (n = 73) | Controls (n = 73) | Unadjusted Odds Ratio | p-value |
|---|---|---|---|---|
| Age (mean ± SD), *in years* | 61.7 | 60.4 | N/A | 0.798 |
| Male | 49 (67.1) | 52 (71.2) | 0.82 | 0.591 |
| Diabetes | 42 (57.5) | 10 (13.7) | 8.53 | < 0.001 |
| Chronic pulmonary disease | 35 (47.9) | 12 (16.4) | 4.68 | < 0.001 |
| Renal insufficiency | 32 (43.8) | 12 (16.4) | 3.97 | < 0.001 |
| Malignancy | 21 (28.8) | 7 (9.6) | 3.81 | 0.005 |
| Corticosteroid intake | 5 (6.8) | 7 (9.6) | 0.69 | 0.55 |
| Urinary catheter in the past 30 days | 62 (84.9) | 58 (79.4) | 1.46 | 0.39 |
| Central venous catheter in the past 30 days | 7 (9.6) | 4 (5.5) | 1.83 | 0.35 |
| Mechanical ventilation in the past 30 days | 43 (58.9) | 39 (53.4) | 1.25 | 0.50 |
| Surgery in the past 30 days | 19 (26.0) | 5 (6.8) | 4.78 | 0.003 |
| Antibiotic use in the past 30 days | 47 (64.3) | 12 (16.4) | 9.19 | < 0.001 |
| All-cause mortality | 34 (46.6) | 27 (37.0) | 1.48 | 0.24 |

All numbers represent no. (%) unless otherwise specified
SD = standard deviation; N/A = not applicable

**Table 2** Complications and outcome in patients with susceptible *Acinetobacter* infection vs. MDR-Ab infection in the case-control study

| Variable | Susceptible *Acinetobacter* infection ($n = 33$) n (%) | MDR-Ab infection ($n = 40$) n (%) |
|---|---|---|
| Sepsis | 15 (45.4) | 17 (42.5) |
| ARDS | 2 (6.1) | 0 |
| Respiratory failure | 4 (12.1) | 8 (20.0) |
| ICU admission | 5 (15.1) | 8 (20.0) |
| AKI | 8 (24.2) | 10 (25.0) |
| Prolonged hospital stay | 27 (81.2) | 31 (77.5) |
| Persistence/progression of infection | 5 (15.1) | 13 (32.5) |
| Recurrence of infection | 6 (18.2 | 8 (20.0) |
| All-cause mortality | 12 (36.4) | 22 (55.0) |

MDR-Ab = multidrug-resistant Acinetobacter; ARDS = adult respiratory distress syndrome; ICU = intensive care unit; AKI = acute kidney injury

**Table 4** Types of MDR-Ab infections in ICU between 2007 and 2014

| Year | CLABSI | VAP | SSI | CAUTI | Others | Total |
|---|---|---|---|---|---|---|
| 2007 | 2 | 11 | 0 | 0 | 3 | 16 |
| 2008 | 3 | 14 | 3 | 3 | 0 | 23 |
| 2009 | 2 | 6 | 3 | 3 | 0 | 14 |
| 2010 | 1 | 8 | 8 | 1 | 0 | 18 |
| 2011 | 3 | 7 | 5 | 0 | 0 | 15 |
| 2012 | 3 | 11 | 3 | 2 | 0 | 19 |
| 2013 | 4 | 5 | 1 | 0 | 0 | 10 |
| 2014 | 2 | 6 | 1 | 4 | 0 | 13 |
| Total number (%) | 20 (15.6) | 68 (53.1) | 24 (18.8) | 13 (10.2) | 3 (2.3) | 128 |

MDR-Ab = multidrug-resistant Acinetobacter; ICU = intensive care unit; CLABSI = central line associated bloodstream infection; VAP = ventilator-associated pneumonia; SSI = surgical site infection; CAUTI = catheter-associated urinary tract infection

262.8–361.6) (Table 5). In addition, the average length of stay for MDR-Ab patients admitted to the ICU was 9.7 days (range 1–150) with the average length of stay till the acquisition of MDR-Ab being 7.3 days (range 2–31). The all-cause mortality rate of patients dying with MDR-Ab infection/colonization was high and ranged between 52% and 66%. Given the fact that the patients were critically ill, calculating the attributable mortality was challenging.

Moreover, the ICPP took several control measures to help break the transmission cycle of the organism. Hand hygiene, universal screening and isolating all newly admitted patients played a key role in containing the outbreaks. Furthermore, the change in cleaning protocols and the extensive focus on educating healthcare workers limited the spread of MDR-Ab to other hospital wards. Didecyldimethylammonium chloride (DDAC) was adopted for cleaning and disinfection of floors,

walls, surfaces, and medical devices. This disinfectant and detergent has bactericidal and fungicidal activity, in addition to being active on HCV, HIV-1, and influenza virus at a dilution of 0.25% (20 ml in 8 l of water).

Table 6 summarizes the clusters and outbreaks encountered throughout the study period along with control measures that were undertaken by the ICPP:

**Environmental cultures**

Sampling environmental culture swabs from patients' environment and equipment was conducted throughout the study period. As a result, positive cultures were recovered from samples taken from the ventilators, the portable X-Ray and the nitric oxide machines. By molecular typing, these isolates were found to be identical to the bacteria isolated from the patients. These pieces of equipment were thought to play a major role in the outbreak. Subsequently, ICPP proposed new protocols for the process of placing patients on assisted respiratory therapy and issued detailed procedures for cleaning and disinfection of ventilators. Cultures were taken from additional environmental sources including the water, the faucets, and the air conditioning outlets in the rooms and failed to yield any Acinetobacter growth. Other sources that were identified during the investigation of later outbreaks included leaking mattresses and pillows, which were thought to be also possible

**Table 3** Characteristics of the patients infected with MDR-Ab in the prospective study of MDR-Ab transmissions in ICU 2007–2014

| Clinical Characteristics | | Number of patients | Percent |
|---|---|---|---|
| Gender | Male | 77 | 60.2 |
| | Female | 51 | 39.8 |
| Age | > 70 years | 54 | 42.2 |
| | ≤ 70 years | 74 | 57.8 |
| Diabetes | | 42 | 32.8 |
| Chronic pulmonary disease | | 86 | 67.2 |
| Hemodialysis | | 21 | 16.4 |
| Malignancy | | 38 | 29.7 |
| Past surgical procedures | | 46 | 36.0 |
| Recent mechanical ventilation | | 73 | 57.0 |
| In-ICU mortality | | 28 | 22.0 |
| Carbapenem susceptibility | Susceptible | 33 | 25.8 |
| | Resistant | 95 | 74.2 |

MDR-Ab = multidrug-resistant Acinetobacter; ICU = intensive care unit

**Table 5** Colonization pressure among patients in ICU during 2012–2014

| Year | 2012 | 2013 | 2014 |
|---|---|---|---|
| MDR-Ab days | 1130 | 814 | 925 |
| Patient days | 3125 | 3097 | 2873 |
| Colonization pressure per 1000 patient days | 361.6 | 262.8 | 322.0 |

ICU = intensive care unit; MDR-Ab = multidrug-resistant Acinetobacter

**Table 6** General characteristics of the reported clusters and outbreaks in ICU

| Timeline | Characteristics | Identified source | Control measures | Recurrence |
|---|---|---|---|---|
| 1995–2007 | Scattered clusters affecting 1–2 patients/month | • Endogenous • Common source | • Hand hygiene compliance • Patient placement on contact isolation | Intermittent |
| 2007–08 | Outbreaks occurring in ICU on periodic basis Incidence rate 5–25/1000 patient-days | Case-control study • Endogenous - Malignancy - Recent surgery • Common source - Water contamination with MDR-Ab | • Targeted intervention - Infection control practices - Enforcing adherence to hand hygiene - Proper use of personal protective equipment - Controlled visitation to patients - Targeted education and guidance - Intensified presence of ICPP team | Frequent |
| 2009–11 | Major outbreaks occurring in ICU on monthly basis Incidence rate 4–30/1000 patient-days | • Endogenous - Underlying diseases - Invasive procedures • Common source - Contaminated ventilators Lack of compliance with IC measures | Key measures • Strict compliance hand hygiene policy • Patient placement on contact precautions until cleared by negative results of screening cultures • Judicious use of antibiotics • $H_2O_2$ decontamination | Ongoing |
| 2012–14 | Alternating endemic clusters and outbreaks occurring on monthly basis Colonization pressure: 2012 284.0 2013 263.0 2014 322.0 | Significant findings for point and propagated sources | Implementation of Drastic measures were implemented - Key revisions of policies and procedures - Key change in cleaning and disinfection methods | Ongoing |

reservoirs for MDR-Ab. All leaking mattresses and pillows were discarded and replaced by new ones.

### Colonization pressure

The program adopted tracking the MDR-Ab colonization pressure (CP) and reporting it on a monthly basis. In fact, during the same study period, MDR-Ab CP was relatively high and correlated with the high crude numbers of MDR-Ab infections and colonizations. By that time, transmissions of MDR-Ab had become endemic.

### Bundles approach

Additional steps that became standard of care in the nursing units included the implementation of the bundles for device-associated infections (VAP, CLABSI, and CAUTI bundles) as recommended by the Institute for Health Care Improvement, proper monthly training for healthcare workers especially in the critical care units, adoption of a "bare below elbow" outfit for all ICU workers, and daily presence of the ICPP team members in the ICUs. All these measures were essential to containing the spread of MDR-Ab inside the ICU. The addition of close-circuit television (CCTV) cameras was also instrumental in identifying health care personnel breaches during the evening and night shifts. These cameras had an additive effect and contributed to the control of the epidemic.

### Discussion

Over the past decade, *Acinetobacter spp.* have been increasingly associated with hospital infections and colonizations. Our study describes several outbreaks caused by MDR-Ab between 2007 and 2014. Our initial case control study of Acinetobacter infections, between 2007 and 2008, revealed that most of the infected patients were elderly, with a male predominance, similar to the study by Abbo et al. [13]. Positive cultures consisted mostly of respiratory secretions, followed by wound, blood, and then urine; findings comparable to an international study [14]. *Acinetobacter baumannii* was the predominant isolated species with only few isolates of *A. junii* and *A. lwoffi*. At the beginning of the study about half of the isolates were carbapenem resistant, of which around half were found to be susceptible to colistin. Most of the infections were considered hospital-acquired with a small percentage being community-acquired infections.

As in previously reported studies [15], patients infected with Acinetobacter had several risk factors including underlying comorbidities such as diabetes mellitus, renal insufficiency, COPD, and malignancy. Furthermore, surgical interventions and prior antibiotic treatment within 30 days before admission were also found to be significant risk factors for developing an Acinetobacter infection in concordance with a study by Playford et al. [16].

In this study, we compared infections with susceptible versus resistant isolates and found that there was a trend towards more sepsis, respiratory failure, ICU admission, and prolonged hospital stay in infections with MDR-Ab strains. However, acute respiratory distress syndrome (ARDS) was seen in both groups. Similar findings were seen in another study in the ICU from China [17].

In the prospective study conducted between 2007 and 2014, there was also a predominance of male gender, with a mean age of 60 years comparable to our case-control study. The mean length of stay in the ICU was around 4 days, however, outliers for patients staying for more than 30 days were documented. During this period, carbapenem resistance among Acinetobacter isolates increased steadily, with prevailing MDR-Ab towards the end of 2014. This was likely due to the significant increase in carbapenem use at AUBMC, in view of the rising incidence of extended spectrum Beta lactamase producing Enterobacteriacae [18]. The most common site of infection among the patients with Acinetobacter infections was found to be the respiratory tract, followed by surgical wound, blood, and urine as reported in other studies [19]. Similarly, the most common colonization site between 2011 and 2014 was the respiratory tract followed by skin colonization.

Acinetobacter infections have been associated with increased mortality in several published reports. In our study, the all-cause mortality rate of patients with MDR-Ab infection/colonization was high, but it was difficult to calculate the attributable mortality due to the fact that many patients were critically ill with multiple comorbid conditions. Higher mortality rates were seen in older patients, those with trauma, cancer, multiple comorbidities, and invasive device use.

In addition, during the study period, the average length of stay for MDR-Ab patients admitted to the ICU increased. Patients with Acinetobacter incurred greater financial costs than those who did not have Acinetobacter transmissions. It is estimated that a single ventilator-associated pneumonia (VAP) or central line-associated bloodstream infection (CLABSI) due to MDR-Ab may result in 2 weeks of additional hospitalization with its incurred added cost. The average cost of ICU stay, at our medical center, for one patient with MDR-Ab infection can reach $1750 per day. For an extended ICU stay of 2 weeks, the patient's bill can be up to $24,000. Because of the poor outcome of the Acinetobacter infections and the incurred increased morbidity, hospital stay and cost of infected patients, the ICPP adopted a series of control measures since December 2012.

For example, in view of published supportive evidence [20], the use of the $H_2O_2$ vaporizer for room disinfection after discharges of colonized or infected patients was initiated in 2013. Although in this report, the Acinetobacter contamination in the ICU environment was found to be a cause of recurrent MDR-Ab clusters or outbreaks, lack of proper hand hygiene and lack of adherence to proper infection control practices were thought to play a major role in the spread of this organism. Audits conducted by the ICPP team as well as anonymous audits led to the identification of several breaches by the health care providers that were promptly addressed. The nursing director and the chief of staff office issued warnings for health care workers with repeated acts of non-compliance. Finally, changes in the reporting of data, namely the introduction of the CP measure as an important predictor of infection and colonization [21], helped in standardization and benchmarking of infection rates.

Our study has limitations. Patient-level antibiotic treatment data were not available. Therefore, patient outcome could not be analyzed based on treatment received. Colonized patients were not followed after discharge from the ICU. The only outcome available for these patients was the overall mortality rate. Attributable mortality was not assessed because of multiple confounding variables such as underlying illnesses, invasive procedures, cancer patients, etc. Another limitation is that some of the data were obtained retrospectively and could not be re-verified. Finally, the fact that multiple interventions were implemented at the same time in an effort to control the epidemic prevented the analysis of the effect of each measure by itself.

## Conclusion

In conclusion, at our center, MDR-Ab infections mostly caused ventilator-associated pneumonia and were associated with a very high mortality rate. Acinetobacter can colonize several environmental sources including respirators, mattresses and others. It is an organism that is difficult to eradicate and easy to spread in the ICU setting. Adherence to proper infection control measures is key in controlling the transmission and spread of these organisms in the ICU.

### Acknowledgements
Not applicable.

### Funding
The study did not require any external funding.

### Authors' contributions
ZK designed the study and analyzed and interpreted the patient data. NZ collected the patient data and obtained the environmental cultures; RT collected the patient data; JS collected the patient data; GA performed the microbiological testing; GM performed the microbiological testing; SK designed and oversaw the conduct of the study. All authors read and approved the final manuscript.

### Author details
[1]Department of Internal Medicine, Division of Infectious Diseases, American University of Beirut, Cairo Street PO Box 11-0236/11D, Riad El Solh, Beirut 1107 2020, Lebanon. [2]Infection Control and Prevention Program, American University of Beirut, Cairo Street PO Box 11-0236/11D, Riad El Solh, Beirut 1107 2020, Lebanon. [3]Department of Pathology and Laboratory Medicine, American University of Beirut, Cairo Street PO Box 11-0236/11D, Riad El Solh, Beirut 1107 2020, Lebanon. [4]Department of Experimental Pathology, Microbiology, and Immunology, American University of Beirut, Cairo Street PO Box 11-0236/11D, Riad El Solh, Beirut 1107 2020, Lebanon.

## References
1. Espinal P, Marti S, Vila J. Effect of biofilm formation on the survival of Acinetobacter Baumannii on dry surfaces. J Hosp Infect. 2012;80(1):56–60.
2. Jawad A, Heritage J, Snelling AM, Gascoyne-Binzi DM, Hawkey PM. Influence of relative humidity and suspending menstrua on survival of Acinetobacter spp. on dry surfaces. J Clin Microbiol. 1996;34(12):2881–7.
3. Sunenshine RH, Wright MO, Maragakis LL, et al. Multidrug-resistant Acinetobacter infection mortality rate and length of hospitalization. Emerg Infect Dis. 2007;13(1):97–103.
4. Caldeira VM, Silva Junior JM, Oliveira AM, et al. Criteria for patient admission to an intensive care unit and related mortality rates. Rev Assoc Med Bras. 1992;56(5):528–34. (2010).
5. Siegel JD, Rhinehart E, Jackson M, Chiarello L. Healthcare Infection Control Practices Advisory C. Management of multidrug-resistant organisms in health care settings, 2006. Am J Infect Control. 35(10 Suppl 2)):S165–93. (2007)
6. Chamoun K, Farah M, Araj G, et al. Surveillance of antimicrobial resistance in Lebanese hospitals: retrospective nationwide compiled data. Int J Infect Dis. 2016;46:64–70.
7. Hammoudi Halat D, Moubareck CA, Sarkis DK. Heterogeneity of Carbapenem resistance mechanisms among gram-negative pathogens in Lebanon: results of the first cross-sectional countrywide study. Microb Drug Resist. 2017;23(6):733–43.
8. Magiorakos AP, Srinivasan A, Carey RB, et al. Multidrug-resistant, extensively drug-resistant and pandrug-resistant bacteria: an international expert proposal for interim standard definitions for acquired resistance. Clin Microbiol Infect. 2012;18(3):268–81.
9. Dudeck MA, Edwards JR, Allen-Bridson K, et al. National Healthcare Safety Network report, data summary for 2013, device-associated module. Am J Infect Control. 2015;43(3):206–21.
10. Edwards JR, Peterson KD, Andrus ML, et al. National healthcare safety network (NHSN) report, data summary for 2006, issued June 2007. Am J Infect Control. 2007;35(5):290–301.
11. Galani I, Kontopidou F, Souli M, et al. Colistin susceptibility testing by Etest and disk diffusion methods. Int J Antimicrob Agents. 2008;31(5):434–9.
12. Nhung PH, Miyoshi-Akiyama T, Phuong DM, et al. Evaluation of the Etest method for detecting colistin susceptibility of multidrug-resistant gram-negative isolates in Vietnam. J Infect Chemother. 2015;21(8):617–9.
13. Abbo A, Navon-Venezia S, Hammer-Muntz O, Krichali T, Siegman-Igra Y, Carmeli Y. Multidrug-resistant Acinetobacter baumannii. Emerg Infect Dis. 2005;11(1):22–9.
14. Maslow JN, Glaze T, Adams P, Lataillade M. Concurrent outbreak of multidrug-resistant and susceptible subclones of Acinetobacter Baumannii affecting different wards of a single hospital. Infect Control Hosp Epidemiol. 2005;26(1):69–75.
15. Dizbay M, Tunccan OG, Sezer BE, Hizel K. Nosocomial imipenem-resistant Acinetobacter Baumannii infections: epidemiology and risk factors. Scand J Infect Dis. 2010;42(10):741–6.
16. Playford EG, Craig JC, Iredell JR. Carbapenem-resistant Acinetobacter Baumannii in intensive care unit patients: risk factors for acquisition, infection and their consequences. J Hosp Infect. 2007;65(3):204–11.
17. Ye JJ, Huang CT, Shie SS, et al. Multidrug resistant Acinetobacter Baumannii: risk factors for appearance of imipenem resistant strains on patients formerly with susceptible strains. PLoS One. 2010;5(4):e9947.
18. Araj GF, Avedissian AZ, Ayyash NS, et al. A reflection on bacterial resistance to antimicrobial agents at a major tertiary care center in Lebanon over a decade. J Med Liban. 2012;60(3):125–35.
19. Bergogne-Berezin E, Towner KJ. Acinetobacter spp. as nosocomial pathogens: microbiological, clinical, and epidemiological features. Clin Microbiol Rev. 1996;9(2):148–65.
20. Blazejewski C, Wallet F, Rouze A, et al. Efficiency of hydrogen peroxide in improving disinfection of ICU rooms. Crit Care. 2015;19:30.
21. Castelo Branco Fortaleza CM. Moreira de Freitas F, da Paz Lauterbach G. Colonization pressure and risk factors for acquisition of imipenem-resistant Acinetobacter Baumannii in a medical surgical intensive care unit in Brazil. Am J Infect Control. 2013;41(3):263–5.

# 11

# Colonization of long term care facility patients with MDR-Gram-negatives during an *Acinetobacter baumannii* outbreak

Ines Zollner-Schwetz[1]*[ID], Elisabeth Zechner[1], Elisabeth Ullrich[2], Josefa Luxner[2], Christian Pux[3], Gerald Pichler[3], Walter Schippinger[3], Robert Krause[1] and Eva Leitner[2]

## Abstract

**Background:** We aimed to determine the prevalence of colonization by multidrug-resistant Gram-negative bacteria including ESBL-producing enterobacteriaceae, carbapenem-resistant enterobacteriaceae, *Pseudomonas aeruginosa* and *Acinetobacter baumannii* at two wards caring long term for patients with disorder of consciousness at the Geriatric Health Centers Graz, Austria. During our study we detected two *A. baumannii* outbreaks.

**Methods:** In August 2015, we conducted a point-prevalence study. Inguinal and perianal swabs were taken from 38 patients and screened for multidrug-resistant Gram-negative rods using standard procedures. Six months after the initial investigation all patients were sampled again and use of antibiotics during the past 6 months and mortality was registered. Genetic relatedness of bacteria was evaluated by DiversiLab system.

**Results:** Fifty percent of patients were colonized by multidrug-resistant Gram-negative isolates. Five patients harboured ESBL-producing enterobacteriaceae. No carbapenem-resistant enterobacteriaceae were detected. 13/38 patients were colonized by *A. baumannii* isolates (resistant to ciprofloxacin but susceptible to carbapenems). There was a significant difference in the prevalence of colonization by *A. baumannii* between ward 2 and ward 1 (60% vs. 5.6%, $p < 0.001$). Two clusters of *A. baumannii* isolates were identified including one isolate detected on a chair in a patient's room.

**Conclusions:** We detected a high prevalence of two multidrug-resistant *A. baumannii* strains in patients with disorder of consciousness at a LTCF in Graz, Austria. Our findings strongly suggest nosocomial cross-transmission between patients. An active surveillance strategy is warranted to avoid missing newly emerging pathogens.

**Keywords:** Acinetobacter Baumannii, Colonization, Long term care facility, Disorder of consciousness

## Background

Long term care facilities (LTCF) play an essential role in contemporary healthcare systems due to an ageing population in the industrialized world. There is increasing evidence suggesting that residents in LTCFs are frequently colonized by multidrug-resistant Gram-negative bacteria [1–3]. Asymptomatic carriage of multidrug-resistant Gram-negative pathogens constitutes a potential source of transmission to other patients. In addition, there is an increased risk of subsequent infection by the multidrug resistant organism [4].

Several organisms are of concern in this setting in particular carbapenemase-producing enterobacteriaceae as well as *Acinetobacter baumannii*. *A. baumannii* has been shown to colonize the skin [5] as well as abiotic surfaces like equipment used in ICUs [6]. The ability of *A. baumannii* to form biofilms is thought to be pivotal for this colonization [6]. Several studies have demonstrated that *A. baumannii* colonizes patients in LTCFs [3, 7, 8].

The aim of our study was to determine the prevalence of colonization by multidrug-resistant Gram-negative bacteria including ESBL-producing enterobacteriaceae, carbapenem-resistant enterobacteriaceae, *P. aeruginosa*

* Correspondence: ines.schwetz@medunigraz.at
[1]Department of Internal Medicine, Section of Infectious Diseases and Tropical Medicine, Medical University of Graz, Auenbruggerplatz 15, A-8036 Graz, Austria
Full list of author information is available at the end of the article

und *A. baumannii* at two wards caring long term for patients with disorders of consciousness (unresponsive wakefulness syndrome and minimally conscious state) at the Geriatric Health Centers Graz, Austria. In the course of this study, an outbreak of *A. baumannii* was discovered and analysed. The results of this analysis are also described in this manuscript.

## Methods

### Setting and study design

We conducted a point-prevalence study in August 2015 at two wards caring long term for patients with disorders of consciousness (unresponsive wakefulness syndrome and minimally conscious state) at the Geriatric Health Centers Graz, Austria. Patients are managed in single or double rooms. The two wards (23 beds each) are located in the same building and are staffed by the same team of health care personnel. Two swabs (Copan, Brescia, Italy) were taken from the perianal region and from skin of the inguinal region (pooled from both sides), respectively. Microbiological sampling was repeated 6 months later in February 2016. Healthcare workers were trained how to obtain microbiological swabs. Sampling was scheduled during the morning ward round before bathing and dressing the patients. Informed written consent was obtained from the legal representatives of all patients.

### Data collection

At the initial survey, structured questionnaires were completed for each patient to document demographic and administrative data as well as data concerning possible risk factors for asymptomatic colonization by multidrug-resistant Gram-negative bacteria. Collected variables included: age, gender, length of stay in the facility, bowel and bladder incontinence, previous hospitalisation or surgery (in past 3 months), previous antibiotic use (in the past 3 months), presence of enteral feeding tubes, tracheostomy and/or urinary catheters, and presence of chronic wounds (decubitus, surgical wounds, and chronic vascular ulcers). Questionnaires for the follow-up survey after 6 months included antibiotic treatment in the past 6 months.

### Microbiological methods

Microbiological samples were transported immediately to the microbiological laboratory of the Institute of Hygiene, Microbiology and Environmental Medicine, Medical University of Graz. Swabs were plated on ChromID ESBL, Chrom ID Carba Smart and MacConkey agar plates (bioMerieux, Marcy l'Etoile, France). The plates were incubated under aerobic conditions at 36 °C and were evaluated for growth after 24 and 48 h. Suspected colonies were further cultivated on blood agar and identified to species level using the automated Vitek MS system (bioMerieux). Antimicrobial susceptibility was tested using Vitek-2 (card AST-N196 and/or N248) with interpretation of the results according to EUCAST breakpoints. All isolates were stored at –70 °C for analysis of genetic relatedness at the end of the study. Automated repetitive PCR with the DiversiLab system (bioMérieux, Nürtingen, Germany) was performed to determine clonal relationships following manufacturer's instructions. Isolates with a similarity index >95% were considered related and with a similarity index >97.5% as indistinguishable.

Multidrug-resistance was defined according to the recommendations of the Robert Koch Institute (RKI) in Germany issued in 2012 [9]. Briefly, isolates resistant to 3 out of 4 relevant antimicrobial classes (acylureidopenicillin, 3rd/4th generation cephalosporins, carbapenems, fluoroquinolones) were classified as 3MRGN. Enterobacteriaceae resistant to carbapenems were classified as 4MRGN even if the isolate remains susceptible to one other antibiotic class. Isolates resistant to all 4 classes were classified as 4MRGN.

### Statistical analysis

Quantitative variables were expressed as mean ± standard deviation. For statistical analysis Student's t-test, Chi Square test and Fisher's exact test were used as appropriate. A *p*-value of less than 0.05 was considered to indicate statistical significance. The statistical software package SPSS 20.0 (Chicago, IL, USA) was used.

## Results

### Patient characteristics

A total of 46 patients was eligible for the study. 38 patients were included in the study (mean age 58.2 ± 13.6 years, 95% CI: 53.7–62.6 years). Eight patients were not included because of a lack of consent of their legal representatives. 21/38 of included patients were male. The mean duration of stay at the ward was 53.6 ± 58 months, 95% CI: 34.2–72.3 months. All patients had enteral feeding tubes. Three patients had suprapubic urinary catheters. None of the patients had chronic wounds/skin defects. Seventeen patients had tracheostomy. None of the patients required mechanical ventilation. None of the patients had been transferred to an acute care hospital within 3 months prior to the study. Five patients had received antibiotic therapy in the 3 months prior to the study.

### Acinetobacter Baumannii outbreak

13/38 patients were found to be colonized by 3MRGN *A. baumannii* isolates. All of these isolates were resistant to ciprofloxacin but susceptible to carbapenems. One patient was co-colonized by an ESBL-producing *E. coli* isolate and a 3MRGN *A. baumannii* isolate. In addition,

5/38 patients were colonized by *A. baumannii* isolates that remained susceptible to carbapenems and ciprofloxacin and were hence not classified as multidrug-resistant. Overall, 18/38 patients were colonized by any *A. baumannii* isolate. Characteristics of patients colonized by 3MRGN *A. baumannii* compared to non-colonized patients are summarized in Table 1. There was a significant difference in the prevalence of colonization by 3MRGN *A. baumannii* between ward 2 and ward 1 (60% vs. 5.6%, $p < 0.001$). Patients colonized by 3MRGN *A. baumannii* had stayed at the ward significantly longer before the study compared to non-colonized patients (91.4 ± 59 months vs. 33.4 ± 47.3 months, $p = 0.002$).

Of 18 patients initially colonized by any *A. baumannii* isolate 10 were still colonized after 6 months (in February 2016), whereas 6 patients were not colonized any longer (Fig. 1). There was no significant difference in mortality and antibiotic use between patients colonized by MRGN bacteria compared to non-colonized patients.

As 18/38 of patients were colonized by any *A. baumannii* isolate a source in the environment of ward 2 was suspected. Several studies documenting *A. baumannii* outbreaks demonstrated that water sources such as sinks and the patients' environment were contaminated by the organism [10–12]. Therefore, swabs were taken from glove boxes, tissue dispensers, sterile filters of a water source, bottles of disinfectant used by cleaning personnel, bedrails, a patient bathtub and a patient elevator into the bathtub, bottles of aromatic oils, sinks in personnel room, a table in personnel room, chairs for visitors in patient rooms. In addition, water drawn from 3 different taps was analysed (source of water for washing patients, kitchen sink, and bathtub). Body care products were not tested as they are used on a single-patient basis. *A. baumannii* was detected on the patient elevator into bathtub (isolate not available for further analysis) and from a chair for visitors in a patient room. The latter was classified as a 3MRGN *A. baumannii* and was included in the Diversilab study. In addition, patients'

charts were reviewed to identify clinical *A. baumannii* isolates during the study period.

**Prevalence of MRGN bacteria**

At the initial survey in August 2015, we detected 19/38 patients harbouring MRGN isolates (overall prevalence 50%, Table 2). Five patients were colonized by 3MRGN enterobacteriaceae (3 by ESBL-producing *E. coli* isolates, 2 by ESBL-producing *Klebsiella pneumoniae* isolates). No carbapenem-resistant enterobacteriaceae were detected. Two patients were colonized by 4MRGN *Pseudomonas aeruginosa* isolates.

The follow-up survey was conducted in February 2016. Four patients died during the study period. No swabs were received from 3 patients. Of 5 patients initially colonized by 3MRGN enterobacteriaceae 3 were still colonized, 1 patient was negative, 1 patient had died during the study period. In contrast, 3 patients were newly colonized by 3MRGN enterobacteriaceae at 6 months. Of 2 patients colonized by 4MRGN *P. aeruginosa* at the beginning of the study, one was negative at 6 months and one patient had died. No patient was newly colonized by 4MRGN *P. aeruginosa* (Table 2). There was no significant difference in mortality and antibiotic use between patients colonized by MRGN bacteria compared to non-colonized patients.

**Genetic relatedness**

Twenty-one 3MRGN *A. baumannii* isolates from patients were included in the DiversiLab analysis as well as the isolate from the environment (chair). One isolate that remained susceptible to ciprofloxacin was also included (patient 9). Two clusters of identical isolates were identified (cluster A and B; Fig. 2). The isolate from the chair was genetically identical to a total of 15 patient isolates and was part of cluster A.

Ten 3MRGN *E.coli* isolates were included in a separate DiversiLab analysis. Two clusters of identical isolates were detected, comprising 6 and 3 isolates, respectively. One isolate was completely different. At the follow-up

**Table 1** Clinical characteristics of 3MRGN *A. baumannii* colonized vs. non-colonized patients

|  | Colonized n = 13 | Non-Colonized n = 25 | p= |
|---|---|---|---|
| Age (years, mean ± SD) | 54 ± 17.6 | 60.4 ± 10.7 | 0.257 |
| Gender (n) |  |  |  |
| Male | 11 | 10 | 0.015 |
| Female | 2 | 15 |  |
| Ward (n) |  |  |  |
| 1 | 1 | 17 | <0.001 |
| 2 | 12 | 8 |  |
| Length of stay (months, mean ± SD) | 91.4 ± 59 | 33.4 ± 47.3 | 0.002 |
| Antibiotic therapy past 3 months (n) | 4 | 3 | 0.203 |

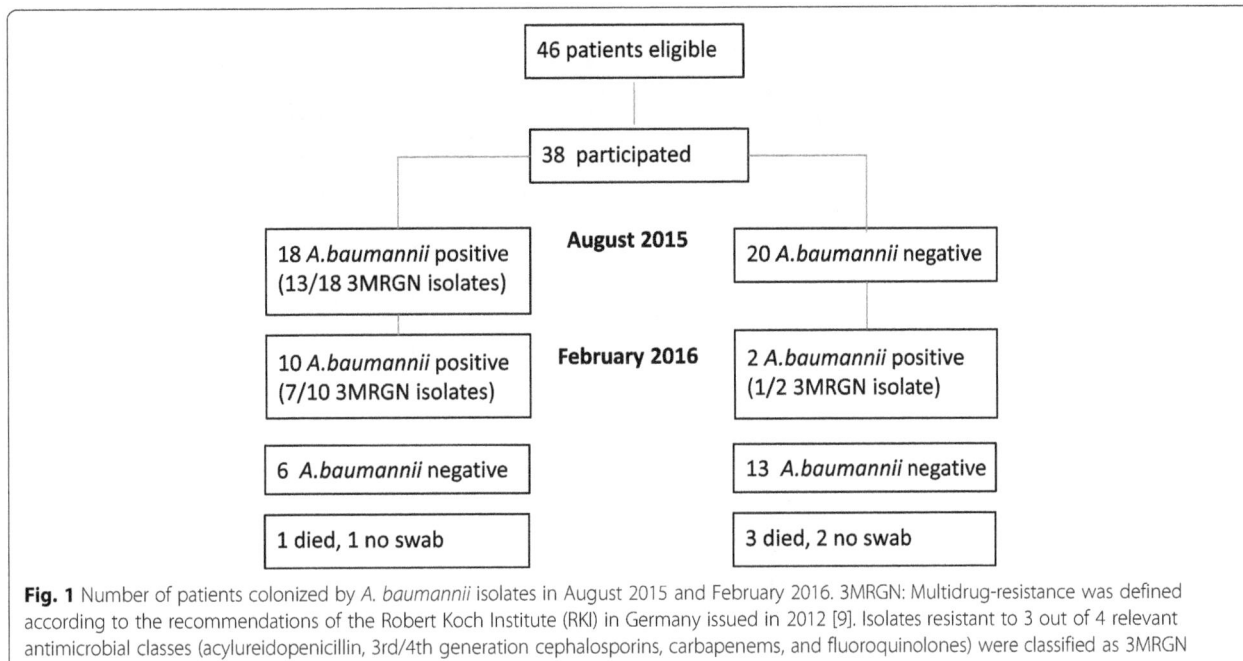

**Fig. 1** Number of patients colonized by *A. baumannii* isolates in August 2015 and February 2016. 3MRGN: Multidrug-resistance was defined according to the recommendations of the Robert Koch Institute (RKI) in Germany issued in 2012 [9]. Isolates resistant to 3 out of 4 relevant antimicrobial classes (acylureidopenicillin, 3rd/4th generation cephalosporins, carbapenems, and fluoroquinolones) were classified as 3MRGN

study (February 2016) 3 patients were found to be newly colonized by 3MRGN *E.coli* isolates. These isolates were all genetically identical and were part of the cluster of six isolates.

## Discussion

This study analyzed the colonization by multidrug-resistant Gram-negative bacteria in patients with disorders of consciousness at a LTCF in Graz, Austria. Notable findings were (1) the prevalence of colonization by multidrug-resistant (3MRGN) *A. baumannii* was unexpectedly high, in particular among patients in ward 2; (2) two clusters of genetically identical *A. baumannii* isolates were identified, including one isolate from the environment; (3) colonization by *A. baumannii* persisted for 6 months in more than half of patients.

*A. baumannii* has emerged as an important pathogen of healthcare-associated infections in critically ill patients in the ICU setting worldwide [10, 13, 14]. In addition, several studies documented that *A. baumannii*

**Table 2** Prevalence of colonization by MRGN bacteria

|  | August 2015 | February 2016 |
|---|---|---|
|  | Number of patients | Number of patients |
| *E. coli* (3MRGN) | 3[a] | 6[b] |
| *K. pneumoniae* (3MRGN) | 2 | 0 |
| *P. aeruginosa* (4MRGN) | 2 | 0 |
| *A. baumannii* (3MRGN) | 13[a] | 7 |

[a]One patient was co-colonized by *E. coli* (3MRGN) and *A. baumannii* (3MRGN)
[b]Three patients were found to be newly colonized by *E. coli* (3MRGN) in February 2016. Four patients died during the study period. No swabs were received from three additional patients

also occurs in patients in LTCFs [3, 7, 8]. In Maryland Thom and colleagues investigated the colonization of patients by *A. baumannii* in LTCFs providing care to mechanically ventilated patients [15]. The authors demonstrated that 63% of patients were colonized by *A. baumannii*. This is comparable to our findings although none of the patients in our study required mechanical ventilation. The high prevalence of colonization by *A. baumannii* could be explained by the fact that 90% of patients are transferred to the LCTF directly from external ICUs. In 2015, one fourth of the newly admitted patients were colonized by a multidrug-resistant pathogen at the time of admission. Although all newly admitted patients are screened for multidrug-resistant pathogens, skin sites were until now only screened for the presence of methicillin-resistant *Staphylococcus aureus*. Screening of the skin for multidrug-resistant Gram-negative rods has been introduced as a consequence of our study (see below).

The prevalence of colonization by *A. baumannii* was unexpectedly high in our study with an accumulation of cases in ward 2. We therefore decided to explore the environment and water sources of this ward to identify a source. *A. baumannii* isolates were detected on the patient elevator into a bathtub (isolate not available for further analysis) and from a chair for visitors in a patient room. The latter isolate was genetically identical to a total of 15 patient isolates. In addition, patients colonized by *A. baumannii* had stayed at the ward significantly longer before the study compared to non-colonized patients. Taken together, these findings

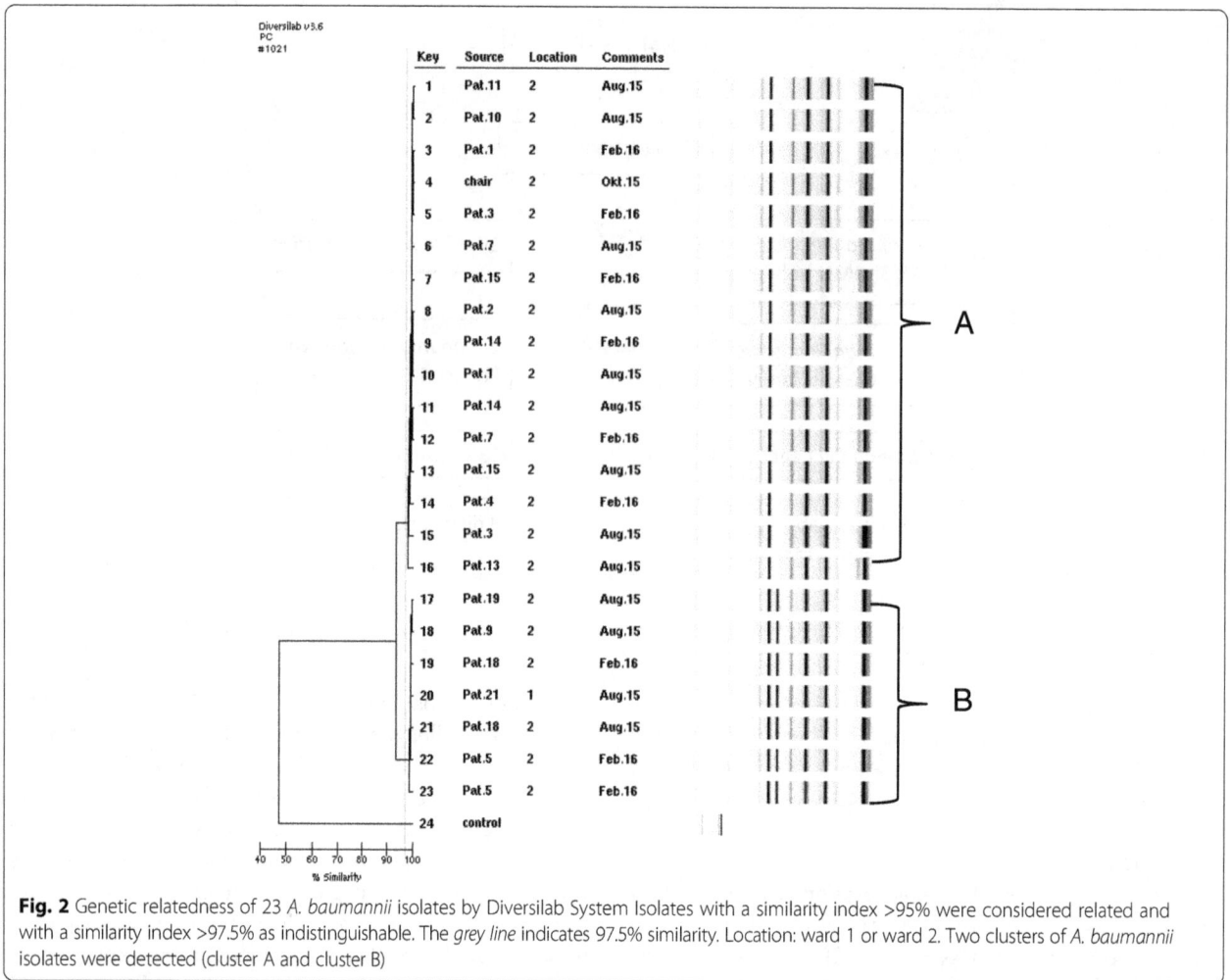

| Key | Source | Location | Comments |
|-----|--------|----------|----------|
| 1 | Pat.11 | 2 | Aug.15 |
| 2 | Pat.10 | 2 | Aug.15 |
| 3 | Pat.1 | 2 | Feb.16 |
| 4 | chair | 2 | Okt.15 |
| 5 | Pat.3 | 2 | Feb.16 |
| 6 | Pat.7 | 2 | Aug.15 |
| 7 | Pat.15 | 2 | Feb.16 |
| 8 | Pat.2 | 2 | Aug.15 |
| 9 | Pat.14 | 2 | Feb.16 |
| 10 | Pat.1 | 2 | Aug.15 |
| 11 | Pat.14 | 2 | Aug.15 |
| 12 | Pat.7 | 2 | Feb.16 |
| 13 | Pat.15 | 2 | Aug.15 |
| 14 | Pat.4 | 2 | Feb.16 |
| 15 | Pat.3 | 2 | Aug.15 |
| 16 | Pat.13 | 2 | Aug.15 |
| 17 | Pat.19 | 2 | Aug.15 |
| 18 | Pat.9 | 2 | Aug.15 |
| 19 | Pat.18 | 2 | Feb.16 |
| 20 | Pat.21 | 1 | Aug.15 |
| 21 | Pat.18 | 2 | Aug.15 |
| 22 | Pat.5 | 2 | Feb.16 |
| 23 | Pat.5 | 2 | Feb.16 |
| 24 | control | | |

**Fig. 2** Genetic relatedness of 23 *A. baumannii* isolates by Diversilab System Isolates with a similarity index >95% were considered related and with a similarity index >97.5% as indistinguishable. The *grey line* indicates 97.5% similarity. Location: ward 1 or ward 2. Two clusters of *A. baumannii* isolates were detected (cluster A and cluster B)

suggest that cross-transmission between patients by staff may have taken place.

As a consequence of our findings a multimodal intervention program was introduced on both wards by the infection control staff at the end of the study period. It included consequent reinforcement of standard hygiene precautions and barrier precautions as well as repeated education for all occupational groups also including visitors. Colonized patients were washed with antiseptic soap once a month. In addition, disinfection protocols were reviewed specifically addressing the patients' environment (including the bathtub and the elevator). The time frame for cleaning personnel on both wards was increased by 1 h per day. Admission screening procedures for new patients were adapted to include multidrug-resistant Gram-negative bacteria also from skin swabs. All patients on both wards will be screened for multidrug-resistant bacteria twice a year. These measures were evaluated in a follow-up survey by the infection control staff in December 2016. Only 4/22 patients (18%) in ward 2 were still colonized by 3MRGN

*A. baumannii.* The long-term effects of these measures will be evaluated by a follow-up study.

Of note *A. baumannii* was identified from a clinical sample only once during the entire study period, indicating that our patients were in fact only colonized but not infected by *A. baumannii.* Using only clinical samples for surveillance purposes would have underestimated the true prevalence of multidrug-resistant organisms in our setting. Our findings favour the implementation of an active surveillance strategy.

In contrast to the high prevalence of colonization by *A. baumannii* the prevalence of multidrug-resistant enterobacteriaceae was moderate (13%). Our findings are comparable to a French study which reported 10% of nursing home residents to be colonized by ESBL-producing enterobacteriaceae [16]. In contrast to an Italian study, in which colonization by carbapenemase-producing enterobacteriaceae has been described in 6.3% of patients, no carbapenemase-producing enterobacteriaceae were detected [1]. Sixty percent of patients were still colonized by 3MRGN *E.coli* isolates at the time of the follow-up study. Our findings are in line with a study by Birgand et al. investigating the gastrointestinal ESBL-colonization in patients after hospital discharge [17]. Median time to clearance was found to be 6.6 months, ranging from 3.4 to 13.4 months [17]. Three patients were found to be newly colonized by 3MRGN *E.coli* isolates at the time of the follow-up study. These 3 isolates were found to be genetically identical, again pointing to a role of institutional cross-transmission in the spread of multidrug resistant bacteria.

Our study has limitations. To fully assess the prevalence of colonization by *A. baumannii* respiratory samples would probably have been a useful addition. However, our study was designed to assess the prevalence of multidrug-resistant Gram-negative pathogens in general. The high prevalence of *A. baumannii* was unexpected.

## Conclusion

We uncovered two clusters of *A. baumannii* colonizing patients with disorder of consciousness at a LTCF in Graz, Austria. Our findings point toward nosocomial cross-transmission as a cause for these outbreaks. Using only clinical samples for surveillance purposes would have underestimated the true prevalence of *A. baumannii* in our setting. Therefore, an active surveillance strategy is warranted to avoid missing newly emerging pathogens at an early stage. In addition, improved infection control measures are necessary in the LTCF setting.

### Abbreviations
3MRGN: multidrug resistant Gram-negative bacteria according to the definition of Robert Koch Institute; ESBL: extended spectrum betalactamases; EUCAST: European Committee on Antimicrobial Susceptibility Testing; ICU: intensive care unit; LTCF: long term care facility

### Acknowledgments
Not applicable.

### Funding
No external funding was received for this study.

### Authors' contributions
EZ, EU and EL processed the swabs and analysed the microbiological data. JL performed DiversiLab analysis and contributed to the manuscript. CP, GP and WS planned the study and contributed to the manuscript. IZS and RK analysed the data and wrote the manuscript. All authors read and approved the final manuscript.

### Competing interests
The authors declare that they have no competing interests.

### Author details
[1]Department of Internal Medicine, Section of Infectious Diseases and Tropical Medicine, Medical University of Graz, Auenbruggerplatz 15, A-8036 Graz, Austria. [2]Institute of Hygiene, Microbiology and Environmental Medicine, Medical University of Graz, Graz, Austria. [3]Geriatric Health Centers of the City of Graz, Graz, Austria.

### References
1. March A, Aschbacher R, Dhanji H, Livermore DM, Bottcher A, Sleghel F, Maggi S, Noale M, Larcher C, Woodford N. Colonization of residents and staff of a long-term-care facility and adjacent acute-care hospital geriatric unit by multiresistant bacteria. Clin Microbiol Infect. 2010;16:934–44.
2. Furuno JP, Hebden JN, Standiford HC, Perencevich EN, Miller RR, Moore AC, Strauss SM, Harris AD. Prevalence of methicillin-resistant *Staphylococcus aureus* and Acinetobacter Baumannii in a long-term acute care facility. Am J Infect Control. 2008;36:468–71.
3. Lim CJ, Cheng AC, Kennon J, Spelman D, Hale D, Melican G, Sidjabat HE, Paterson DL, Kong DC, Peleg AY. Prevalence of multidrug-resistant organisms and risk factors for carriage in long-term care facilities: a nested case–control study. J Antimicrob Chemother. 2014;69:1972–80.
4. Reddy P, Malczynski M, Obias A, Reiner S, Jin N, Huang J, Noskin GA, Zembower T. Screening for extended-spectrum beta-lactamase-producing Enterobacteriaceae among high-risk patients and rates of subsequent bacteremia. Clin Infect Dis. 2007;45:846–52.
5. Sebeny PJ, Riddle MS, Petersen K. Acinetobacter Baumannii skin and soft-tissue infection associated with war trauma. Clin Infect Dis. 2008;47:444–9.
6. Gaddy JA, Actis LA. Regulation of Acinetobacter Baumannii biofilm formation. Future Microbiol. 2009;4:273–8.
7. Sengstock DM, Thyagarajan R, Apalara J, Mira A, Chopra T, Kaye KS. Multidrug-resistant Acinetobacter Baumannii: an emerging pathogen among older adults in community hospitals and nursing homes. Clin Infect Dis. 2010;50:1611–6.
8. Mortensen E, Trivedi KK, Rosenberg J, Cody SH, Long J, Jensen BJ, Vugia DJ. Multidrug-resistant Acinetobacter Baumannii infection, colonization, and transmission related to a long-term care facility providing subacute care. Infect Control Hosp Epidemiol. 2014;35:406–11.
9. Hygienemaßnahmen bei Infektionen oder Besiedlung mit multiresistenten gramnegativen Stäbchen. Bundesgesundheitsblatt: Springer; 2012;55:1311–1354.
10. Wang SH, Sheng WH, Chang YY, Wang LH, Lin HC, Chen ML, Pan HJ, Ko WJ, Chang SC, Lin FY. Healthcare-associated outbreak due to pan-drug resistant Acinetobacter Baumannii in a surgical intensive care unit. J Hosp Infect. 2003;53:97–102.
11. Umezawa K, Asai S, Ohshima T, Iwashita H, Ohashi M, Sasaki M, Kaneko A, Inokuchi S, Miyachi H. Outbreak of drug-resistant Acinetobacter Baumannii ST219 caused by oral care using tap water from contaminated hand hygiene sinks as a reservoir. Am J Infect Control. 2015;43:1249–51.
12. Hong KB, Oh HS, Song JS, Lim JH, Kang DK, Son IS, Park JD, Kim EC, Lee HJ, Choi EH. Investigation and control of an outbreak of imipenem-resistant Acinetobacter Baumannii infection in a pediatric intensive care unit. Pediatr Infect Dis J. 2012;31:685–90.
13. Enoch DA, Summers C, Brown NM, Moore L, Gillham MI, Burnstein RM, Thaxter R, Enoch LM, Matta B, Sule O. Investigation and management of an outbreak of multidrug-carbapenem-resistant Acinetobacter Baumannii in Cambridge, UK. J Hosp Infect. 2008;70:109–18.
14. Frickmann H, Crusius S, Walter U, Podbielski A. Management of an Outbreak with cases of Nosocomial pneumonia caused by a novel multi-drug-resistant Acinetobacter Baumannii clone. Pneumologie. 2010;64:686–93.
15. Thom KA, Maragakis LL, Richards K, Johnson JK, Roup B, Lawson P, Harris AD, Fuss EP, Pass MA, Blythe D, et al. Assessing the burden of Acinetobacter Baumannii in Maryland: a statewide cross-sectional period prevalence survey. Infect Control Hosp Epidemiol. 2012;33:883–8.
16. Cochard H, Aubier B, Quentin R, van der Mee-Marquet N, Reseau des Hygienistes du C. Extended-spectrum beta-lactamase-producing Enterobacteriaceae in French nursing homes: an association between high carriage rate among residents, environmental contamination, poor conformity with good hygiene practice, and putative resident-to-resident transmission. Infect Control Hosp Epidemiol. 2014;35:384–9.
17. Birgand G, Armand-Lefevre L, Lolom I, Ruppe E, Andremont A, Lucet JC. Duration of colonization by extended-spectrum beta-lactamase-producing Enterobacteriaceae after hospital discharge. Am J Infect Control. 2013;41:443–7.

# 12

# Variability in contact precautions to control the nosocomial spread of multi-drug resistant organisms in the endemic setting

Danielle Vuichard Gysin[1,5], Barry Cookson[2], Henri Saenz[3], Markus Dettenkofer[4], Andreas F. Widmer[1*] and for the ESCMID Study Group for Nosocomial Infections (ESGNI)

## Abstract

**Background:** Definitions and practices regarding use of contact precautions and isolation to prevent the spread of gram-positive and gram-negative multidrug-resistant organisms (MDRO) are not uniform.

**Methods:** We conducted an on-site survey during the European Congress on Clinical Microbiology and Infectious Diseases 2014 to assess specific details on contact precaution and implementation barriers.

**Results:** Attendants from 32 European (EU) and 24 non-EU countries participated ($n = 213$). In EU-respondents adherence to contact precautions and isolation was high for Methicillin-resistant *Staphylococcus aureus* (MRSA), carbapenem-resistant Enterobacteriaceae, and MDR *A. baumannii* (84.7, 85.7, and 80%, respectively) whereas only 68% of EU-respondents considered any contact precaution measures for extended-spectrum-beta-lactamase (ESBL) producing non-*E. coli*. Between 30 and 45% of all EU and non-EU respondents did not require health-care workers (HCW) to wear gowns and gloves at all times when entering the room of a patient in contact isolation. Between 10 and 20% of respondents did not consider any rooming specifications or isolation for gram-positive MDRO and up to 30% of respondents abstain from such interventions in gram-negative MDRO, especially non-*E. coli* ESBL. Understaffing and lack of sufficient isolation rooms were the most commonly encountered barriers amongst EU and non-EU respondents.

**Conclusion:** The effectiveness of contact precautions and isolation is difficult to assess due to great variation in components of the specific measures and mixed levels of implementation. The lack of uniform positive effects of contact isolation to prevent transmission may be explained by the variability of interpretation of this term. Indications for contact isolation require a global definition and further sound studies.

**Keywords:** Contact precaution, Isolation, Multi-drug resistant organisms, Implementation, Barriers

## Background

The European Society of Clinical Microbiology and Infectious Diseases (ESCMID) and Healthcare Infection Control Practices Advisory Committee (HICPAC) have defined multidrug-resistant organisms (MDRO) that qualify for contact precautions and isolation [1]. According to HICPAC, contact precaution measures are indicated if transmission of an infectious agent is not interrupted by the use of standard precautions alone due to environmental contamination and, therefore, requires HCW to wear gloves and gowns upon room entry, not only if contact with blood or body fluid is anticipated. HICPAC also recommends that such patients should be placed preferably in a single room [2]. Similarly, the guidelines on prevention of transmission of gram-negative MDRO issued by ESCMID require contact precaution for patients colonized or infected with an epidemiologically targeted organism, that includes wearing gloves and gowns upon entry to the room and the use of

* Correspondence: andreas.widmer@usb.ch
[1]Department of Infectious Diseases and Hospital Epidemiology, University Hospital Basel, 4051 Basel, Switzerland
Full list of author information is available at the end of the article

patient-dedicated or single-use disposable non-critical equipment [3] (Table 1).

However, there is no uniform definition of multidrug resistance in gram-negative bacteria and the indications to implement isolation precaution measures for MDRO vary substantially [4]. Reasons for this are not well understood. The variability in practices and the strictness of implementation (e.g. whether gowns and gloves are worn upon room entry or only if contact with blood or bodily fluid is anticipated, or whether implementation of contact precaution and isolation depends on the presence or absence of patient risk factors), has not been well studied amongst health-care professionals. This is of major relevance when examining the success of prevention and control of the spread of MDRO and when designing studies to look at the effectiveness of such interventions. Interestingly, comparison of national MRSA guidelines of 13 European (EU) countries has also shown divergent implementation regarding donning of gloves and gowns [5].

## Methods

Our main survey aims were to explore the diversity in adopting contact precaution and isolation practices for gram-positive and gram-negative MDRO and to assess barriers to their implementation.

After an in-depth discussion amongst the ESCMID nosocomial infection study group (ESGNI) committee members we decided to focus on the indication, circumstances and implementation of contact precautions and isolation for MRSA, glycopeptide-resistant enterococci (GRE), extended-spectrum-beta-lactamase-producing Enterobacteriaceae (ESBL-E) and carbapenem-resistant Enterobacteriaceae (CRE), MDR *P. aeruginosa*, and MDR *A. baumannii*.

A questionnaire survey was developed by the authors and distributed amongst the ESGNI committee members for revision. Levels of agreement on barriers frequently encountered during implementation were measured on a 5-point Likert scale (3 being neutrality) [6]. The survey was then transferred onto Survey Monkey® [7] and pilot-tested among a broader group including five infection control nurses and five infectious diseases physicians from Switzerland, Germany and the USA.

The online survey was applied to attendees of the 2014 ECCMID in Barcelona, Spain. On-site participant recruitment was by study team members during the regular opening hours. Individuals were invited to complete the survey at a booth. Study team members addressed any issues of comprehension. As a recruitment incentive, there was a lottery with three prizes. In addition, the online survey was open to all ESCMID members for six weeks after the congress.

### Statistical analyses

Numbers, percentages, median and interquartile range (IQR) were used for descriptive statistics. Countries were categorised into EU and non-EU in compliance with a reference classification system [8]. We regrouped the transcontinental Eurasian countries, e.g. Turkey, as belonging to the Southern EU Area rather than Western Asia to be consistent with other publications [9]. We compared differences in proportions among EU and non-EU responders using Chi-square or Fisher's exact test. Missing answers were removed from the respective analysis on a case-by-case basis. In our primary analysis, we considered all non-missing responses equivalently without taking potential nesting into account. In order to evaluate a possible overestimation of effects due to nested data, we eliminated

**Table 1** Core elements of contact precautions (CP) recommended by recent ESCMID and HICPAC/CDC guidelines

|  | ESCMID 2014 (3) | HICPAC/CDC 2007 (2) |
|---|---|---|
| Indication for CP | Colonization or infection with MDRO | Colonization or infection with MDRO |
| Donning and wearing of gloves and gowns | Gown and gloves are donned upon entry to a room | Gown and gloves are donned upon room entry Gown and gloves are indicated for all interactions that may involve contact with the patient or potentially contaminated areas in the patient's environment. |
| Disposal of gowns and gloves | Not stated | Gown and gloves are discarded before exiting the patient room |
| Additional requirements & recommendations | Use of disposable single-use or patient-dedicated non-critical care equipment (e.g. blood pressure cuffs and stethoscopes). | Use of patient-dedicated or single-use disposable noncritical equipment |
| Placement of patients | Special isolation wards Nursing cohort with separate rooms on general wards Single room or cohort in same room without dedicated personnel Placement in a room with patients unaffected by MDROs but maintaining CP by use of gowns and gloves based on the patient's extent of MDRO carriage | Single patient room preferred Cohort patients with same MDRO Multi-bed rooms with non-infected/non-colonized patients: at least 3 ft spatial separation between beds |

*CDC* centers for disease control and prevention, *CP* contact precaution, *ESCMID* european society of clinical microbiology and infectious diseases, *HICPAC* healthcare infection control practices advisory committee, *MDRO* multidrug resistant organism

all duplicates that we defined as respondents from the same country and from the same hospital size. We then repeated the primary analysis with the de-duplicated dataset. All analyses were performed using SPSS statistical software version 23.0 [10].

## Results

Overall, 213 individuals from 32 EU and 28 non-EU countries participated in the survey. The majority were European and had their workplace in either the Southern European Area (31%), in Western (22%), Northern (16%), or Eastern Europe (7%); about a quarter of the respondents came from countries out-side Europe (Asia and The Middle East 11%, South America 8%, Africa 5%). A total of 77 (36.1%) respondents were specialized in infection control and prevention and 108 respondents (50.7%) had either a background in microbiology and/or infectious diseases. The median experience in infection control was 8 (IQR: 3–15) years. There were 159 (74.6%) medical doctors and the majority (71.8%) worked in acute care. Details on the participants' country of workplace and professional responsibilities are listed in the supplementary appendix. Numbers (%) of completely missing answers to questions concerning indications of contact precautions were: 14 (6.6) for MRSA, 38 (17.8) for GRE, 27 (12.7) for $E.\ coli$ ESBL, 14 (6.6) for non-$E.\ coli$ ESBL, 14 (6.6) for CR $E.\ coli$, 17 (8.0) for CRE (other than $E.\ coli$), 14 (6.6) for MDR $P.\ aeruginosa$, and 14 (6.6) for MDR $A.\ baumannii$. The proportion of EU-respondents reporting any form of contact precautions/isolation, irrespective whether a patient was colonized or infected, was high ($\geq 80\%$) for MRSA, CRE (other than $E.\ coli$), and MDR $A.\ baumannii$ (84.7, 85.7, and 80%, respectively) with lower, but still similar percentages among non-EU respondents (Table 2). The proportions amongst EU-respondents who would apply any form of contact precaution were markedly lower for ESBL-producing $E.\ coli$ and non-$E.\ coli$ ESBL (59.4 and 68%, respectively). Answers from EU and non-EU responders differed significantly regarding overall contact precaution indications for ESBL-E other than $E.\ coli$ ($p = 0.044$) in that approximately one third of non-EU responders either did not consider any contact precaution measures or did not determine the presence of ESBL. Amongst those who implemented contact precautions more non-EU responders than EU-responders did so if the patient was only colonized (Table 2).

The majority (> 56%) of EU responders reported donning of gowns and gloves upon entry into the room *at all times* for all MDRO except ESBL-E. However, only non-EU responders followed this practice in ESBL-E in contrast to EU responders, where a majority (55 and 53%, for $E.\ coli$ and non-$E.\ coli$, respectively) indicated that donning of gowns and gloves was required only when

patient-care was likely. The differences in proportions of EU and non-EU responders were statistically significant for ESBL-E other than $E.\ coli$ ($p = 0.046$) (Table 2). After removing potential duplicate answers, the discrepancy became even more evident with statistically significant lower proportions of responders from EU countries that had strict gowning and gloving at all times implemented for ESBL-producing $E.\ coli$ ($p = 0.017$) and other Enterobacteriaceae ($p = 0.005$) (Additional file 1).

A majority of EU and non-EU country participants preferred single room placement for MRSA (62.5 and 63.8%) and GRE (59.4 and 56.3%) (Table 2). The answers, however, were less consistent for gram-negative MDRO. Only about one third of EU and non-EU responders advocated single room placement for ESBL-$E$. major differences between responses from participants from EU and non-EU countries were encountered for rooming specifications in CR $E.\ coli$ and CRE (other than $E.\ coli$), where EU responders compared to non-EU responders favoured single room placement (64.1% vs. 41.7 and 71.6% vs. 47.9%, respectively) over cohorting or spatial separation, whereas responses from non-EU participants were more divergent among the different placement options. Differences in placements of patients with MDRO among EU and non-EU responders, however, were not statistically significant in the sensitivity analysis (see Additional file 1).

The answers were highly consistent among all participants and for any MDRO, except for MRSA, that pre-emptive contact precautions/isolation had a significant value, whereas only a minority considered limiting implementation of contact precautions to patients with certain risk factors (e.g. diarrhoea or urinary incontinence) in their local practice (Table 3). None of the differences between responses from EU and non-EU countries were significant after deduplication (Additional file 1). When comparing the responses between infection control practitioners (ICP) and non-ICPs, as well as the responses between clinicians and non-clinicians, we also detected significantly different approaches to infection control measures across different pathogens (Additional file 1: Tables S3-S10). However, the results also demonstrated large incongruities amongst ICPs as well as amongst clinicians as to what strictness level of contact precaution is pursued.

Most respondents demonstrating poor knowledge were either no medical doctors, were not working in hospitals or had fewer years of experience in infection control (Additional file 1 Table S13).

### Most commonly encountered barriers

Of the 213 participants, 15 (10%) Europeans and 4 (7%) non-Europeans did not respond to these questions. Respondents from EU- and non-EU countries largely agreed that the major obstacles to implement appropriate contact

**Table 2** Indication and specification for contact precautions (CP) and isolation[a]

| | MRSA | | | GRE | | | E. coli ESBL | | | Non-E. coli ESBL | | |
|---|---|---|---|---|---|---|---|---|---|---|---|---|
| | EU | Non EU | p-value[b] | EU | Non EU | p-value[b] | EU | Non EU | p-value[b] | EU | Non EU | p-value[b] |
| No CP | 12.7 | 24.5 | 0.165 | 30.0 | 32.7 | 0.396 | 32.7 | 34.7 | 0.636 | 23.3 | 34.7 | 0.044 |
| CP only if infected | 16.7 | 10.2 | | 54.7 | 44.9 | | 14.7 | 10.2 | | 17.3 | 6.1 | |
| CP if colonised and/or infected | 68.0 | 65.3 | | 15.3 | 22.4 | | 44.7 | 40.8 | | 50.7 | 40.8 | |
| Unknown | 42.7 | 0 | | 0 | 0 | | 5.3 | 10.2 | | 6.0 | 14.3 | |
| ESBL not determined | n.a. | n.a. | | n.a. | n.a. | | 2.7 | 4.1 | | 2.7 | 33.3 | |
| Total no. responses (%) | 150 (75.4) | 49 (24.6) | | 131 (74.9) | 44 (24.1) | | 150 (75.4) | 47 (24.6) | | 150 (75.4) | 49 (24.6) | |
| Gowns and gloves whenever entering the room | 57.3 | 62.9 | 0.398 | 59.0 | 56.7 | 0.623 | 44.9 | 59.1 | 0.234 | 47.3 | 71.4 | 0.046 |
| Gowns and gloves if direct contact is anticipated | 37.9 | 37.1 | | 37.1 | 43.3 | | 55.1 | 40.9 | | 52.7 | 28.6 | |
| Other procedures (e.g. standard precautions only) | 4.8 | 0.0 | | 3.8 | 0.0 | | 0 | 0 | | 0 | 0 | |
| Total no. responses (%) | 124 (78.0) | 35 (22.0) | | 105 (77.8) | 30 (22.2) | | 89 (80.2) | 22 (19.8) | | 93 (81.6) | 21 (18.4) | |
| Single room | 62.5 | 63.8 | | 59.4 | 56.3 | 0.703 | 31.4 | 31.3 | 0.960 | 36.4 | 27.1 | 0.494 |
| Cohorting | 17.4 | 10.6 | | 16.1 | 16.7 | | 19.3 | 18. | | 20.7 | 18.8 | |
| Spatial separation[c] | 10.4 | 6.4 | 0.235 | 9.8 | 6.3 | | 13.6 | 16.7 | | 13.6 | 20.8 | |
| No specific measures | 9.7 | 19.1 | | 14.7 | 20.8 | | 35.7 | 33.3 | | 29.3 | 33.3 | |
| Total no. responses (%) | 144 (75.4) | 47 (24.6) | | 143 (74.9) | 48 (25.1) | | 140 (74.5) | 48 (25.5) | | 140 (74.5) | 48 (25.5) | |

| | Carbapenem resistant E. coli | | | Carbapenem resistant non-E. coli | | | MDR P. aeruginosa | | | MDR A. baumannii | | |
|---|---|---|---|---|---|---|---|---|---|---|---|---|
| | EU | Non EU | p-value[b] | EU | Non EU | p-value[b] | EU | Non EU | p-value[b] | EU | Non EU | p-value[b] |
| No CP | 11.3 | 16.3 | 0.745 | 8.2 | 18.4 | 0.246 | 13.3 | 20.4 | 0.597 | 9.3 | 20.4 | 0.171 |
| CP only if infected | 14.0 | 10.2 | | 13.6 | 10.2 | | 17.3 | 14.3 | | 17.3 | 20.4 | |
| CP if colonised and/or infected | 65.3 | 63.3 | | 72.1 | 65.3 | | 60.0 | 59.2 | | 62.7 | 51.0 | |
| Unknown | 9.3 | 10.2 | | 6.1 | 6.1 | | 9.3 | 6.1 | | 10.7 | 8.2) | |
| Total no. responses (%) | 150 (75.4) | 49 (24.6) | | 147 (75.0) | 49 (25.0) | | 150 (75.4) | 49 (24.6) | | 150 (75.4) | 49 (24.6) | |
| Gowns and gloves whenever entering the room | 61.3 | 68.8 | 0.440 | 63.5 | 60.6 | 0.763 | 56.3 | 64.7 | 0.389 | 58.7 | 61.3 | 0.797 |
| Gowns and gloves if direct contact is anticipated | 38.7 | 31.3 | | 36.5 | 39.4 | | 43.7 | 35.3 | | 41.3 | 38.7 | |
| Total no. responses (%) | 111 (77.6) | 32 (22.4) | | 115 (77.7) | 33 (22.3) | | 103 (75.2) | 34 (24.8) | | 109 (77.9) | 31 (22.1) | |
| Single room | 64.1 | 41.7 | 0.029 | 71.6 | 47.9 | 0.026 | 56.7 | 43.8 | 0.156 | 61.6 | 45.8 | 0.067 |
| Cohorting | 13.4) | 14.6 | | 12.1 | 18.8 | | 18.7 | 14.6 | | 18.1 | 14.6 | |
| Spatial separation[c] | 9.9 | 20.8 | | 7.1 | 14.6 | | 12.7 | 18.8 | | 8.7 | 18.8 | |
| No specific measures | 12.7 | 22.9 | | 9.2 | 18.8 | | 11.9 | 22.9 | | 11.6 | 20.8 | |
| Total no. responses (%) | 142 (74.7) | 48 (25.3) | | 141 (74.6) | 48 (25.4) | | 134 (73.6) | 48 (26.4) | | 138 (74.2) | 48 (25.8) | |

[a]Values are percentages (related to the corresponding total respondents) unless indicated otherwise
[b]A two-sided p-value of < 0.05 was considered statistically significant
[c]Shared room with MDRO-negative patients but with optical barrier (e.g. red margin on the floor) or separated by screen/curtains

precaution/isolation measures were shortage of personnel (EU-respondents: 67%; non-EU respondents: 80%) and lack of rooms for isolation (77 and 84%, respectively). The opinions were more divergent between EU- and non-EU-respondents regarding lack of environmental cleanliness (EU-respondents: 38%, non-EU respondents: 61%), support from administration (27 and 41%, respectively) or microbiology (14 and 30%, respectively), and

**Table 3** Other specific requirements and conditions for contact precaution (CP)

| MDRO | Origin of responses | Total responses | Additional pre-emptive CP based on patient's history[a] | CP only required if specific risk factors present[b] | Additional pre-emptive CP but only if specific risk factors | None applicable | p-value[c] |
|------|------|------|------|------|------|------|------|
| MRSA | EU | 126 | 117 (92.9) | 1 (0.8) | 1 (0.8) | 7 (5.6) | 0.038 |
|      | Non EU | 38 | 30 (78.9) | 1 (2.6) | 2 (5.3) | 5 (13.2) | |
| GRE | EU | 94 | 81 (86.2) | 3 (3.2) | 1 (1.1) | 9 (9.6) | 0.265 |
|     | Non EU | 30 | 24 (80.00) | 2 (6.7) | 2 (6.7) | 2 (6.7) | |
| ESBL *E. coli* | EU | 91 | 74 (81.3) | 8 (8.8) | 4 (4.7) | 5 (4.7) | 0.812 |
|                | Non EU | 26 | 22 (84.6) | 1 (3.8) | 2 (7.7) | 1 (3.8) | |
| ESBL non-*E. coli* | EU | 101 | 86 (85.1) | 5 (5.0) | 3 (3.0) | 7 (6.9) | 0.131 |
|                    | Non EU | 23 | 18 (78.3) | 3 (13.0) | 2 (8.7) | 0 (0.0) | |
| Carbapenem resistant *E. coli* | EU | 120 | 103 (85.8) | 4 (3.3) | 4 (3.3) | 9 (7.5) | 0.465 |
|                                | Non EU | 36 | 33 (91.7) | 0 (0.0) | 2 (5.6) | 1 (2.8) | |
| Carbapenem resistant Enterobacteriaceae (non-*E. coli*) | EU | 126 | 111 (88.1) | 2 (1.6) | 4 (3.2) | 9 (7.1) | 0.560 |
|                                | Non EU | 37 | 33 (89.2) | 1 (2.7) | 2 (5.4) | 1 (2.7) | |
| MDR *P. aeruginosa* | EU | 112 | 96 (85.7) | 3 (2.7) | 4 (3.6) | 9 (8.0) | 0.178 |
|                     | Non EU | 35 | 31 (88.6) | 1 (2.9) | 3 (8.6) | 0 (0.0) | |
| MDR *A. baumannii* | EU | 120 | 107 (89.2) | 1 (0.8) | 5 (4.2) | 7 (5.8) | 0.758 |
|                    | Non EU | 33 | 31 (91.2) | 0 (0.0) | 2 (5.9) | 1 (2.9) | |

[a]Formerly positive for respective MDRO or presumptive infection/colonization with respective MDRO
[b]CP only when certain risk factors present e.g. incontinence, diarrhoea, draining wounds
[c]A two-sided p-value of < 0.05 was considered statistically significant

provision of supplies (25 and 38%, respectively), where non-EU respondents perceived more frequent constraints than EU respondents (Fig. 1).

## Discussion

MDRO comprise a global threat [11] causing economic damage comparable to the 2008 financial crisis [12]. International experts rated their control the highest priority [13]. Surprisingly, to the best of our knowledge, this is the first multinational survey addressing specifically potential differences and major hindrances in practical implementation of contact precaution/isolation measures in MDROs. Representatives from most European countries and from a large number of non-EU countries across Africa, Asia, and South America participated. The results have confirmed our suspicions that indications and practical implementation of contact precautions including isolation measures vary considerably. This study also showed there were major inconsistencies particularly in the handling of ESBL-E, CR *E. coli*, and CREs.

Firstly, in contrast to ESCMID [3] recommendations, 23.3% of EU-respondents did not consider any contact precaution measures in non-*E. coli* ESBL; the proportion was even higher amongst non-EU respondents (34.7%). Secondly, we found between 30 and 45% of all respondents neither followed the HICPAC nor the ESCMID recommendations requiring HCW to wear gowns and

gloves at all times when entering the room of a patient in contact isolation [14]. In clinical practice it seems sufficient not to don a gown (and gloves) if no contact with blood or bodily fluid is anticipated, rendering more time urgently needed for care and treatment. In any case, the emphasis has to be on thorough education and proper implementation of standard precautions and hand hygiene as their integral component because they constitute the mainstay of controlling the spread of all micro-organisms (including MDROs).

Thirdly, contrary to these recommendations, between 10 and 20% of respondents from all countries did not consider any rooming specifications, e.g. cohorting or isolation for gram-positive MDRO. Up to 30% of all respondents abstained from such interventions in gram-negative MDRO, especially non-*E. coli* ESBL. These deficits seem somewhat alarming, since omitting such control measures is likely to facilitate the nosocomial spread of these organisms [15].

Our survey found the inability to separate patients colonized or infected with MDRO was due to the lack of personnel and insufficient single rooms, rather than a consequence of guideline scepticism or evidence-base paucity. Isolation practices implementation barriers were similar to those found for MRSA interventions in USA HCW interviews [16]. These findings underpin the view that the greatest challenge to implement contact precautions/isolation is the need for more staffing and isolation

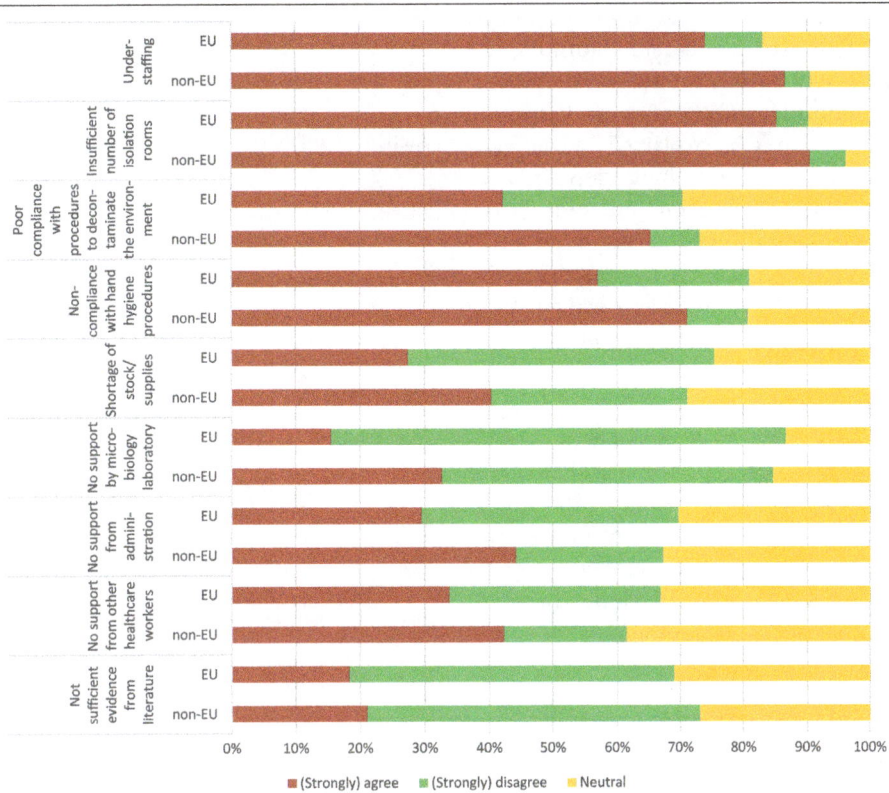

**Fig. 1** Most commonly encountered barriers when trying to implement contact precaution and isolation measures from the survey respondents' perspective (*n* = 194, 4 missing from non-EU and 15 missing from EU countries)

facilities, reinforced by a strong infection prevention ethos amongst HCWs and supported by a skilled infection control team as outlined in a previous European project [17].

A more recent survey among members of the Society for Healthcare Epidemiology of America (SHEA) on contact precaution use for MRSA and GRE revealed that over 60% of respondents were interested in alternative approaches, such as enhanced standard precautions and environmental cleaning/disinfection or targeted contact precautions and isolation (e.g., in conditions enhancing horizontal spread, such as diarrhoea or urinary incontinence) [18]. Our survey underlines that risk-stratified precautions are implemented for ESBL-E in few institutions or countries, respectively.

However, whether limiting contact precaution to those who have diarrhoea or urinary incontinence is equally effective in reducing transmission than application of contact precautions irrespective of the presence of risk factors, and whether this newer approach may be considered for gram-positive as well as gram-negative MDROs, remains to be determined in future studies and are matters of some urgency.

The strengths of this survey were its comprehensiveness about use of personal protective equipment and augmenting the response with on-site recruitment using a booth at ECCMID. Compared to other surveys we explicitly differentiated between *E. coli* and other Enterobacteriaceae, since the transmission risk of ESBL *E. coli* is deemed to be lower compared to non-*E. coli* ESBL, at least in the acute care setting [3, 19, 20]. The survey encompassed a broad geographical area across the world, including 32 EU and 28 non-EU countries.

Our study has some limitations. The online survey was potentially available to approx. 7000 ESCMID members and the ECCMID attendance was 10,839. Thus, the response rate was very poor, but still of significant size to draw interesting conclusions. Also, ECCMID attendants may have differed from other infection control experts and 10% of participants, though mostly non-clinicians with less experience in infection control and infectious diseases, showed unexpectedly poor knowledge about their local practice.

We therefore would urge some caution in generalising from these results, but they are a worrying potential indicator of variability in recommended practices, and are surely causes for concern which cannot be ignored. Larger studies, perhaps by individual countries, are required and measures to relieve recognised hindrances to improvement reflected upon and implemented.

The need for more rigorous studies comparing standard precautions to contact precautions/isolation in reducing the spread of MDRO has been previously highlighted [18]. These are essential to informing the best prevention strategies to combat spread of MDRO. The lack of uniform positive effects of contact isolation to prevent transmission may be explained by the variability of interpretation of this term. Indications for contact isolation require a global definition and further sound studies. ESCMID, HICPAC and any other MDR guidelines could perhaps add a score to the current infection control guidelines that would allow estimation of the level of implementation of contact precautions.

## Conclusion

We discovered great variation in components of the specific measures of contact precaution and isolation and mixed levels of implementation.

Our findings should inform the design of future trials ensuring that the methodology and different levels of contact precautions need to be described clearly to enhance comparability between studies.

## Additional files

**Additional file 1: Table S1.** Country of workplace of the 213 survey participants (number of respondents per country). **Table S2.** Survey respondents affiliations (*n* = 213). **Table S3.** MRSA contact precaution measures according to professional background. **Table S4.** GRE contact precaution measures according to professional background. **Table S5.** ESBL-*E. coli* contact precaution measures according to professional background. **Table S6.** ESBL-non-*E. coli* contact precaution measures according to professional background. **Table S7.** CR-*E. coli* contact precaution measures according to professional background. **Table S8.** CRE contact precaution measures according to professional background. **Table S9.** MRD *P. aeruginosa* contact precaution measures according to professional background. **Table S10.** MRD A. baumannii contact precaution measures according to professional background. **Table S11.** Indication and specification for contact precautions (CP) and isolation (cont. Next page) after deduplication*. **Table S12.** Other specific requirements for CP, results after deduplication*. **Table S13.** Characteristics of respondents that indicated "unknown" compared to respondents that provided any other answer.

## Abbreviations

CRE: Carbapenem-resistant enterobacteriaceae; ECCMID: European congress on clinical microbiology and infectious diseases; ESBL: Extended-spectrum-beta-lactamase; ESCMID: European society of clinical microbiology and infectious diseases; ESGNI: ESCMID nosocomial infection study group; EU: European; GRE: Glycopeptide-resistant enterococci; HCW: Health-care workers; HICPAC: Healthcare infection control practices advisory committee; ICP: Infection control practitioner; IQR: Interquartile range; MDRO: Multidrug resistant organism; MRSA: Methicillin resistant *Staphylococcus aureus*

## Acknowledgements

We would like to acknowledge the European Study Group for Nosocomial Infections and its Executive Committee members for their commitment.

## Funding

The study has not been funded.

## Declarations

Preliminary results have been presented as a poster (P0847) at the ECCMID 2015 in Copenhagen, Denmark.

## Authors' contributions

DVG developed the survey, collected and analysed the data and drafted the manuscript. MD, HS, and BC offered essential expertise during the survey development and critically revised the manuscript, HS further helped with technical and logistical issues regarding survey deployment. AFW conceived the idea of the survey, gave important inputs and critically revised the content of the manuscript. All authors read and approved the final manuscript.

## Competing interests

All authors declare to have no conflict of interests with regard to this manuscript.

## Author details

[1]Department of Infectious Diseases and Hospital Epidemiology, University Hospital Basel, 4051 Basel, Switzerland. [2]Division of Infection and Immunity, University College London, London, UK. [3]ESCMID Executive Office, Basel, Switzerland. [4]Institute of Hospital Hygiene and Infection Prevention, Gesundheitsverbund Landkreis Konstanz, Radolfzell, Germany. [5]Present address: Department of Internal Medicine, Cantonal Hospital Thurgau, Muensterlingen, Switzerland.

## References

1. Magiorakos AP, Srinivasan A, Carey RB, et al. Multidrug-resistant, extensively drug-resistant and pandrug-resistant bacteria: an international expert proposal for interim standard definitions for acquired resistance. Clin Microbiol Infect. 2012;18:268–81.
2. Siegel JD, Rhinehart E, Jackson M, et al. 2007 guideline for isolation precautions: preventing transmission of infectious agents in health care settings. Am J Infect Control. 2007;35:S65–164.
3. Tacconelli E, Cataldo MA, Dancer SJ, et al. ESCMID guidelines for the management of the infection control measures to reduce transmission of multidrug-resistant gram-negative bacteria in hospitalized patients. Clin Microbiol Infect. 2014;20(Suppl 1):1–55.
4. Drees M, Pineles L, Harris AD, Morgan DJ. Variation in definitions and isolation procedures for multidrug-resistant gram-negative bacteria: a survey of the Society for Healthcare Epidemiology of America research network. Infect Control Hosp Epidemiol. 2014;35:362–6.
5. Kalenic S, Cookson B, Gh R, et al. Comparison of recommendations in national/regional guidelines for prevention and control of MRSA in thirteen European countries. International Journal of Infection Control. 2010;6:1–10.
6. Likert R. A technique for the measurement of attitudes. Arch Psychol. 1932; 20(140):5–55.
7. Survey Monkey Europe UC. Dublin. Theatr Irel. www.surveymonkey.com. Accessed 20 Aug 2014.
8. Population Reference Bureau. World Population Data Sheet. Washington, DC; 2016. p. 10–4. https://www.prb.org/2016-world-population-data-sheet. Accessed 05 Nov 2017.
9. MacKenzie FM, Bruce J, Van Looveren M, et al. Antimicrobial susceptibility testing in European hospitals: report from the ARPAC study. Clin Microbiol Infect. 2006;12:1185–92.
10. IBM Corp. Released 2015. IBM SPSS Statistics for Windows, Version 23.0. Armonk: IBM Corp; 2015.
11. WHO. Antimicrobial resistance: global report on surveillance. 2014. http://www.who.int/drugresistance/documents/surveillancereport/en/. Accessed 11 June 2018.
12. The World Bank. Drug-resistant infections: A Threat to Our Economic Future. Washington, DC; 2017. http://documents.worldbank.org/curated/en/323311493396993758/final-report. Accessed 05 Nov 2017.
13. Dettenkofer M, Humphreys H, Saenz H, et al. Key priorities in the prevention and control of healthcare-associated infection: a survey of European and other international infection prevention experts. Infection. 2016;44:719–24.

Variability in contact precautions to control the nosocomial spread of multi-drug resistant organisms...

83

14. Clock SA, Cohen B, Behta M, et al. Contact precautions for multidrug-resistant organisms: current recommendations and actual practice. Am J Infect Control. 2010;38:105–11.

15. Paterson DL, Ko WC, Von Gottberg A, et al. International prospective study of Klebsiella pneumoniae bacteremia: implications of extended-spectrum beta-lactamase production in nosocomial infections. Ann Intern Med. 2004; 140:26–32.

16. Seibert DJ, Speroni KG, Oh KM, et al. Knowledge, perceptions, and practices of methicillin-resistant Staphylococcus aureus transmission prevention among health care workers in acute-care settings. Am J Infect Control. 2014;42:254–9.

17. Brusaferro S, Cookson B, Kalenic S, et al. Training infection control and hospital hygiene professionals in Europe, 2010: agreed core competencies among 33 European countries. Euro Surveill. 2014;19:45-54.

18. Morgan DJ, Murthy R, Munoz-Price LS, et al. Reconsidering contact precautions for endemic methicillin-resistant Staphylococcus aureus and vancomycin-resistant enterococcus. Infect Control Hosp Epidemiol. 2015;36:1163–72.

19. Tschudin-Sutter S, Frei R, Dangel M, et al. Rate of transmission of extended-spectrum beta-lactamase-producing enterobacteriaceae without contact isolation. Clin Infect Dis. 2012;55:1505–11.

20. Tschudin-Sutter S, Frei R, Schwahn F, et al. Prospective validation of cessation of contact precautions for extended-Spectrum beta-lactamase-producing Escherichia coli. Emerg Infect Dis. 2016;22:1094–7.

# Efficacy of intravenous plus intrathecal/intracerebral ventricle injection of polymyxin B for post-neurosurgical intracranial infections due to MDR/XDR *Acinectobacter baumannii*

Sijun Pan[1,2†], Xiaofang Huang[1†], Yesong Wang[1†], Li Li[3], Changyun Zhao[3], Zhongxiang Yao[2], Wei Cui[1] and Gensheng Zhang[1*]

## Abstract

**Background:** Post-neurosurgical intracranial infections caused by multidrug-resistant or extensively drug-resistant *Acinetobacter baumannii* are difficult to treat and associated with high mortality. In this study, we analyzed the therapeutic efficacy of intravenous combined with intrathecal/intracerebral ventricle injection of polymyxin B for this type of intracranial infection.

**Methods:** This retrospective study was conducted from January 2013 to September 2017 at the Second Affiliated Hospital, Zhejiang University School of Medicine (Hangzhou,China) and included 61 cases for which cerebrospinal fluid (CSF) cultures were positive for multidrug-resistant or extensively drug-resistant *A. baumannii* after a neurosurgical operation. Patients treated with intravenous and intrathecal/intracerebral ventricle injection of polymyxin B were assigned to the intrathecal/intracerebral group, and patients treated with other antibiotics without intrathecal/intracerebral injection were assigned to the intravenous group. Data for general information, treatment history, and the results of routine tests and biochemistry indicators in CSF, clinical efficiency, microbiological clearance rate, and the 28-day mortality were collected and analyzed.

**Results:** The rate of multidrug-resistant or extensively drug-resistant *A. baumannii* infection among patients who experienced an intracranial infection after a neurosurgical operation was 33.64% in our hospital. The isolated *A. baumannii* were resistant to various antibiotics, and most seriously to carbapenems (100.00% resistance rate to imipenem and meropenem), cephalosporins (resistance rates of 98.38% to cefazolin, 100.00% to ceftazidime, 100.00% to cefatriaxone, and 98.39% to cefepime). However, the isolated *A. baumannii* were completely sensitive to polymyxin B (sensitivity rate of 100.00%), followed by tigecycline (60.66%) and amikacin (49.18%). No significant differences in basic clinical data were observed between the two groups. Compared with the intravenous group, the intrathecal/intracerebral group had a significantly lower 28-day mortality (55.26% vs. 8.70%, $P = 0.01$) and higher rates of clinical efficacy and microbiological clearance (95.65% vs. 23.68%, $P < 0.001$; 91.30% vs. 18.42%, $P < 0.001$, respectively).

(Continued on next page)

* Correspondence: genshengzhang@zju.edu.cn
†Equal contributors
[1]Department of Critical Care Medicine, Second Affiliated Hospital, Zhejiang University School of Medicine, Hangzhou, Zhejiang 310009, People's Republic of China
Full list of author information is available at the end of the article

(Continued from previous page)

**Conclusions:** Intravenous plus intrathecal/intracerebral ventricle injection of polymyxin B is an effective regimen for treating intracranial infections caused by multidrug-resistant or extensively drug-resistant *A. baumannii.*

**Keywords:** *Acinetobacter Baumannii*, Polymyxin B, Intrathecal injection, Intracerebral ventricle injection, Multidrug resistance

## Background

Postoperative nervous system infection is a common complication of neurosurgery and accounts for 0.8–7% of intracranial infections [1]. The most common pathogens are Gram-negative *Bacilli* and *Staphylococcus aureus*, but the percentage of post-neurosurgical intracranial infections caused by *Acinetobacter baumannii* is still high at 15–21.74% [2, 3] with a high associated mortality rate ranging from 20 to 40% [4, 5]. A previous study reported a frequency of nosocomial, post-neurosurgical meningitis caused by *A. baumannii* as high as 10.9% with a mortality rate of 33.3% [6]. An urgent clinical problem that has arisen in recent years is the high prevalence of intracranial infections with multidrug-resistant (MDR)/extensively drug-resistant (XDR) *A. baumannii* (MDR/XDR-Ab) due to the widespread use of broad-spectrum antibiotics. Thus, effective treatments for MDR/XDR-Ab intracranial infections are needed.

Although MDR/XDR-Ab is resistant to multiple antibiotics, it is still currently susceptible to polymyxins. The high molecular weight of polymyxins and the existence of the blood–brain barrier have forced the use of "intravenous combined with intrathecal/intracerebral ventricle injection" in order to achieve an effective therapeutic concentration [7, 8]. This method has been used clinically to treat intracranial infections caused by MDR/XDR-Ab, but the outcomes have been described in mostly case reports or case series [9, 10]. To further confirm the efficacy of this treatment strategy and provide more solid evidence, we retrospectively analyzed the effects of intravenous antibiotics without polymyxin B and intravenous plus intrathecal/intraventricular injection of polymyxin B in 61 cases of intracranial infection with MDR/XDR-Ab after neurosurgery.

## Methods

### Patients

This single-center retrospective cohort study was conducted from January 2013 to September 2017 at the Second Affiliated Hospital, Zhejiang University School of Medicine (Hangzhou, China), and consecutive, unselected adult patients (age > 18 years) with a diagnosis of intracranial infection due to MDR/XDR-Ab after a neurosurgery were enrolled. The exclusion criteria were: a polymicrobial result from cerebrospinal fluid (CSF) culture; non-MDR/XDR-Ab intracranial infection; MDR/XDR-Ab

intracranial infection not occurring as a complication after neurosurgery; or intracranial colonization due to MDR/XDR-Ab. Patients also were excluded from the study if they were pregnant or had a malignancy outside of the nervous system. Figure 1 outlines the selection of the patients. Sixty-one patients were assessed as eligible for inclusion in this study, including 38 in the intravenous only group and 23 in the intravenous plus intrathecal/intracerebral group. The diagnostic criteria for post-neurosurgical intracranial infection due to MDR/XDR-Ab were as reported [11, 12]: (1) a positive CSF culture for MDR/XDR-Ab. MDR was defined as resistance to at least one agent in three or more antimicrobial categories (such as carbapenems, aminoglycosides, and cephalosporins); XDR was defined as resistance to all other antimicrobial agents, except one or two antimicrobials (such as tigecycline and polymyxins) [13]. The antibiotic susceptibilities were determined using a Vitek 2 compact automated system (bioMerieux, Marcy-l'Etoile, France) or the disk diffusion method according to the Clinical Laboratory Standards Institute (CLSI) criteria in our microbiology laboratory, and the results were interpreted according to the CLSI 2016 criteria [14]. (2) At least two of the following symptoms with no other recognized cause: fever > 38 ° C or headache, meningeal signs, or cranial nerve signs. (3) CSF/serum glucose ratio < 0.5, CSF nucleated cells > 10 × $10^6$ /L, or protein level > 0.45 g/L. A positive CSF culture was defined by colonization or contamination if the patient had no clinical symptoms or had normal levels of glucose, nucleated cells and protein [12].

### Treatment protocol

The patients treated with intravenous and intrathecal/intracerebral ventricle injection of polymyxin B (Fresenius Kabi USA) were assigned to the intrathecal/intracerebral group, and patients treated with intravenous antibiotics only were assigned to the intravenous group. In the intrathecal/intracerebral group, 450,000 units per 12 h were administered intravenously and 50,000 units/day were simultaneously administered via the lumbar cistern drainage tube or ventricular drainage tube twice daily [9–11]. The drainage tube was removed and replaced upon diagnosis of infection. The process of intrathecal/intracerebral injection was as follows: we withdrew 2 mL CSF via the tube and discarded it; then we injected 50,000 units/day of polymyxin B; and then we kept the

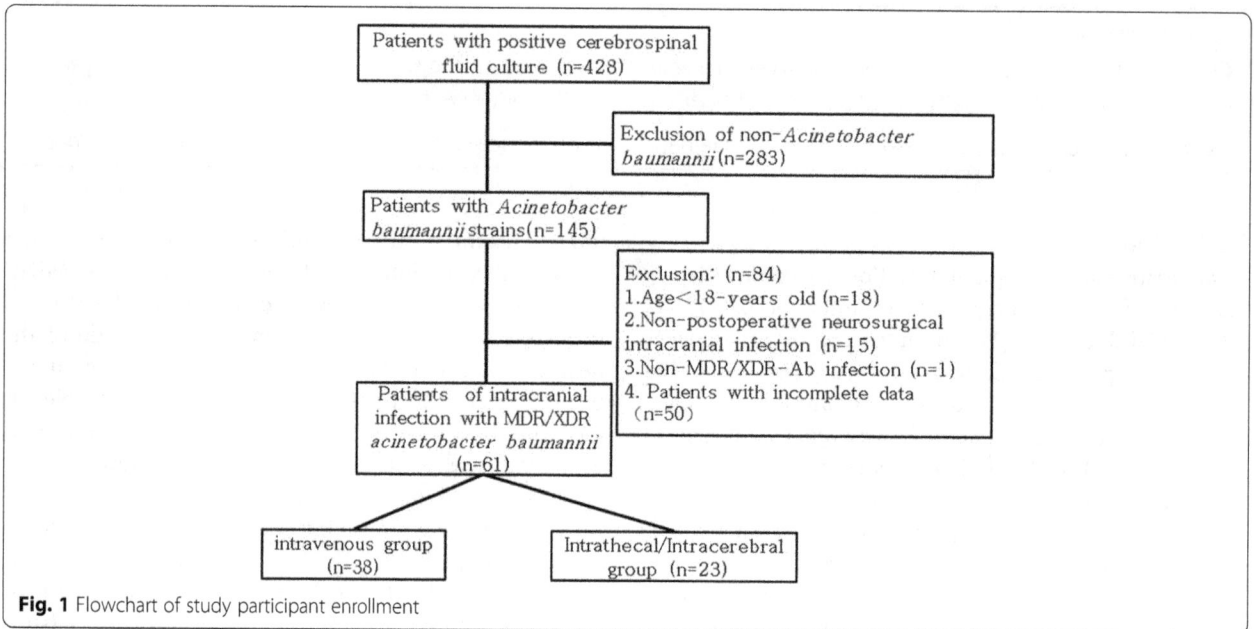

**Fig. 1** Flowchart of study participant enrollment

tube closed for 2 h [9, 11]. In the intravenous group, patients were treated with other antibiotics without intrathecal/intracerebral injection.

## Data collection

Demographic characteristics including age, sex, underlying disease, co-morbidities, operation method, co-infections, and liver and kidney function were reviewed, and the acute physiology and chronic health evaluation (APACHE) II score, sequential organ failure assessment (SOFA) score, and the general history of initial antimicrobial use were also recorded. Symptoms of intracranial infection like temperature and meningeal stimulation, routine and biochemistry indicators in CSF, culture results for CSF, the use of antibiotics, and treatment efficacy were also recorded (Table 1). Evaluation of treatment efficacy was based on the above clinical and microbiologic parameters. Clinical efficiency was defined as the disappearance or improvement of symptoms. Microbiological efficiency was defined as disappearance/clearance of *A. baumannii* from three consecutive CSF cultures after treatment. The primary end point of this study was 28-day mortality, and secondary end points were clinical efficiency and microbiological efficiency.

## Statistical analysis

Statistical analysis was performed with SPSS 19.0 (SPSS, IBM Company, Chicago, IL) software. Continuous variables are presented as mean ± standard deviation if normally distributed, and as median and interquartile range if non-normally distributed. The Student's t-test was performed for comparison of continuous variables, and chi-square test

for categorical variables. A two-tailed $P < 0.05$ was considered statistically significant.

## Results

### Study participants and demographic characteristics

A total of 428 cases with positive CSF cultures were retrospectively reviewed, including infections by *A. baumannii* ($n = 145$, 33.88%), *Klebsiella pneumonia* ($n = 81$, 18.93%), *Staphylococcus epidermidis* ($n = 33$, 7.71%), *Staphylococcus aureus* ($n = 16$, 3.74%), *Pseudomonas aeruginosa* ($n = 11$, 2.57%), and others such as *Klebsiella oxytoca*, *Cryptococcus neoformans*. Among the 145 cases with *A. baumannii*-positive CSF cultures, 84 subjects were excluded, and a total of 61 patients with intracranial infection due to MDR/XDR-Ab after neurosurgery were finally enrolled. There were 38 cases in the intravenous group and 23 cases in the intrathecal/intracerebral group. The baseline characteristics of these patients according to the two groups are summarized in Table 1, and no significant differences were observed in characteristics including age, sex, underlying disease, surgical history, use of external CSF drainage tube, APACHE II score, or SOFA score.

### Susceptibility testing and antimicrobial therapies

The detailed testing of the susceptibility of MDR/XDR-Ab to different antibiotics in these patients with intracranial infection after neurosurgery is described in Table 2. Among the most common antibiotics, MDR/XDR-Ab was most resistant to carbapenems (resistance rate of 100% to imipenem and to meropenem), cephalosporins (98.38% resistant to cefazolin, 100% to ceftazidime, 100% to ceftriaxone, and 98.38% to cefepime), whereas in no cases

**Table 1** Baseline characteristics of patients enrolled in the study

| Characteristic | ITV group ($n = 38$) | ITV + ITC group ($n = 23$) | $P$ |
|---|---|---|---|
| Sex (male) (n, %) | 20, 52.63% | 10, 43.48% | 0.488 |
| Age (years) | 53.50 ± 15.17 | 55.00 ± 15.08 | 0.761 |
| Primary disease (n, %) | | | 0.091 |
|   Cerebral hemorrhage | 30, 78.95% | 14, 60.87% | |
|   Craniocerebral trauma | 4, 10.53% | 2, 8.70% | |
|   Benign Intracranial tumor | 4, 10.53% | 7, 30.43% | |
| Comorbidities (n, %) | | | 0.833 |
|   Diabetes | 3, 7.89% | 4, 17.39% | |
|   Cardiovascular disease | 11, 28.95% | 9, 39.13% | |
|   Pulmonary disease | 0, 0.00% | 1, 4.35% | |
|   Nervous system disease | 1, 2.63% | 1, 4.35% | |
| Surgeries (n, %) | | | 0.396 |
|   Craniotomy evacuation of hematoma + decompressivecraniectomy | 32, 84.21% | 21, 91.27% | |
|   Intracranial tumor resection | 3, 7.89% | 2, 8.70% | |
|   Craniotomy aneurysm clipping | 12, 31.58% | 9, 39.13% | |
|   Drainage of intracranial hematoma | 9, 23.68% | 7, 30.43% | |
|   Ventricle peritoneal shunt | 6, 15.79% | 5, 21.74% | |
|   Lumbar cistern drainage | 26, 68.42% | 15, 65.22% | |
|   Ommaya reservoir | 2, 5.26% | 2, 8.70% | |
| Coinfection (n, %) | | | 0.727 |
|   Lung | 29, 76.32% | 18, 78.26% | |
|   Bloodstream | 5, 13.16% | 4, 17.39% | |
| SOFA score | 5.34 ± 3.02 | 5.08 ± 2.23 | 0.707 |
| APACHE II score | 18.55 ± 5.62 | 17.65 ± 4.90 | 0.513 |
| Clinical symptoms | | | |
|   Fever (°C) | 39.02 ± 0.53 | 39.17 ± 0.48 | 0.256 |

*SOFA* sequential organ failure assessment, *APACHE* acute physiology and chronic health evaluation. *ITV* intravenous, *ITV + ITC* intrathecal/intracerebral

was MDR/XDR-Ab resistant to polymyxins. No significant differences in the results of susceptibility testing were observed between the two groups.

The most common antimicrobial regime used for the initially empirical therapy was meropenem/imipenem plus vancomycin (efficacy of 37.70%), followed by meropenem/imipenem only (18.03%), tigecycline plus cefperazone-sulbactam (16.39%), and meropenem/imipenem plus linezolid (14.75%; Table 3). Empirical antimicrobial use did not differ significantly between the two groups before intracranial infection ($P = 0.684$; Table 3). After MDR/XDR-Ab infection was confirmed, the most commonly employed antimicrobial regimes shifted to the combination of tigecycline plus cefperazone-sulbactam (31.15%), meropenem/imipenem plus tigecycline (19.67%), meropenem/ imipenem alone (18.03%) or cefperazone-sulbactam alone (13.11%) in the intravenous group.

### Microbiological clearance and biochemistry indicators of CSF

The intrathecal/intracerebral group achieved a significantly higher microbiological clearance rate (91.30%, 21/23) than in the intravenous group (18.42%, 7/38; $P < 0.01$). Before treatment, there were no significant differences in the nuclei counts, chlorine, glucose, adenosine deaminase (ADA), and protein levels in CSF between the two groups. In comparison with the intravenous group, the intrathecal/intracerebral group showed a significantly decreased body temperature (39.20 ± 0.48 °C vs. 37.48 ± 0.56 °C, $P < 0.01$), a reduced number of nucleated cells in the CSF (4242.82 ± 3100.17 vs. 106.45 ± 120.00 × 10$^6$/L, $P < 0.01$), greater recovery of the glucose level in CSF (0.56 ± 1.27 mmol/L vs. 3.20 ± 0.95 mmol/L, $P < 0.01$), a decreased level of ADA in the CSF (19.18 ± 10.02 U/L vs. 8.18 ± 6.78 U/L, $P < 0.001$), and reduced levels of total protein in CSF (207.10 ± 77.40 mg/dL vs. 87.81 ± 45.47 mg/dL, $P = 0.012$; Fig. 2).

**Table 2** Susceptibility testing results for isolated *A. baumannii*

| | MIC Break-point (mg/L) | Total (*n* = 61) | ITV group (*n* = 38) | ITV + ITC group (*n* = 23) | *P* |
|---|---|---|---|---|---|
| Antibiotic resistance (n, %) | | | | | 0.402 |
| Amikacin | $R \geq 32$ | 25, 40.98% | 12, 31.58% | 13, 56.52% | |
| Tigecycline | $R \geq 8$ | 3, 2.92% | 2, 5.26% | 1, 4.35% | |
| Carbapenems | | | | | |
| Imipenem | $R \geq 8$ | 60, 98.36% | 37, 97.36% | 23, 100.00% | |
| Meropenem | $R \geq 8$ | 60, 98.36% | 37, 97.36% | 23, 100.00% | |
| Cephalosporins | | | | | |
| Cefazolin | $R \geq 32$ | 60, 98.36% | 38, 100.00% | 22, 95.65% | |
| Ceftazidime | $R \geq 32$ | 60, 98.36% | 37, 97.36% | 23, 100.00% | |
| Cefatriaxone | $R \geq 64$ | 61, 100.00% | 38, 100.00% | 23, 100.00% | |
| Cefepime | $R \geq 32$ | 60, 98.36% | 37, 97.36% | 23, 100.00% | |
| Polymyxin B | $R \geq 4$ | 0, 0.00% | 0, 0.00% | 0, 0.00% | |

*ITV* intravenous, *ITV + ITC* intrathecal/intracerebral

## Clinical outcomes

Among the 61 patients with *A. baumannii* infection, the earliest death occurred on day two, and the total mortality rate was 37.70%. In the intravenous group, the mortality rate was 55.26% (21/38), while in the intrathecal/intracerebral group, the mortality rate was 8.70% (2/23; *P* = 0.01).

## Safety analysis

As renal function impairment is one of the side effects of polymyxin B treatment, we analyzed the changes in serum creatinine from before to after polymyxin B treatment. The mean creatinine level was 41.09 ± 11.46 μmol/L at 48 h after polymyxin B injection, which did not differ significantly from the baseline level (41.09 ± 11.46 μmol/L; *P* = 0.799).

**Table 3** The initially applied empirical antimicrobial therapies

| | Total (*n* = 61) | ITV group (*n* = 38) | ITV + ITC group (*n* = 23) | *P* |
|---|---|---|---|---|
| Before infection (n, %) | | | | 0.684 |
| M/I + vancomycin | 23, 37.70% | 15, 39.47% | 8, 34.78% | |
| M/I + linezolid | 9, 14.75% | 7, 18.42% | 2, 8.70% | |
| M/I + cefperazone-sulbactam | 2, 3.28% | 2, 5.26% | 0, 0.00% | |
| M/I | 11, 18.03% | 7, 18.42% | 4, 17.39% | |
| Tigecycline + cefperazone-sulbactam | 10, 16.39% | 6, 15.78% | 4, 17.39% | |
| Tigecycline | 2, 3.28% | 1, 2.63% | 1, 4.34% | |
| Ceftriaxone | 4, 6.56% | 4, 10.53% | 0, 0.00% | |
| Cefperazone-sulbactam + vancomycin | 1, 1.64% | 1, 2.63% | 0, 0.00% | |
| Cefperazone-sulbactam | 3, 4.92% | 3, 7.89% | 3, 13.04% | |
| Piperacillin-tazobactam | 6, 9.84% | 6, 15.79% | 7, 30.43% | |
| After infection (n, %) | | | | 0.723 |
| M/I + amikacin | 3, 4.92% | 3, 7.89% | 0, 0.00% | |
| M/I + tigecycline | 12, 19.67% | 8, 21.05% | 4, 17.39% | |
| M/I + cefperazone-sulbactam | 7, 11.48% | 4, 10.52% | 3, 13.04% | |
| M/I | 11, 18.03% | 8, 21.05% | 3, 13.04% | |
| Tigecycline+cefperazone-sulbactam | 19, 31.15% | 10, 6.32% | 9, 39.13% | |
| Cefperazone-sulbactam | 8, 13.11% | 4, 10.53% | 4, 17.39% | |
| Cefperazone-sulbactam + amikacin | 1, 1.64% | 1, 2.63% | 0, 0.00% | |

*ITV* intravenous, *ITV + ITC* intrathecal/intracerebral, */I* meropenem/imipenem

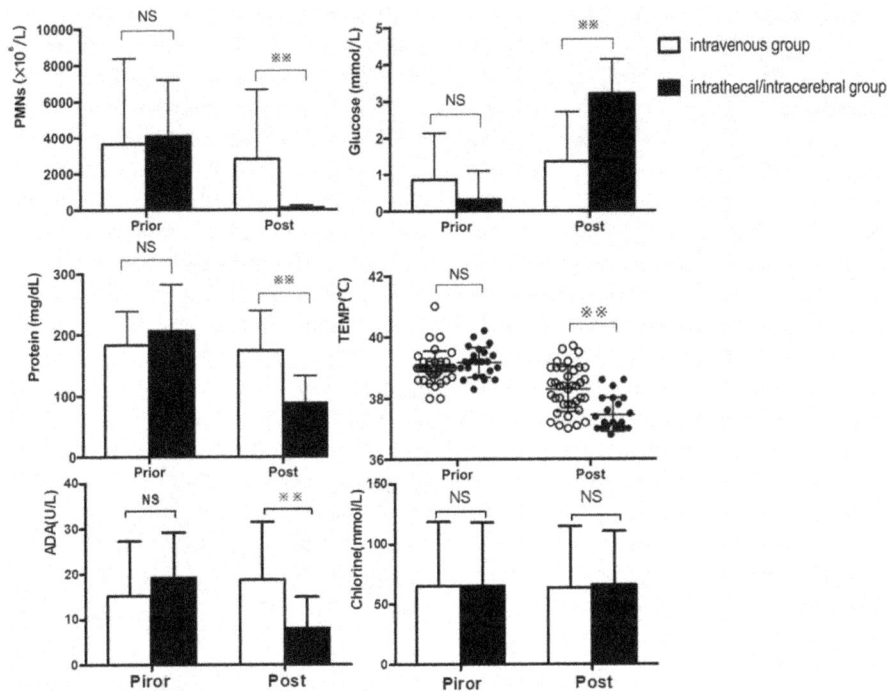

**Fig. 2** Laboratory indicators for CSF and body temperature before and after treatment in the two groups. PMNs: polymorph nuclear neutrophils; TEMP: temperature. ADA: adenosine deaminase. NS: not significant; **$P < 0.01$

## Discussion

*A. baumannii* is an opportunistic pathogen. The CHI-NET surveillance of bacterial resistance (2005–2014) [15] reported that *A. baumannii* accounts for 8.7–12.1% of clinical isolates in China, with the total number of bacterial isolates was ranging from 22,774–84,572 annually. In the current study, *A. baumannii* accounted for 33.88% of all isolates, which was considerably higher than the frequency noted in the 2005–2014 CHINET surveillance report. The reasons might be as follows: first, the incidence of *A. baumannii* infection is increasing; second, most of the patients recovering from neurosurgery were in an immune compromised state. Some had acquired artificial devices such as an external ventricular drain or intraventricular catheter, and some had hospitalized for a long time and had already received broad-spectrum antibiotics. All of these conditions are known risk factors for developing *A. baumannii* infection [16].

*A. baumannii* tends to quickly develop resistance to multiple antimicrobial agents through various mechanisms, such as through degrading enzymes targeting β-lactams, modifying enzymes targeting aminoglycosides, and alteration to the binding sites for quinolones [17]. A report from the SENTRY antimicrobial surveillance program (2001–2004) [18] showed that the resistance rates of *A. baumannii* exceeded 25% for imipenem and meropenem, 40% for cefepime and ceftazidime, 35% for

amikacin, and 45% for ciprofloxacin. The CHINET surveillance report (2005–2014) from China [15] showed the resistance rate of *A. baumannii* for imipenem approximately doubled from 31% in 2005 to 62.4% in 2014, while that for meropenem increased from 39% in 2005 to 66.7% in 2014. Cefepime and ceftazidime resistance levels ranged from 54.8%–67.6% and 52.4%–71.9%, respectively, and amikacin and ciprofloxacin resistance levels ranged from 40.2%–61% and 60%–68.3%, respectively. In the present study, we found that 49.36% of *A. baumannii* isolates were MDR and 28.47% were XDR, with resistance to carbapenems (resistance rate of 100% for both imipenem and meropenem), cephalosporins (98.38% for cefazolin, 100% for ceftazidime, 100% for cefatriaxone, and 98.38% for cefepime). In comparison to the findings of the SENTRY antimicrobial surveillance report (2001–2004) and CHINET surveillance report (2005–2014), we observed major increases in the resistance of *A. baumannii* to these antibiotics. These results suggest that the treatment of *A. baumannii* is becoming more complicated, especially in the intensive care unit (ICU) where broad spectrum antimicrobials are commonly used.

For the initial empirical antimicrobial therapy, carbapenems, as broad-spectrum β-lactam antibiotics, have remained the first-line agents for patients who are immunocompromised or have had a prolonged period of hospitalization even though the prevalence of carbapenem-resistant bacteria is increasing [11]. Meropenem/imipenem is active against carbapenemase-negative *A. baumannii* isolates, but inactive against *A. baumannii* isolates that express plasmid-mediated carbapenemases [19]. Sulbactam is a β-lactamase inhibitor with intrinsic antibacterial activity against many *Acinectobacter* isolates, which is related to its affinity for penicillin-binding proteins [20]. It can be effective against infections caused by moderately imipenem-resistant isolates [21]. Because the combination of sulbactam and carbapenems showed better results than carbapenems alone for MDR-Ab infections [22], the combination of meropenem/imipenem and other antibiotics have been used as initial empirical therapy in our hospital. Considering that polymyxins are expensive and not easily accessible in China, after confirmation of MDR/XDR-Ab, most of the patients in the intravenous group received tigecycline together with cefperazone-sulbactam or meropenem/imipenem, but this did not effectively reduce mortality, which we attribute to the weak dispersion of tigecycline in CSF [23].

Consistent with the results of the CHINET report [15], the results of the present study demonstrate that *A. baumannii* is highly sensitive to polymyxins (100.00%), tigecycline (60.66%), and amikacin (49.18%). Thus, polymyxins may be an ideal antibiotic for the treatment of MDR/XDR-Ab, as they effectively and rapidly kill most Gram-negative microorganisms. The 2017 Infectious Diseases Society of America (IDSA) Clinical Practice Guide recommends that colistin or polymyxin B be administered intravenously and intraventricularly for the treatment of intracranial infections caused by carbapenem-resistant *Acinetobacter* species [11], but the quality of evidence is moderate as is mentioned in the Guide. In a retrospective study, Moon et al. [24] found that colistimethate-containing regimens could cure post-neurosurgical meningitis caused by carbapenem-resistant *A. baumannii*. Fotakopoulos et al. [25] reported that the combination of intravenous and intraventricular colistin may improve outcomes in patients with meningitis/ventriculitis due to multidrug resistance infections, especially that attributed to *A. baumannii*. Guardado et al. [6] studied intracranial infections caused by MDR/XDR-Ab after neurosurgery and found that intravenous injection along with intrathecal/intraventricular injection of polymyxin resulted in a significant reduction in mortality [0 vs. 80%, *P* = 0.04, odds ratio [OR]: 1.69 (1.32–2.16)]. Although a satisfactory result was achieved by intrathecal/intracerebral ventricle injection of polymyxins, the evidence remains rather weak as it stems from clinical studies or case series with small sample numbers. To our knowledge, our current study is the largest cohort study to date to compare the efficacy of intravenous combined with intrathecal/intracerebral ventricle injection of polymyxin B for intracranial infection due to MDR/XDR-Ab in post-neurosurgical patients. The intrathecal/intraventricular group showed significant improvement in microbiological

eradication, biochemistry indicators of CSF, clinical efficiency, and 28-day mortality compared with the intravenous group. A retrospective case-control study analyzed the efficacy of intravenous plus intrathecal injection of colistin in 18 cases with XDR-Ab meningitis in the past 11 years [9]. It showed that the CSF sterilization rate was only 33.3% after treatment with intravenous administration of colistin alone, but reached complete sterilization with a rate of 100% after combination treatment with intravenous plus intraventricular injection of colistin (*P* = 0.009). These sterilization rates were similar to ours calculated in the present study. In Karaiskos' study [26], the all-cause mortality rate of patients with intracranial infection caused by MDR/XDR-Ab was 71%, while the all-cause mortality rate in our study was only 47.54% (29/61). This could partially explain why intrathecal/intraventricular injection of polymyxin B significantly improved the survival rate, although it is impossible to discern the definitive cause of mortality. Evidence has revealed that the level of colistin in CSF is only 5–10% of that in blood when using intravenous administration only [27]. Moreover, the administration of polymyxin with direct intrathecal/intraventricular injection could increase the penetration of polymyxins into the central nervous system. Together with our study, all these findings suggest that a combination treatment with intravenous and intrathecal/intraventricular polymyxins be superior to routine intravenous antibiotics for the treatment of patients with an intracranial infection due to MDR/XDR-Ab.

A last-line treatment for infections that are resistant to other available antibiotics, the polymyxins antibiotics (including colistin and polymyxin B) are potentially nephrotoxic, but the relative risk of this adverse effect is still unclear [28]. Early reports revealed that use of more than the recommended dosage of colistin (2.5–5 mg/kg/day) was associated with an adverse renal reaction [29–31]. Additional research suggested that the incidence of nephrotoxic effects is higher with colistimethate than with polymyxin B [32]. In the present study, 61 patients received polymyxin B at a dose of 450,000 units per 12 h intravenously and at the same time received intrathecal/intraventricular injection of polymyxin B at 50,000 units/day. No cases of acute kidney injury were observed among the study participants according to the KDIGO guidelines [33], and several studies have shown that intravenous polymyxins is not associated with serious renal toxicity if the dosage is proper [34, 35]. Thus, the method of polymyxin B administration in the current study might be relatively safe for renal function. Notably, since the kidney is the primary route of elimination for polymyxins, the dosage must be carefully monitored [36].

Intravenous along with intrathecal/intracerebral injection of polymyxins might not only be effective for MDR/XDR-Ab but also have significant effects on other multidrug-resistant gram-negative bacteria. Macedo et al. [37] reported that intraventricular therapy with polymyxins improved outcomes in patients presenting with meningoencephalitis due to multidrug-resistant Gram-negative bacteria infections (*A. baumannii, P. aeruginosa*, etc.), with no cases of neurotoxicity and nephrotoxicity. In the study by Falagas et al. [35], intraventricular and intrathecal polymyxins (alone or with systemic antibiotics) were effective for Gram-negative meningitis *(P. aeruginosa, A. baumannii, etc)*, and that toxicity is not uncommon but is usually dose-dependent and reversible. Therefore, taken together, these results suggest that intrathecal/intracerebral of polymyxins is an effective treatment strategy against intracranial infection by MDR/XDR-Ab or other MDR/XDR gram-negative bacteria without toxicity.

There were some limitations in this study. (1) This was a single-center retrospective study, and thus, further multi-center randomized controlled studies (prospective or retrospective) are needed. (2) The sample size in our current study ($n = 61$) was still small and needs to be expanded. (3) The most significant adverse effects of intraventricular or intrathecal injection that have been reported are chemical ventriculitis and meningitis. This study did not evaluate the neurotoxicity of polymyxin B nor obtain any dynamic records on changes in consciousness (such as the Glasgow Coma Scale score) and other clinical indicators due to the retrospective nature of the study. (4) Polymyxins must be bought from outside China, and they are too expensive for some patients.

## Conclusions

Intravenous plus intrathecal/intraventricular injection of polymyxin B can effectively improve levels of CSF indicators and support clinical efficiency, microbiologic eradication, and 28-day mortality without adverse effects, which might be a promising strategy to treat intracranial infections due to MDR/XDR-Ab.

## Acknowledgements
Not applicable.

## Funding
This work was supported in part by grants from the National Natural Science Foundation of China (No. 81570017 to GS Zhang), the Medical and Health Research Program of Zhejiang Province (Core Talents Plan) of Zhejiang Province (No. 2016RCA014 to GS Zhang), and the Medical and Health Research Program of Zhejiang Province (No. 2017KY371 to GS Zhang).

## Authors' contributions
SJ, XF and YS contributed to the acquisition and analysis of the data and writing the initial draft of this paper. LL, CY, ZX and CW contributed to the collection and interpretation of data. GS contributed to the concept of the study, the revision of this paper, and the final approval of the version to be published. SJ, XF and YS contributed equally to this work. All authors read and approved the final manuscript.

## Competing interests
The authors declare that they have no competing interests.

## Author details
[1]Department of Critical Care Medicine, Second Affiliated Hospital, Zhejiang University School of Medicine, Hangzhou, Zhejiang 310009, People's Republic of China. [2]Department of Critical Care Medicine, Anji County People's Hospital, Huzhou, Zhejiang Province 313300, China. [3]Department of Critical Care Medicine, Zhejiang Hospital, Hangzhou 310013, China.

## References
1. Ruan L, Wu D, Li X, et al. Analysis of microbial community composition and diversity in postoperative intracranial infection using high-throughput sequencing. Mol Med Rep. 2017;16(4):3938–46.
2. Dettenkofer M, Ebner W, Els T, Babikir R, Lucking C, Pelz K, Ruden H, Daschner F. Surveillance of nosocomial infections in a neurology intensive care unit. J Neurol. 2001;248(11):959–64.
3. Jiang L, Guo L, Li R, Wang S. Targeted surveillance and infection-related risk factors of nosocomial infection in patients after neurosurgical operation. Pak J Pharm Sci. 2017;30(3(Special)):1053–6.
4. Kasiakou SK, Rafailidis PI, Liaropoulos K, Falagas ME. Cure of post-traumatic recurrent multiresistant gram-negative rod meningitis with intraventricular colistin. J Inf Secur. 2005;50(4):348–52.
5. Bergogne-Berezin E, Towner KJ. Acinetobacter spp. as nosocomial pathogens: microbiological, clinical, and epidemiological features. Clin Microbiol Rev. 1996;9(2):148–65.
6. Rodriguez Guardado A, Blanco A, Asensi V, Perez F, Rial JC, Pintado V, Bustillo E, Lantero M, Tenza E, Alvarez M, et al. Multidrug-resistant Acinetobacter meningitis in neurosurgical patients with intraventricular catheters: assessment of different treatments. J Antimicrob Chemother. 2008;61(4):908–13.
7. Imberti R, Cusato M, Accetta G, Marino V, Procaccio F, Del Gaudio A, Iotti GA, Regazzi M. Pharmacokinetics of colistin in cerebrospinal fluid after intraventricular administration of colistin methanesulfonate. Antimicrob Agents Chemother. 2012;56(8):4416–21.
8. Lonsdale DO, Udy AA, Roberts JA, Lipman J. Antibacterial therapeutic drug monitoring in cerebrospinal fluid: difficulty in achieving adequate drug concentrations. J Neurosurg. 2013;118(2):297–301.
9. De Bonis P, Lofrese G, Scoppettuolo G, Spanu T, Cultrera R, Labonia M, Cavallo MA, Mangiola A, Anile C, Pompucci A. Intraventricular versus intravenous colistin for the treatment of extensively drug resistant Acinetobacter Baumannii meningitis. Eur J Neurol. 2016;23(1):68–75.
10. Sandri AM, Landersdorfer CB, Jacob J, et al. Population pharmacokinetics of intravenous polymyxin B in critically ill patients: implications for selection of dosage regimens. Clin Infect Dis. 2013;57(4):524–31.
11. Tunkel AR, Hasbun R, Bhimraj A, Byers K, Kaplan SL, Michael Scheld W, van de Beek D, Bleck TP, Garton HJ, Zunt JR. Infectious Diseases Society of America's clinical practice guidelines for healthcare-associated Ventriculitis and meningitis. Clin Infect Dis. 2017; https://doi.org/10.1093/cid/ciw861. Epub ahead of print.
12. Durand ML, Calderwood SB, Weber DJ, Miller SI, Southwick FS, Caviness VS Jr, Swartz MN. Acute bacterial meningitis in adults. A review of 493 episodes. N Engl J Med. 1993;328(1):21–8.
13. Magiorakos AP, Srinivasan A, Carey RB, Carmeli Y, Falagas ME, Giske CG, Harbarth S, Hindler JF, Kahlmeter G, Olsson-Liljequist B, et al. Multidrug-resistant, extensively drug-resistant and pandrug-resistant bacteria: an international expert proposal for interim standard definitions for acquired resistance. Clin Microbiol Infect. 2012;18(3):268–81.
14. Clinical and Laboratory Standards Institute. Performance standards for antimicrobial susceptibility testing: 26st informational supplement M100-S26. Wayne: CLSI; 2016.
15. Hu FP, Guo Y, Zhu DM, Wang F, Jiang XF, Xu YC, Zhang XJ, Zhang CX, Ji P, Xie Y, et al. Resistance trends among clinical isolates in China reported from CHINET surveillance of bacterial resistance, 2005-2014. Clin Microbiol Infect. 2016;22(Suppl 1):S9–14.
16. Howard A, O'Donoghue M, Feeney A, Sleator RD. Acinetobacter Baumannii: an emerging opportunistic pathogen. Virulence. 2012;3(3):243–50.
17. Peleg AY, Seifert H, Paterson DL. Acinetobacter Baumannii: emergence of a successful pathogen. Clin Microbial Rev. 2008;21(3):538–82.

18. Gales AC, Jones RN, Sader HS. Global assessment of the antimicrobial activity of polymyxin B against 54 731 clinical isolates of gram-negative bacilli: report from the SENTRY antimicrobial surveillance programme (2001-2004). Clin Microbiol Infect. 2006;12(4):315–21.

19. Jones RN, Huynh HK, Biedenbach DJ. Activities of doripenem (S-4661) against drug-resistant clinical pathogens. Antimicrob Agents Chemother. 2004;48(8):3136–40.

20. Bassetti M, Righi E, Esposito S, Petrosillo N, Nicolini L. Drug treatment for multidrug-resistant Acinetobacter Baumannii infections. Future Microbiol. 2008;3(6):649–60.

21. Corbella X, Ariza J, Ardanuy C, Vuelta M, Tubau F, Sora M, Pujol M, Gudiol F. Efficacy of sulbactam alone and in combination with ampicillin in nosocomial infections caused by multiresistant Acinetobacter Baumannii. J Antimicrob Chemother. 1998;42(6):793–802.

22. Lee NY, Wang CL, Chuang YC, Yu WL, Lee HC, Chang CM, Wang LR, Ko WC. Combination carbapenem-sulbactam therapy for critically ill patients with multidrug-resistant Acinetobacter Baumannii bacteremia: four case reports and an in vitro combination synergy study. Pharmacotherapy. 2007;27(11):1506–11.

23. Ceylan B, Arslan F, Sipahi OR, et al. Variables determining mortality in patients with Acinetobacter Baumannii meningitis/ventriculitis treated with intrathecal colistin. Clin Neurol Neurosurg. 2017;153:43–9.

24. Moon C, Kwak YG, Kim BN, Kim ES, Lee CS. Implications of postneurosurgical meningitis caused by carbapenem-resistant Acinetobacter Baumannii. J Infect Chemother. 2013;19(5):916–9.

25. Fotakopoulos G, Makris D, Chatzi M, Tsimitrea E, Zakynthinos E, Fountas K. Outcomes in meningitis/ventriculitis treated with intravenous or intraventricular plus intravenous colistin. Acta Neurochir. 2016;158(3):603–10. discussion 610

26. Karaiskos I, Galani L, Baziaka F, Giamarellou H. Intraventricular and intrathecal colistin as the last therapeutic resort for the treatment of multidrug-resistant and extensively drug-resistant Acinetobacter Baumannii ventriculitis and meningitis: a literature review. Int J Antimicrob Agents. 2013;41(6):499–508.

27. Markantonis SL, Markou N, Fousteri M, Sakellaridis N, Karatzas S, Alamanos I, Dimopoulou E, Baltopoulos G. Penetration of colistin into cerebrospinal fluid. Antimicrob Agents Chemother. 2009;53(11):4907–10.

28. Nation RL, Li J, Cars O, et al. Framework for optimisation of the clinical use of colistin and polymyxin B: the Prato polymyxin consensus. Lancet Infect Dis. 2015;15(2):225–34.

29. Randall RE, Bridi GS, Setter JG, Brackett NC. Recovery from colistimethate nephrotoxicity. Ann Intern Med. 1970;73(3):491–2.

30. Price DJ, Graham DI. Effects of large doses of colistin sulphomethate sodium on renal function. Br Med J. 1970;4(5734):525–7.

31. Koch-Weser J, Sidel VW, Federman EB, Kanarek P, Finer DC, Eaton AE. Adverse effects of sodium colistimethate. Manifestations and specific reaction rates during 317 courses of therapy. Ann Intern Med. 1970;72(6):857–68.

32. Akajagbor DS, Wilson SL, Shere-Wolfe KD, Dakum P, Charurat ME, Gilliam BL. Higher incidence of acute kidney injury with intravenous colistimethate sodium compared with polymyxin b in critically ill patients at a tertiary care medical center. Clin Infect Dis. 2013;57(9):1300–3.

33. Khwaja A. KDIGO clinical practice guidelines for acute kidney injury. Nephron Clin Pract. 2012;120(4):c179–84.

34. Reina R, Estensssoro E, Saenz G, Canales HS, Gonzalvo R, Vidal G, Martins G, Das Neves A, Santander O, Ramos C. Safety and efficacy of colistin in Acinetobacter and pseudomonas infections: a prospective cohort study. Intensive Care Med. 2005;31(8):1058–65.

35. Falagas ME, Rizos M, Bliziotis IA, Rellos K, Kasiakou SK, Michalopoulos A. Toxicity after prolonged (more than four weeks) administration of intravenous colistin. BMC Infect Dis. 2005;5:1.

36. Evans ME, Feola DJ, Rapp RP. Polymyxin B sulfate and colistin: old antibiotics for emerging multiresistant gram-negative bacteria. Ann Pharmacother. 1999;33(9):960–7.

37. Macedo S, Gonçalves I, Bispo G, et al. Intrathecal (intraventricular) polymyxin B in the treatment of patients with meningoencephalitis by Acinetobacter baumanii and Pseudomonas Aeruginosa. Crit Care. 2011;15(S1):P235.

# 14

# Clonal diversity and detection of carbapenem resistance encoding genes among multidrug-resistant *Acinetobacter baumannii* isolates recovered from patients and environment in two intensive care units in a Moroccan hospital

Jean Uwingabiye[1*], Abdelhay Lemnouer[1], Ignasi Roca[2], Tarek Alouane[3], Mohammed Frikh[1], Bouchra Belefquih[1], Fatna Bssaibis[1], Adil Maleb[1], Yassine Benlahlou[1], Jalal Kassouati[1], Nawfal Doghmi[4], Abdelouahed Bait[4], Charki Haimeur[4], Lhoussain Louzi[1], Azeddine Ibrahimi[3], Jordi Vila[2] and Mostafa Elouennass[1]

## Abstract

**Background:** Carbapenem-resistant *Acinetobacter baumannii* has recently been defined by the World Health Organization as a critical pathogen. The aim of this study was to compare clonal diversity and carbapenemase-encoding genes of *A. baumannii* isolates collected from colonized or infected patients and hospital environment in two intensive care units (ICUs) in Morocco.

**Methods:** The patient and environmental sampling was carried out in the medical and surgical ICUs of Mohammed V Military teaching hospital from March to August 2015. All *A. baumannii* isolates recovered from clinical and environmental samples, were identified using routine microbiological techniques and Matrix-Assisted Laser Desorption/Ionization Time-of-Flight Mass Spectrometry. Antimicrobial susceptibility testing was performed using disc diffusion method. The carbapenemase-encoding genes were screened for by PCR. Clonal relatedness was analyzed by digestion of the DNA with low frequency restriction enzymes and pulsed field gel electrophoresis (PFGE) and the multi locus sequence typing (MLST) was performed on two selected isolates from two major pulsotypes.

**Results:** A total of 83 multidrug-resistant *A. baumannii* isolates were collected: 47 clinical isolates and 36 environmental isolates. All isolates were positive for the $bla_{OXA51-like}$ and $bla_{OXA23-like}$ genes. The coexistence of $bla_{NDM-1}/bla_{OXA-23-like}$ and $bla_{OXA\ 24-like}/bla_{OXA-23-like}$ were detected in 27 (32.5%) and 2 (2.4%) of *A. baumannii* isolates, respectively. The environmental samples and the fecally-colonized patients were significantly identified ($p < 0.05$) as the most common sites of isolation of NDM-1-harboring isolates. PFGE grouped all isolates into 9 distinct clusters with two major groups (0007 and 0008) containing up to 59% of the isolates. The pulsotype 0008 corresponds to sequence type (ST) 195 while pulsotype 0007 corresponds to ST 1089.The genetic similarity between the clinical and environmental isolates was observed in 80/83 = 96.4% of all isolates, belonging to 7 pulsotypes.

(Continued on next page)

* Correspondence: uwije2020@yahoo.fr
[1]Department of Clinical Bacteriology, Mohammed V Military Teaching Hospital, Research Team of Epidemiology and Bacterial Resistance, Faculty of Medicine and Pharmacy, Mohammed V University, Rabat, Morocco
Full list of author information is available at the end of the article

(Continued from previous page)

**Conclusion:** This study shows that the clonal spread of environmental *A. baumannii* isolates is related to that of clinical isolates recovered from colonized or infected patients, being both associated with a high prevalence of the $bla_{OXA23-like}$ and $bla_{NDM-1}$genes. These findings emphasize the need for prioritizing the bio-cleaning of the hospital environment to control and prevent the dissemination of *A. baumannii* clonal lineages.

**Keywords:** *Acinetobacter Baumannii*, Multidrug-resistant, Pulsed-field gel electrophoresis, OXA genes, $bla_{NDM-1}$ gene, Intensive care unit

## Background

Multidrug-resistant (MDR) *Acinetobacter baumannii* is recognized to be responsible for nosocomial outbreaks in severely ill patients and it is predominantly isolated in intensive care units (ICUs) around the world [1]. This microorganism colonizes certain areas of the body such as the skin, the oropharynx and the gastrointestinal tract [1]. The prevalence of digestive tract colonization varies from 8.3 to 41% in ICU patients [2, 3] but this pathogen is also the causative agent of serious infections including pneumonia, septicemia, urinary tract infection, wound infection and meningitis with mortality rates varying from 7.8 to 75% [1]. Risk factors for *Acinetobacter* colonization and infection are linked to the presence of underlying disease, long-term hospitalization, ICU stay, administration of broad spectrum antibiotics and invasive procedures such as mechanical ventilation or catheters [1, 4]. This bacterium displays an outstanding ability to survive in the environment, with some studies reporting up to 48% of environmental samples being contaminated with *Acinetobacter* [5, 6]. Environmental sites most likely to be contaminated include bed sheets, bed railings, touch pads of ventilator equipment, trolleys, surfaces of respiratory monitors as well as the hands and uniforms of healthcare workers [5–7].

*A. baumannii* has also the capacity to develop resistance to multiple antibiotics, which limits the therapeutic options to treat these infections [1, 4]. A recent Moroccan study showed that the resistance rate of *Acinetobacter* isolates to ciprofloxacin, imipenem, amikacin netilmicin, and colistin was 87%, 86%, 52%, 33% and 1.7%,respectively [8]. Resistance to carbapenems among *A. baumannii* isolates all over the world is mostly linked to the carriage of the $bla_{OXA-23-like}$, $bla_{OXA-24-like}$, and $bla_{OXA-58-like}$ genes, encoding carbapenem hydrolyzing class D β-lactamases (OXA-type), but also to the recent dissemination of the $bla_{NDM}$ gene, encoding a class B metallo-β-lactamase [9–14]. Since 2010, NDM-producing *A. baumannii* isolates have been found in different countries including Kenya, Ethiopia, Algeria, Egypt, Germany, France, Spain, Turkey, India,Vietnam, China and Nepal [14, 15].

Overall, the clonal dissemination of carbapenem-resistant *A. baumannii* isolates has been documented in different countries [6, 7, 9–11] but only a few studies have focused on the clonal relationships between clinical and environmental isolates [5, 16, 17].

To our knowledge, there are no previous studies regarding the prevalence of carbapenemase encoding genes or the clonal diversity of *A. baumannii* isolates in Morocco.

The objective of this study was to characterize the carbapenemase-encoding genes and molecular diversity of clinical and environmental carbapenem-resistant *A. baumannii* isolates recovered from two ICUs of a Moroccan hospital.

## Methods

This study was carried out in the clinical bacteriology laboratory of Mohammed V Military teaching hospital in collaboration with Barcelona Institute for Global Health (IS global)-Hospital Clínic, Universitat de Barcelona.

### Sampling strategies

The patient and environmental sampling was carried out from March to August 2015 in the medical and surgical ICUs of Mohammed V Military teaching hospital, a teaching hospital with 700-beds, located in Rabat in the Kingdom of Morocco, and which contains 2 ICUs (medical and surgical) with 10 beds each, a center for burns, surgical and medical units, and laboratory and imagery departments.

The clinical isolates were recovered from the mouth, the anal margin and the groin for colonized patients and from the respiratory tract and blood cultures for infected patients. The criteria of colonization or infection were assessed according to the Centers for Disease Control and Prevention guidelines [18]. Screening samples were collected at the time of ICU admission and weekly during hospitalization. Collected clinical data included demographic characteristics, hospital wards, underlying diseases, invasive procedures, specimen types, antibiotic use, ICU length of stay and clinical outcome.

Environmental samples were collected from the patients' rooms. At each site, an area of 10 cm$^2$ was sampled using a sterile swab moistened with physiological saline [19, 20]. The sampled sites were: floors, bed sheets, medical ventilators, pillows, monitors, patient trolleys and intravenous solution stand.

All swabs were then immersed in brain heart infusion broth, incubated overnight at 37 °C and further subcultured on bromocresol purple lactose agar for the isolation of *Acinetobacter*.

All *Acinetobacter spp.* isolates were identified using routine microbiological techniques (direct examination, biochemical test of orientation, API20NE) and species identification was confirmed by matrix-assisted laser desorption/ionization time-of-flight mass spectrometry (MALDI-TOF-MS) [21].

### Antibiotic susceptibility testing
Antimicrobial susceptibility testing was performed by the disc diffusion method on Mueller-Hinton agar plates in accordance with the French Society of Microbiology in their 2015 recommendations guidelines. MDR *A. baumannii* isolates were defined as resistant to three or more classes of antibiotics represented by piperacillin/tazobactam,ceftazidime, imipenem, ciprofloxacin, aminoglycosides and colistin [22].

### PCR assays for detection of carbapenemase-encoding genes
DNA extractions from overnight cultures were performed using PureLink® Genomic DNA Kit (Invitrogen, Carlsbad, USA) and DNA IQ™ System (Promega Corporation, Madison, WI, USA) according to the manufacturer's instructions. PCR analysis was carried out as described previously [23, 24] using the thermocycler (Biometra, Göttingen, Germany) with the primers listed in Table 1.

Multiplex PCR assays were used to detect four carbapenemase-encoding genes ($bla_{OXA-51-like}$, $bla_{OXA-23-like}$, $bla_{OXA-24-like}$ and $bla_{OXA-58-like}$). PCR amplifications for $bla_{OXA}$ genes were performed in a final volume of 50 µl, reaction mixtures contained 5 µl of 10× PCR buffer, 25 mmol/µL of MgCI2, 2.5 Mm of deoxynucleoside triphosphates (dNTPs), 0.5 µl of each primer, 1 U Taq DNA polymerase (New England BioLabs Inc., Beverly, MA, USA) and 3 µl of DNA template. The amplification conditions were initial denaturation at 94 °C for 5 min, followed by 30 cycles of 94 °C for 25 s, 52 °C for 40s and 72 °C for 50s, with final extension for 6 min at 72 °C.

**Table 1** Primers used for amplification of carbapenemase genes [23, 24]

| Primer | Sequence (5'→3') | Amplicon size (bp) |
|---|---|---|
| OXA-51 | F: TAATGCTTTGATCGGCCTTG R: TGGATTGCACTTCATCTTGG | 353 |
| OXA-23 | F: GATCGGATTGGAGAACCAGA R: ATTTCTGACCGCATTTCCA | 501 |
| OXA-24 | F: GGTTAGTTGGCCCCCCTTAAA R: AGTTGAGCGAAAAGGGGATT | 246 |
| OXA-58 | F: AAGTATTGGGGGCTTGTGCTG R: CCCCTCTGCGCTCTACATAC | 599 |
| NDM-1 | F:CATTTGCGGGGTTTTTAATG R:CTGGGTCGAGGTCAGGATAG | 998 |

Uniplex PCR was used for detection of NDM-1 gene. PCR reaction for $bla_{NDM-1}$ gene was carried out by adding 0.5 µl of each primer, 5 µl of 10Xbuffer, 3 µl of MgCl2, 1.25 µl of dNTP's, and 0.25 µl of Taq polymerase in a final volume of 50 µl. PCR conditions were as follows: initial denaturation at 94 °C for 10 min, followed by 32 cycles consisting of denaturation at 94 °C for 30 s, 40 s annealing at 57 °C, 50 s extension at 72 °C, followed by a final extension step at 72 °C for 5 min.

Hyperladder 100 bp (Bioline, London, UK) was used as a molecular weight marker. PCR amplification products were analyzed by gel electrophoresis in a 1.5% *w/v* Agarose gel stained with SYBR safe.

### Molecular typing using pulsed-field gel electrophoresis
The clonal relationship of all isolates was analyzed by PFGE as previously described with minor modifications [25]. An overnight culture on blood agar was suspended in 120 µl of cell suspension buffer (100 mM Tris-HCl, 100 mM EDTA, pH 8.0) and then, the bacterial suspension was mixed with an equal volume of 2% InCert™ Agarose (Lonza,Rockland,ME,USA) and dispensed in a plug mould. Genomic DNA in agarose plugs was lysed in the cell lysis solution (50 Mm Tris-HCl, 1% sarcosil, 100 µg/ml proteinase K), washed and digested with ApaI (New England BioLabs Inc., Beverly, MA, USA). Electrophoresis was performed in 1% InCert™ Agarose (Lonza, Rockland,ME,USA) and 0.5X TBE Buffer (PH 8.0) containing 0.02 g of thiourea using either a CHEF-DR III system (Bio-Rad Laboratories) or a CHEF-Mapper TM apparatus (Bio-Rad Laboratories) at 6 V/cm2 with switch times ranging from 5 s to 35 s at an angle of 120°, at temperature of 14 °C, for 20 h.

A standard molecular weight Lambda DNA ladder (Bio-Rad Laboratories) was included at least twice per gel to allow normalization of all fingerprints. The Info-Quest™FP v.4.5 software (Bio-Rad Laboratories) was used for dendrogram construction by the UPGMA (Unweighted Pair Group Method with Arithmetic Mean) method, based on Dice's similarity coefficient. Isolates were considered to belong to the same PFGE cluster (pulsotype) if their Dice similarity index was ≥ 85% [26].

On the basis of the number of isolates, PFGE pulsotypes were divided into major pulsotypes (more than ten isolates/PFGE types), intermediate pulsotypes (five to nine isolates/PFGE types) and minor pulsotypes (less than five isolates/PFGE types) (Table 2).

### Multi locus sequence typing (MLST)
The whole-genome sequencing was performed on the extracted genomic DNA of the two selected strains of major pulsotypes by using the Nextera XT DNA library preparation kit (Illumina), with dual indexing adapters, and sequenced using an Illumina MiSeq sequencer with

**Table 2** Distribution of PFGE pulsotypes according to the source of samples and status of pulsotypes

| PFGE pulsotype | Clinical isolates (N = 47) | Environmental isolates (N = 36) | Total (N = 83) | Status of pulsotypes |
|---|---|---|---|---|
| | N (%) | N (%) | N (%) | |
| 0001 | 7(14.9) | 1(2.8) | 8(9.6) | Intermediate pulsotype |
| 0002 | 1(2.1) | 2(5.6) | 3(3.6) | Minor pulsotype |
| 0003 | 1(2.1) | 4(11.1) | 5(6) | Intermediate pulsotype |
| 0004 | 2(2.4) | 0 | 2(4.3) | Minor pulsotype |
| 0005 | 3(6.4) | 4(11.1) | 7(8.4) | Intermediate pulsotype |
| 0006 | 1(2.1) | 0 | 1(1.2) | Minor pulsotype (Singleton) |
| 0007 | 16(34) | 3(8.3) | 19(22.9) | Major pulsotype |
| 0008 | 14(29.8) | 16(44.4) | 30(36.1) | Major pulsotype |
| 0009 | 2(4.3) | 6(16.7) | 8(9.6) | Intermediate pulsotype |

a 2 × 251-bp paired-end configuration. The Next Generation Sequencing Data (FASTA format) were then used for further MLST analysis, carried out using MLST Oxford scheme (https://pubmlst.org/abaumannii/).

## Statistical analysis

Statistical analysis was performed using SPSS Statistics for Windows, version 10.0. The results were expressed as effective and percentages for qualitative variables and as mean (standard deviation) or median (interquartile range: IQR) for quantitative variables. The chi-square and Fisher exact tests were used to compare the qualitative variables. A comparison between the two quantitative variables was performed using the Mann–Whitney U test for non-normal distributed variables, whereas Student's $t$-test was used for normally distributed variables. $P$ values less than 0.05 were considered significant.

## Results

### Bacterial isolates and epidemiological data

A total of 83 non-duplicate *A. baumannii* isolates were collected: 47 clinical isolates from 40 colonized or infected patients and 36 isolates from 72 environmental specimens.

Among 40 patients, 32 (80%) were colonized and 8 (20%) were infected. The epidemiological and clinical characteristics of patients are shown in Table 3. The average age was 54.38 ± 15.22 years and 30 (75%) were males representing a sex ratio M/F of 3:1. The crude mortality rate was 54.2%. The crude mortality rate was 43.8% in colonized patients and 87.5% in infected ones ($p$ = 0.031). Clinical isolates were recovered from 39 screening samples including anal margin (22/47 = 46.8%), mouth (10/47 = 21.3%), groin (7/47 = 14.9%) and from 8 diagnosis samples composed of blood culture (3/47 = 6.4%), protected distal sampling (3/47 = 6.4%) and bronchial aspiration (2/47 = 4.2%).

Of the 72 environmental samples, 36 (50%) yielded *A. baumannii* isolates. Surgical ICU samples were more contaminated (22/31 = 71%) than those from the medical ICU (14/41 = 34.1%) ($p$ = 0.004). The environmental *A. baumannii* isolates were obtained from bed sheets (14/36 = 38.9%), floors (13/36 = 36.1%), medical ventilators (4/36 = 11.1%), patient trolleys (2/36 = 5.5%), pillows (1/36 = 2.8%), monitors (1/36 = 2.8%), and intravenous solution stands (1/36 = 2.8%).

### Antimicrobial susceptibility profile

All isolates were MDR. The difference in resistance rates between the clinical isolates and the environmental ones was not statistically significant except for gentamicin (85.1% vs 100% respectively, $p$ = 0.015).

### Distribution of carbapenemase genes

The intrinsic chromosomally encoded $bla_{OXA-51\ like}$ gene characteristic of *A. baumannii* was detected in all isolates. All isolates were positive for $bla_{OXA-23-like}$. The coexistence of $bla_{NDM-1}$ with $bla_{OXA-23-like}$ and $bla_{OXA\ 24-like}$ with $bla_{OXA-23}$ was detected in 27 (32.5%) and 2 (2.4%) of *A. baumannii* isolates, respectively. The $bla_{OXA-58-like}$ gene was not detected. The percentage of NDM-1 carriage was significantly higher in environmental isolates than in clinical ones (18/36 = 50% vs 9/47 = 19.1%, $p$ = 0.004). NDM-1 producing clinical isolates were recovered from: anal margin (88.9%) and mouth (11.1%). The NDM-1 harboring isolates were significantly ($p$ = 0.006) more frequently isolated from anal margin samples than from other clinical specimens. The distribution of NDM-1 positive isolates among hospital environment samples is as follows: bed sheets (38.9%), floor (16.7%), medical ventilators (16.7%), intravenous solution stands (5.5%), monitors (5.5%), patient trolleys (5.5%) and pillows (5.5%). No significant differences ($p$ = 0.432) in the number of NDM-1 positive isolates were found between different environmental sampling sites.

### PFGE and MLST analyses

The isolates were classified into 9 PFGE pulsotypes (0001–0009) with two major pulsotypes (0008, 0007),

**Table 3** Epidemiological and clinical features of colonized or infected patients

| Variable | Total N = 40 |
| --- | --- |
| Number of Male patients(%) | 30(75) |
| Mean Age (years) (Mean ± Standard deviation) | 52.45 ± 16.5 |
| Median length of ICU stay (days) [IQR] | 10 [5–16] |
| Patients with lenght of ICU stay ≥7 days (%) | 26(65) |
| Median duration of ICU stay prior to Colonization/infection(days) [IQR] | 6[1.5–16.5] |
| Respiratory distress | 7(17.5) |
| postoperative care | 10(25) |
| Cerebrovascular accidents | 13(32.5) |
| Severe polytrauma | 6(15) |
| Underlyning disease | N (%) |
| Diabetes | 7(17.5) |
| Chronic renal failure | 5(12.5) |
| Arterial hypertension | 6(15) |
| Chronic heart failure | 7(17.5) |
| Chronic obstructive pulmonary disease | 6(15) |
| Chronic smoking | 6(15) |
| Solid tumor | 7(17.5) |
| Invasive procedure | N (%) |
| Venous catheter | 11(27.5) |
| Arterial catheter | 4(10) |
| Urinary catheter | 26(65) |
| Mechanical ventilation | 24(60) |
| Nasogastric tube | 3(7.5) |
| Abdominal drain | 4(10) |
| Recent surgery | 4(10) |
| Parenteral nutrition | 30(77.5) |
| Dialysis | 3(7.5) |
| Septic shock N (%) | 14(76) |
| Previous antibiotic treatment N (%) | 35(87.5) |
| Amoxicillin/clavulanic acid N (%) | 10(25) |
| Ceftriaxone N (%) | 7(17.5) |
| Imipenem N (%) | 23(57.5) |
| Aminoglycosides N (%) | 19(47.5) |
| Colistin | 9(22.5) |
| Ciprofloxacin | 3(7.5) |
| Corticosteroid therapy N (%) | 19(47.5) |
| Death rate N (%) | 21(52.5) |

ICU Intensive care unit, IQR Interquartile rang

containing up to 59% of all isolates. The strains of pulsotype 0008 belonged to sequence type (ST) 195 while those of pulsotype 0007 belonged to ST 1089. Clinical isolates were found in all 9 different pulsotypes while

environmental isolates were only present in 7 pulsotypes, as they were missing from pulsotypes 0004 and 0006 which included just 2 and 1 isolates, respectively (Table 2) (Fig. 1) (Additional file 1) .

## Discussion

In the present study we have analyzed the clonal relatedness and resistance characteristics of A. baumannii isolates recovered. The clinical isolates were commonly isolated from the anal margin (46.8%) followed by the mouth (24%). The digestive tract of patients hospitalized in the ICU, has been identified as an important site for Acinetobacter colonization which can lead to severe infections, with a prevalence of 8.3% in Saudi Arabia [2] and 41% in Spain [3]. A study conducted in Spain by Corbella et al. showed that MDR A. baumannii infections occurred more frequently in patients with fecal colonization than in those without fecal colonization [3]. The crude mortality found in this study (50%) was comparable to that reported in colonized or infected patients in Italy (58%) [27] but significantly higher than that of Spanish hospitals (18.9%) [4].The mortality rate of patients depends on clinical significance of A. baumannii. In the current study, the mortality rate was significantly higher in infected patients than in colonized ones (87.5% vs 43.8%, $p = 0.031$). This result is similar to that of Rodríguez-Baño J et al. in Spain who showed that crude mortality was higher in infected (27%) than in colonized patients (10%) [4].

Our findings show a higher environmental contamination around infected or colonized patients in our ICU. The presence of A. baumannii among environmental specimens (50%) was higher than that observed in similar studies: 7.7% in Algeria [7], 9.9% in the United States of America [19], 13.1% in China [16] and between 2% and 18% in two different studies in Turkey [5, 6]. This can be attributed to the lack of hospital decontamination procedures and hand hygiene in our region. This study also shows that the surgical ICU samples were more contaminated than those of medical ICU (71% vs 37.2%, $p = 0.004$) and the sites frequently touched by both the health-care workers and patients were the most contaminated as the majority of environmental isolates were recovered from floors (42.1%) followed by bed sheets (34.2%) and medical ventilators (10.5%). These findings are in agreement with that of other researchers who reported that this pathogen was isolated from near-patient surfaces, medical equipment, airborne samples and healthcare workers' hands [5–7, 19].

In the current study, all isolates were resistant to imipinem. Carbapenem-resistance among A. baumannii isolates has shown a steady increase in our region since 2001, when it was reported around 23.6% [28] and then increased to 76.19% in 2012–2014 [8]. This can be explained by the excessive use of inadequate empirical

Dice (Opt: 1.50%) (Tol 1.5%-1.5%) (H>0.0% S>0.0%) [0.0%-100%]

| Strain | Source | Unit | Pulsetype | Carbapenemase |
|---|---|---|---|---|
| 46 | C | M-ICU | 0001 | OXA-23 |
| 8 | C | M-ICU | 0001 | OXA-23 |
| 9 | E | M-ICU | 0001 | OXA-23 |
| 26 | C | S-ICU | 0001 | OXA-23/NDM-1 |
| 35 | C | S-ICU | 0001 | OXA-23/NDM-1 |
| 25 | C | S-ICU | 0001 | OXA-23/NDM-1 |
| 21 | C | S-ICU | 0001 | OXA-23 |
| 20 | C | S-ICU | 0001 | OXA-23 |
| 39 | C | S-ICU | 0002 | OXA-23/NDM-1 |
| 11 | E | M-ICU | 0002 | OXA-23/NDM-1 |
| 17 | E | S-ICU | 0002 | OXA-23/NDM-1 |
| 28 | E | M-ICU | 0003 | OXA-23 |
| 30 | E | M-ICU | 0003 | OXA-23 |
| 34 | E | S-ICU | 0003 | OXA-23 |
| 29 | E | S-ICU | 0003 | OXA-23 |
| 36 | C | M-ICU | 0003 | OXA-23 |
| 42 | C | S-ICU | 0004 | OXA-23 |
| 44 | C | M-ICU | 0004 | OXA-23 |
| 2 | C | S-ICU | 0005 | OXA-23 |
| 4 | E | S-ICU | 0005 | OXA-23 |
| 12 | E | M-ICU | 0005 | OXA-23 |
| 14 | E | M-ICU | 0005 | OXA-23 |
| 20 | E | S-ICU | 0005 | OXA-23 |
| 14 | C | M-ICU | 0005 | OXA-23 |
| 4 | C | S-ICU | 0006 | OXA-23 |
| 33 | C | M-ICU | 0006 | OXA-23 |
| 16 | C | S-ICU | 0007 | OXA-23/OXA-24 |
| 18 | C | S-ICU | 0007 | OXA-23/OXA-24 |
| 17 | C | S-ICU | 0007 | OXA-23 |
| 15 | C | M-ICU | 0007 | OXA-23 |
| 22 | C | S-ICU | 0007 | OXA-23 |
| 24 | C | M-ICU | 0007 | OXA-23 |
| 10 | C | M-ICU | 0007 | OXA-23 |
| 5 | C | S-ICU | 0007 | OXA-23 |
| 6 | C | M-ICU | 0007 | OXA-23 |
| 27 | E | M-ICU | 0007 | OXA-23/NDM-1 |
| 43 | C | S-ICU | 0007 | OXA-23 |
| 40 | C | M-ICU | 0007 | OXA-23 |
| 15 | E | M-ICU | 0007 | OXA-23 |
| 16 | E | S-ICU | 0007 | OXA-23 |
| 7 | C | S-ICU | 0007 | OXA-23 |
| 30 | C | M-ICU | 0007 | OXA-23/NDM-1 |
| 29 | C | S-ICU | 0007 | OXA-23/NDM-1 |
| 27 | C | S-ICU | 0007 | OXA-23/NDM-1 |
| 28 | C | M-ICU | 0007 | OXA-23/NDM-1 |
| 47 | C | S-ICU | 0008 | OXA-23 |
| 3 | C | S-ICU | 0008 | OXA-23 |
| 25 | E | S-ICU | 0008 | OXA-23/NDM-1 |
| 32 | C | M-ICU | 0008 | OXA-23 |
| 38 | C | S-ICU | 0008 | OXA-23 |
| 37 | C | M-ICU | 0008 | OXA-23 |
| 34 | C | S-ICU | 0008 | OXA-23 |
| 19 | C | S-ICU | 0008 | OXA-23 |
| 45 | C | S-ICU | 0008 | OXA-23 |
| 1 | C | S-ICU | 0008 | OXA-23 |
| 31 | C | S-ICU | 0008 | OXA-23 |
| 7 | E | M-ICU | 0008 | OXA-23/NDM-1 |
| 24 | E | S-ICU | 0008 | OXA-23 |
| 13 | E | S-ICU | 0008 | OXA-23/NDM-1 |
| 12 | C | M-ICU | 0008 | OXA-23/NDM-1 |
| 1 | E | S-ICU | 0008 | OXA-23/NDM-1 |
| 2 | E | S-ICU | 0008 | OXA-23/NDM-1 |
| 3 | E | S-ICU | 0008 | OXA-23/NDM-1 |
| 5 | E | S-ICU | 0008 | OXA-23/NDM-1 |
| 6 | E | S-ICU | 0008 | OXA-23/NDM-1 |
| 8 | E | S-ICU | 0008 | OXA-23/NDM-1 |
| 10 | E | M-ICU | 0008 | OXA-23/NDM-1 |
| 18 | E | S-ICU | 0008 | OXA-23/NDM-1 |
| 19 | E | S-ICU | 0008 | OXA-23/NDM-1 |
| 21 | E | M-ICU | 0008 | OXA-23/NDM-1 |
| 22 | E | M-ICU | 0008 | OXA-23/NDM-1 |
| 13 | C | M-ICU | 0008 | OXA-23 |
| 9 | C | S-ICU | 0008 | OXA-23 |
| 11 | C | M-ICU | 0008 | OXA-23 |
| 26 | E | S-ICU | 0008 | OXA-23/NDM-1 |
| 32 | E | S-ICU | 0009 | OXA-23 |
| 33 | E | S-ICU | 0009 | OXA-23 |
| 23 | C | M-ICU | 0009 | OXA-23 |
| 31 | E | M-ICU | 0009 | OXA-23 |
| 35 | E | M-ICU | 0009 | OXA-23 |
| 36 | E | S-ICU | 0009 | OXA-23 |
| 41 | C | S-ICU | 0009 | OXA-23 |
| 23 | E | M-ICU | 0009 | OXA-23 |

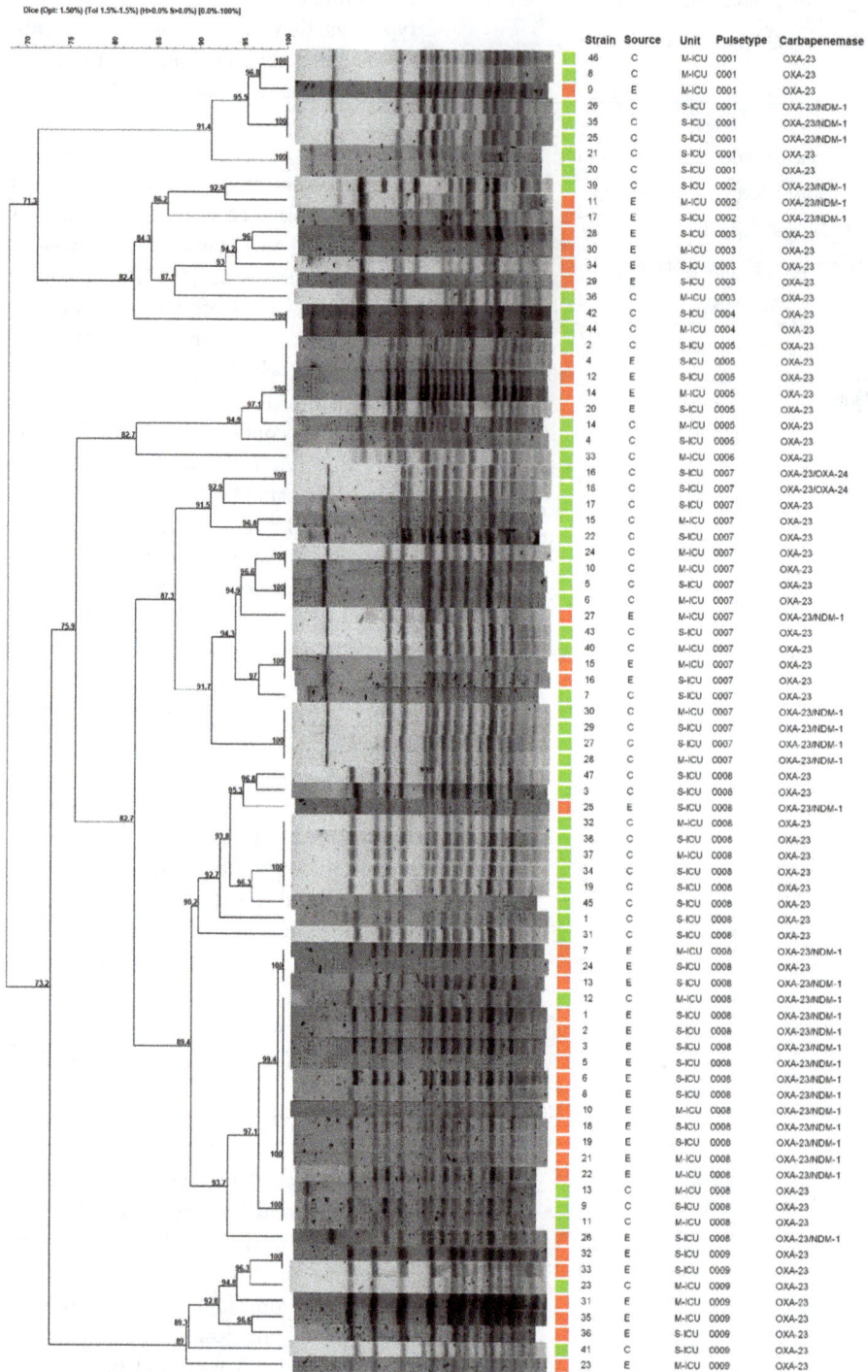

**Fig. 1** PFGE dendrogram of Clinical and environmental *A.baumannii* isolates (M-ICU: Medical intensive care unit, S-ICU: Surgical intensive care unit)

antimicrobial treatment including carbapenems, poor infection control practices, poor antimicrobial stewardship governance and widespread dissemination of carbapenem-resistant strains in the community.

In the present study, carbapenem-resistance was mainly attributed to the carriage of the $bla_{OXA-23-like}$ gene that was present in all isolates (100%). This prevalence is similar to that reported in Turkey (100%) [11] and Egypt (100%) [12] but higher than that observed in Brazil (95.4%) [29], Asian pacific countries (95%) [9], France (82%) [30], South Africa (77%) [31] and Italy (71.7%) [10]. During the past decades, outbreak or sporadic *A. baumannii* clones producing OXA-

23 have disseminated around the world [32] but such dissemination has been particularly relevant among Mediterranean countries, where the $bla_{OXA-23-like}$ gene has replaced previously predominant blaOXA genes such as $bla_{OXA-24-like}$ and $bla_{OXA-58-like}$ [33]. In our study, only 2 clinical isolates also harbored the $bla_{OXA-24-like}$ gene (4.25%) but this gene was not detected among the environmental isolates and all isolates were negative for the $bla_{OXA-58-like}$ gene. The high prevalence of $bla_{OXA-23-like}$ gene is probably associated with horizontal gene transfer by mobile genetic elements such as plasmids, transposable elements and integron systems. It has been reported that the spread of $bla_{OXA-23-like}$ genes is associated with the Tn2006, Tn2007, Tn2008, and Tn2009 transposons, which can be further located on the chromosome or on conjugative plasmids [32, 34, 35].

Likewise, 32.5% of all isolates also presented the $bla_{NDM-1}$ gene and this is the first time that NDM-producing A. baumannii isolates are reported in Morocco. Our results indicate that NDM-1-producing A. baumannii isolates are widely circulating in the hospital environment and they were found in all environmental sampling sites. Moreover, the NDM-1-producing A. baumannii isolates were more frequently recovered ($p$ = 0.004) from environmental isolates (50%) than from clinical isolates (19.1%). The environmental NDM-1 producing A. baumannii isolates have also been reported in Algeria [7] and in China [36]. The high rate of environmental $bla_{NDM-1}$ contamination is alarming as the hospital environment may become a potential reservoir for A. baumannii isolates carrying NDM-1 which could result in transfer the $bla_{NDM-1}$ gene to other bacterial species.

Among clinical isolates, the anal margin samples were identified ($p$ = 0.006) as the most common sites of isolation of NDM-1-producing A. baumannii isolates. These findings also highlight the role played by fecally-colonized patients as reservoirs for carbapenem-resistant nosocomial A. baumannii isolates.

In the current study, the genetic similarity between clinical and environmental isolates was observed in (80/83 = 96.4%) of all isolates, classified into 7 pulsotypes (0001, 0002, 0003, 0005, 0007, 0008 and 0009). These results suggest a dynamic exchange of A. baumannii isolates between patients and their environmental surroundings. These pathogens can be transmitted from patient-to-patient, patient to a health care worker, patient to environment and vice versa. In our study, three clinical isolates belonging to the pulsotypes (0004 and 0006) which were not detected in environmental isolates, may be exclusively transmitted through direct contact between an infected or colonized patient and another person or they may come from other environmental reservoirs which are either rare or not identified in our study.

Our results also show that the most frequent pulsotype was PFGE type 0008 (30/83 = 36.1%). Among the two major pulsotypes, clinical isolates were predominant within pulsotype 0007 (16/47 = 34%) while environmental isolates were a majority within pulsotype 0008 (16/36 = 44.4%). Overall, however, both major pulsotypes were closely related (Dice similarity >82%) and contained up to 59% of all isolates, they were found in all sampling sites and it is clear that they have become endemic in this particular setting. The PFGE cluster 0008 corresponds to ST195 (Oxford MLST) which has been previously reported from Asian countries, European nations and Egypt [37–39] while the strains from pulsotype 0007 were assigned to ST 1089(Oxford MLST) which is very rare ST and according to "the profile history for A. baumannii MLST (Oxford) database", the ST 1089 has been found for the first time in India in 2015.

## Conclusion

This study shows that the clonal spread of environmental A. baumannii isolates is related to that of clinical isolates recovered from colonized or infected patients. Our results have also shown that OXA-23 is the most common carbapenemase among A. baumannii isolates in our hospital but the prevalence of isolates producing both OXA-23 and NDM-1 is also alarming.

Effective control measures are urgently needed to prevent the transmission of endemic lineages of MDR A. baumannii and they should take into account the decontamination of the patients' environmental surroundings.

### Abbreviation

DNA: Deoxyribonucleic acid; dNTPs: deoxynucleoside triphosphates; ICU: Intensive care unit; IQR: Interquartile range; MALDI-TOF-MS: Matrix-assisted laser desorption/ionization time-of-flight mass spectrometry; MDR: Multidrug-resistant; MLST: Multi locus sequence typing; PCR: Polymerase chain reaction; PFGE: Pulsed-field gel electrophoresis; ST: Sequence type; UPGMA: Unweighted Pair Group Method with Arithmetic Mean

### Acknowledgements

Not applicable.

### Funding

This work was supported by a grant from Mohammed V Military Teaching Hospital and from the Ministry of Higher education of Morocco.
This study was also supported by grant 2014SGR0653 from the Departament de Universitats, Recerca i Societat de la Informació de la Generalitat de Catalunya, by the Ministerio de Economía y Competitividad, Instituto de Salud Carlos III, co-financed by European Regional Development Fund (ERDF) "A Way to Achieve Europe," the Spanish Network for Research in Infectious Diseases (REIPI RD12/0015).
The research leading to these results has also received funding from the People Programme (Marie Curie Actions) of the European Union's seventh Framework Programme FP7/2007–2013 under REA grant agreement n° 612,216.

### Authors' contributions

UJ, EM, JV and IG participated in study design, interpreted the results and wrote the manuscript. UJ, MF, BB and FB involved in data acquisition and in laboratory work. YB, JK, TA, ND, AB, CH, LL participated in the review of literature. LA and AI provided critical revision of the manuscript. All authors approved final version of manuscript.

## Competing interests

The authors declare that they have no competing interests.

## Author details

[1]Department of Clinical Bacteriology, Mohammed V Military Teaching Hospital, Research Team of Epidemiology and Bacterial Resistance, Faculty of Medicine and Pharmacy, Mohammed V University, Rabat, Morocco. [2]Department of Clinical Microbiology and ISGlobal- Barcelona Ctr. Int. Health Res. CRESIB, Hospital Clínic - Universitat de Barcelona, Barcelona, Spain. [3]Medical Biotechnology Laboratory (Medbiotech), Faculty of Medicine and Pharmacy, Mohammed V University, Rabat, Morocco. [4]Department of Intensive Care Units , Mohammed V Military Teaching Hospital, Faculty of Medicine and Pharmacy, Mohammed V University, Rabat, Morocco.

## References

1. Manchanda V, Sanchaita S, Singh N. Multidrug Resistant Acinetobacter. J Glob Infect Dis. 2010;2(3):291–304.
2. Aljindan R, Bukharie H, Alomar A, Abdalhamid B. Prevalence of digestive tract colonization of Carbapenem-Resistant acinetobacter baumannii in hospitals in Saudi Arabia. J Med Microbiol. 2015;64(Pt 4):400–6.
3. Corbella X, Pujol M, Ayats J, Sendra M, Ardanuy C, Domínguez MA, Liñares J, Ariza J, Gudiol F. Relevance of digestive tract colonization in the epidemiology of nosocomial infections due to multiresistant Acinetobacter baumannii. Clin Infect Dis. 1996;23(2):329–34.
4. Rodríguez-Baño J, Cisneros JM, Fernández-Cuenca F, Ribera A, Vila J, Pascual A, Martínez-Martínez L, Bou G, Pachón J, Grupo de Estudio de Infección Hospitalaria (GEIH). Clinical Features and Epidemiology of Acinetobacter baumannii Colonization and Infection in Spanish Hospitals. Infect Control Hosp Epidemiol. 2004;25(10):819–24.
5. Kirkgoz E, Zer Y. Clonal comparison of Acinetobacter strains isolated from intensive care patients and the intensive care unit environment. Turk J Med Sci. 2014;44(4):643–8.
6. Ertürk A, Çiçek AÇ, Gümüş A, Cüre E, Şen A, Kurt A, Karagöz A, Aydoğan N, Sandallı C, Durmaz R. Molecular characterisation and control of Acinetobacter baumannii isolates resistant to multi-drugs emerging in inter-intensive care units. Ann Clin Microbiol Antimicrob. 2014;13:36.
7. Zenati K, Touati A, Bakour S, Sahli F, Rolain JM. Characterization of NDM-1- and OXA-23-producing Acinetobacter baumannii isolates from inanimate surfaces in a hospital environment in Algeria. J Hosp Infect. 2016;92(1):19–26.
8. Uwingabiye J, Frikh M, Lemnouer A, Bssaibis F, Belefquih B, Maleb A, Dahraoui S, Belyamani L, Bait A, Haimeur C, Louzi L, Ibrahimi A, Elouennass M. Acinetobacter infections prevalence and frequency of the antibiotics resistance: comparative study of intensive care units versus other hospital units. Pan Afr Med J. 2016;23:191.
9. Mendes RE, Bell JM, Turnidge JD, Castanheira M, Jones RN. Emergence and widespread dissemination of OXA-23, −24/40 and −58 carbapenemases among Acinetobacter spp. in Asia-Pacific nations: report from the SENTRY Surveillance Program. J Antimicrob Chemother. 2009;63(1):55–9.
10. D'Arezzo S, Principe L, Capone A, Petrosillo N, Petrucca A, Visca P. Changing carbapenemase gene pattern in an epidemic multidrug-resistant Acinetobacter baumannii lineage causing multiple outbreaks in central Italy. J Antimicrob Chemother. 2011;66(1):54–61.
11. Aksoy MD, Çavuşlu Ş, Tuğrul HM. Investigation of metallo beta lactamases and oxacillinases in carbapenem resistant Acinetobacter baumannii strains isolated from inpatients. Balkan Med J. 2015;32(1):79–83.
12. Fouad M, Attia AS, Tawakkol WM, Hashem AM. Emergence of carbapenem-resistant Acinetobacter baumannii harboring the OXA-23 carbapenemase in intensive care units of Egyptian hospitals. Int J Infect Dis. 2013;17(12):e1252–4.
13. Mesli E, Berrazeg M, Drissi M, Bekkhoucha SN, Rolain JM. Prevalence of carbapenemase-encoding genes including New Delhi metallo-β-lactamase in Acinetobacter species. Algeria Int J Infect Dis. 2013;17(9):e739–43.
14. Berrazeg M, Diene S, Medjahed L, Parola P, Drissi M, Raoult D, Rolain J. New Delhi Metallo-beta-lactamase around the world : An eReview using Google Maps. Euro Surveill. 2014;19(20):20809.
15. Wei WJ, Yang HF, Ye Y, Li JB. New Delhi Metallo-β-Lactamase-Mediated Carbapenem Resistance: Origin, Diagnosis, Treatment and Public Health Concern. Chin Med J. 2015;128(14):1969–76.
16. Ying C, Li Y, Wang Y, Zheng B, Yang C. Investigation of the molecular epidemiology of Acinetobacter baumannii isolated from patients and environmental contamination. J Antibiot (Tokyo). 2015;68(9):562–7.
17. Tjoa E, Moehario LH, Rukmana A, Rohsiswatmo R. Acinetobacter baumannii: Role in blood stream infection in Neonatal Unit, Dr. Cipto Mangunkusumo Hospital, Jakarta, Indonesia. Int. J Microbiol. 2013;2013:180763.
18. Horan TC, Andrus M, Dudeck MA. CDC/NHSN surveillance definition of health care-associated infection and criteria for specific types of infections in the acute care setting. Am J Infect Control. 2008;36(5):309–32.
19. Thom KA, Johnson JK, Lee MS, Harris AD. Environmental contamination because of multidrug-resistant Acinetobacter baumannii surrounding colonized or infected patients. Am J Infect Control. 2011;39(9):711–5.
20. Sehulster L, Chinn RY, CDC; HICPAC. Guidelines for environmental infection control in health-care facilities. Recommendations of CDC and the Healthcare Infection Control Practices Advisory Committee (HICPAC). MMWR Recomm Rep. 2003;52(RR-10):1–42.
21. Marí-Almirall M, Cosgaya C, Higgins PG, Van Assche A, Telli M, Huys G, Lievens B, Seifert H, Dijkshoorn L, Roca I, Vila J. MALDI-TOF/MS identification of species from the Acinetobacter baumannii (Ab) group revisited: inclusion of the novel A. seifertii and A. dijkshoorniae species. Clin Microbiol Infect. 2017;23(3):210.e1–9.
22. Magiorakos AP, Srinivasan A, Carey RB, Carmeli Y, Falagas ME, Giske CG, Harbarth S, Hindler JF, Kahlmeter G, Olsson-Liljequist B, Paterson DL, Rice LB, Stelling J, Struelens MJ, Vatopoulos A, Weber JT, Monnet DL. Multidrug-resistant, extensively drug-resistant and pandrug-resistant bacteria: an international expert proposal for interim standard definitions for acquired resistance. Clin Microbiol Infect. 2012;18(3):268–81.
23. Woodford N, Ellington MJ, Coelho JM, Turton JF, Ward ME, Brown S, Amyes SG, Livermore DM. Multiplex PCR for genes encoding prevalent OXA carbapenemases in Acinetobacter spp. Int J Antimicrob Agents. 2006;27(4):351–3.
24. Diene SM, Bruder N, Raoult D, Rolain JM. Real-time PCR assay allows detection of the New Delhi metallo-β-lactamase (NDM-1)-encoding gene in France. Int J Antimicrob Agents. 2011;37(6):544–6.
25. Seifert H, Dolzani L, Bressan R, van der Reijden T, van Strijen B, Stefanik D, Heersma H, Dijkshoorn L. Standardization and interlaboratory reproducibility assessment of pulsed-field gel electrophoresis-generated fingerprints of Acinetobacter baumannii. J Clin Microbiol. 2005;43(9):4328–35.
26. Durmaz R, Otlu B, Koksal F, Hosoglu S, Ozturk R, Ersoy Y, Aktas E, Gursoy NC, Caliskan A. The optimization of a rapid pulsed-field gel electrophoresis protocol for the typing of Acinetobacter baumannii, Escherichia coli and Klebsiella spp. Jpn J Infect Dis. 2009;62(5):372–7.
27. Zarrilli R, Casillo R, Di Popolo A, Tripodi MF, Bagattini M, Cuccurullo S, Crivaro V, Ragone E, Mattei A, Galdieri N, Triassi M, Utili R. Molecular epidemiology of a clonal outbreak of multidrug-resistant Acinetobacter baumannii in a university hospital in Italy. Clin Microbiol Infect. 2007;13(5):481–9.
28. Elouennass M, Bajou T, Lemnouer AH, Foissaud V, Hervé VBA. Acinetobacter baumannii : étude de la sensibilité des souches isolées à l'hôpital militaire d'instruction MohammedV, Rabat, Maroc. Med Mal Infect. 2003;33:361–4.
29. Corrêa LL, Botelho LA, Barbosa LC, Mattos CS, Carballido JM, de Castro CL, Mondino PJ, de Paula GR, de Mondino SS, de Mendonça-Souza CR. Detection of bla(OXA-23) in Acinetobacter spp. isolated from patients of a university hospital. Braz J Infect Dis. 2012;16(6):521–6.
30. Jeannot K, Diancourt L, Vaux S, Thouverez M, Ribeiro A, Coignard B, Courvalin P, Brisse S. Molecular epidemiology of carbapenem non-susceptible Acinetobacter baumannii in France. PLoS One. 2014;9(12):e115452.
31. Lowings M, Ehlers MM, Dreyer AW, Kock MM. High prevalence of oxacillinases in clinical multidrug-resistant Acinetobacter baumannii isolates from the Tshwane region, South Africa - an update. BMC Infect Dis. 2015 Nov 14;15:521.
32. Mugnier PD, Poirel L, Naas T, Nordmann P. Worldwide dissemination of the blaOXA-23 Carbapenemase gene of Acinetobacter baumannii. Emerg Infect Dis. 2010;16(1):35–40.
33. Djahmi N, Dunyach-Remy C, Pantel A, Dekhil M, Sotto A, Lavigne JP. Epidemiology of Carbapenemase-Producing Enterobacteriaceae and Acinetobacter baumannii in Mediterranean Countries. Biomed Res Int. 2014;2014:305784.
34. Liu LL, Ji SJ, Ruan Z, Fu Y, Fu YQ, Wang YF, Yu YS. Dissemination of blaOXA-23 in Acinetobacter spp. in China: Main Roles of Conjugative Plasmid pAZJ221 and Transposon Tn2009. Antimicrob Agents Chemother. 2015;59(4):1998–2005.

35.  Guerrero-Lozano I, Fernández-Cuenca F, Galán-Sánchez F, Egea P,
     Rodríguez-Iglesias M, Pascual Á. Description of the OXA-23 β-lactamase
     gene located within Tn2007 in a clinical isolate of Acinetobacter baumannii
     from Spain. Microb Drug Resist. 2015;21(2):215–7.
36.  Zhang C, Qiu S, Wang Y, Qi L, Hao R, Liu X, Shi Y, Hu X, An D, Li Z, Li P,
     Wang L, Cui J, Wang P, Huang L, Klena JD, Song H. Higher Isolation of
     NDM-1 Producing Acinetobacter baumannii from the Sewage of the
     Hospitals in Beijing. PLoS One PLoS One. 2013;8(6):e64857.
37.  Ghaith DM, Zafer MM, Al-Agamy MH, Alyamani EJ, Booq RY, Almoazzamy O.
     The emergence of a novel sequence type of MDR Acinetobacter baumannii
     from the intensive care unit of an Egyptian tertiary care hospital. Ann Clin
     Microbiol Antimicrob. 2017;16(1):34.
38.  Hammerum AM, Hansen F, Skov MN, Stegger M, Andersen PS, Holm A,
     Jakobsen L, Justesen US. Investigation of a possible outbreak of
     carbapenem-resistant Acinetobacter baumannii in Odense, Denmark using
     PFGE, MLST and whole-genome-based SNPs. J Antimicrob Chemother.
     2015;70(7):1965–8.
39.  Rieber H, Frontzek A, Pfeifer Y. Molecular Investigation of Carbapenem-
     Resistant Acinetobacter spp. from Hospitals in North Rhine-Westphalia,
     Germany. Microb Drug Resist. 2017;23(1):25–31.

# 15

# Multidrug-resistant gram-negative bacterial infections in a teaching hospital in Ghana

Nicholas Agyepong[1], Usha Govinden[1], Alex Owusu-Ofori[2*] ⓘ and Sabiha Yusuf Essack[1]

## Abstract

**Background:** Multidrug-resistant Gram-negative bacteria have emerged as major clinical and therapeutic dilemma in hospitals in Ghana.
To describe the prevalence and profile of infections attributable to multidrug-resistant Gram-negative bacteria among patients at the Komfo Anokye Teaching Hospital in the Ashanti region of Ghana.

**Methods:** Bacterial cultures were randomly selected from the microbiology laboratory from February to August, 2015. Bacterial identification and minimum inhibitory concentrations were conducted using standard microbiological techniques and the Vitek-2 automated system. Patient information was retrieved from the hospital data.

**Results:** Of the 200 isolates, consisting of *K. pneumoniae*, *A. baumannii*, *P. aeruginosa*, *Enterobacter spp.*, *E. coli*, *Yersinia spp.*, *Proteus mirabilis*, *Pasteurella spp.*, *Chromobacterium violaceum*, *Salmomella enterica*, *Vibrio spp.*, *Citrobacter koseri*, *Pantoea spp.*, *Serratia spp.*, *Providencia rettgeri Burkholderia cepacia*, *Aeromonas spp.*, *Cadecea lapagei* and *Sphingomonas paucimobilis*, 101 (50.5%) and 99 (49.5%) recovered from male and female patients respectively The largest proportion of patients were from age-group ≥60 years (24.5%) followed by < 10 years (24.0%) and least 10–19 years (9.5%) with a mean patient age of 35.95 ± 27.11 (0.2–91) years. The decreasing order of specimen source was urine 97 (48.5%), wound swabs 47 (23.5%), sputum 22 (11.0%) bronchial lavage, nasal and pleural swabs 1 (0.50%). Urinary tract infection was diagnosed in 34.5% of patients, sepsis in 14.5%, wound infections (surgical and chronic wounds) in 11.0%, pulmonary tuberculosis in 9.0% and appendicitis, bacteremia and cystitis in 0.50%. The isolates showed high resistance to ampicillin (94.4%), trimethoprim/sulfamethoxazole (84.5%), cefuroxime (79.0%) and cefotaxime (71.3%) but low resistance to ertapenem (1.5%), meropenem (3%) and amikacin (11%). The average multi-drug resistance was 89.5%, and ranged from 53.8% in *Enterobacter* spp. to 100.0% in *Acinetobacter* spp. and *P. aeruginosa*.

**Conclusion:** Bacterial infections caused by multi-drug resistant (isolates resistant to at least one agent in three or more antibiotic classes) Gram-negative pathogens among patients at Komfo Anokye Teaching Hospital in Kumasi, Ghana are rife and interventions are necessary for their containment.

**Keywords:** Antibiotic resistance, Infections, Multidrug resistance, Pathogens

## Background

The emergence of multidrug-resistant Gram-negative bacteria is a major concern in hospital settings in many parts of the world. Infections caused by these pathogens have become significantly challenging over the past two decades, particularly in the developing countries, and are associated with high morbidity and mortality rates as well as protracted hospital stay [1]. Enterobacteriaceae including *Klebsiella pneumoniae*, *Escherichia coli* as well as *Enterobacter spp.* and non-lactose fermenting bacteria such as *Pseudomonas aeruginosa* and *Acinetobacter spp.* have been identified as major cause of multi-drug resistant bacterial infections [2–4].

Studies conducted in many developing countries including Africa, have indicated high antibiotic resistance among Gram-negative bacteria to commonly used antibiotics, leading to a loss of efficacy for treatment of common infections [5–7]. These resistant bacterial pathogens are a major cause of both community and hospital-acquired infections. Respiratory tract, urinary tract, bloodstream (septic), post-surgical (wound) infections and pneumonia are among

* Correspondence: owusu_ofori@hotmail.com
[2]School of Medical Sciences, Kwame Nkrumah University of Science and Technology, Kumasi, Ghana
Full list of author information is available at the end of the article

most commonly reported infections attributable to these pathogens in many hospitals [8].

Although, the impact of antibiotic resistance caused by multidrug resistant Gram-negative bacteria has been recognised in hospitals in Ghana, measures such as surveillance studies that provide reliable data to mitigate the problem are not in place. Therefore studies to establish the prevalence and extent of resistance are necessary to bridge the information gap and provide the basis to guide empiric therapy. This study aimed to assess multidrug-resistance among Gram-negative bacteria in Komfo Anokye Teaching Hospital in Ghana to guide treatment protocols. The data further provides a baseline for future comparative studies.

## Materials
### Setting of study
The study was conducted between February and August 2015, in Komfo Anokye Teaching Hospital (KATH) in Kumasi, in the Ashanti region of Ghana. The facility is a 1000-bed tertiary care government hospital. The average daily primary care and specialist outpatient attendance was 169 and 954 patients respectively, during the period of study. The population of the region is concentrated in a few districts, with the Kumasi metropolis accounting for nearly one-third of the region's population of 4,780,380 [9]. KATH is the only regional and referral hospital that takes care of about 80% of both emergencies and regular medical cases in the region and serves as referral hospital for part of Brong Ahafo, Western, Eastern and the Northern regions of Ghana.

### Bacterial collection and identification
Two hundred (200) clinical, non-duplicate Gram-negative bacteria were randomly selected from urine, pus, wound swab, pleural fluid endotracheal tubes, gastric lavage and blood specimens processed by the diagnostic microbiological laboratory in the hospital from both in-patients and out-patients. Information on diagnosis, sex, age and ward type were obtained from patients records. The isolates were maintained on nutrient agar slants, frozen in lyophilizing medium at − 70 °C and subsequently transported to National Health Laboratory Services in South Africa to confirm identification and ascertain antibiotic susceptibility profiles using Vitek-2 (Biomerieux, France) Automated Systems with *P. aeruginosa* ATCC27853 and *E.coli* ATCC35218 as control strains. Multidrug-resistance in this study was defined as isolates that were resistant to at least one agent in three or more antibiotic classes.

## Results
Of the 200 resistant Gram-negative bacterial isolates obtained, *E. coli* was most frequent pathogen 49 (24.5%), followed by *P. aeruginosa* 39 (19.5%), *K. pneumoniae* 38 (19.0%), *Enterobacter spp.* 12 (6.0%) *Serratia spp.* 8

(4.0%), *Sphingimonas spp.* 10 (5.0%) and *Acinetobacter spp.* 8 (4.0%). The remaining 36 (18%) (Table 1) consisted of *Yersinia spp.* (5) *Proteus mirabilis* (1), *Salmonella enterica* (1), *Vibrio spp.* (5), *Citrobacter koseri* (3), *Pantoea* spp. (5), *Providencia rettgeri* (4), *Pasteurella spp.* (2) *Chromobacterium violaceum* (2), *Burkholderia cepacia* (2), *Aeromonas spp.* (5), *Cadecea lapagei* (1). The distribution of the specimen types showed highest proportion of isolates, were from urine specimens 94 (47.0%), followed by wound swabs 45 (22.5%) and sputum 24 (12.0%) with just 1 (0.5%) from each of bronchial lavage, nasal and pleural swabs respectively. A higher proportion of isolates were recovered from in-patients 161 (80.5%) compared to the out-patients 39 (19.5%). The number of isolates from the medical intensive care unit (ICU) 78 (39.0%) was highest, followed by Child Health 39 (19.5%) and the Obstetrics and Gynecology wards 17 (8.5%) with the smallest number of 10 (5.0%) isolated in the Accident and Emergency Unit. *E. coli* 49 (24.5%), *P. aeruginosa* 39 (19.5%) and *K. pneumoniae* 38 (19.0%) (Table 1) were the most predominant pathogens implicated in 63.0% of all infections. The distribution of bacterial pathogens among clinical diagnosis showed urinary tract infection (UTI) 69 (34.5%) as the most prevalent, followed by sepsis 29 (14.5%), tuberculosis 18 (9.0%) and wound infections 12 (6.0%) with the least prevalence in appendicitis, bacteremia, cystitis and prostitis 1 (0.5%) (Table 1). *E. coli* 24 (34.8) was identified as most common cause of UTI, followed by *K. pneumoniae* 17 (24.6%) and *P. aeruginosa* 9 (13.04%) implicated in 72.4% of all UTI pathogens.

### Demographic characteristics of patients with bacterial infections
The patients' ages ranged between 2 months to 90 years and mean age was $35.95 \pm 27.11$ years with the gender distribution of 101 (50.5%) males and 99 (49.5%) females. Samples from outpatients (OPD) made up 19.5% of the total samples. All the other samples (80.5%) from Accident and Emergency, Child Health, Medical ICU, Surgery and Obstetrics and Gynaecology departments were inpatient samples (Table 1). The prevalence of infections were highest among the patients of age-group ≥60 years 49 (24.5%) followed by < 10 years 48 (24.0%), 20–29 years 26 (13.0), 30–39 years and least in 50–59 years 17 (8.5%) (Table 2). UTI was highest among the age-group < 10 years 23 (33.3%) followed by 30–39 years 12 (17.4%) and least 50–59 years 4 (5.8%). Septic infection was highest in patients within the age-group < 10 years 8 (40.0%), followed by ≥60 years 5 (25.0%) least in 10–19 years 3 (15.0%) (Table 2). Among the different types of wound infections, diabetic foot ulcer showed high proportion within age-groups 50–59 and ≥60 years of patients.

**Table 1** Distribution of isolates among clinical specimen, wards and diagnosis

| | Isolates (N) | | | | | | | | |
| --- | --- | --- | --- | --- | --- | --- | --- | --- | --- |
| | Acinetobacter spp | E. coli | Enterobacter spp | K. pneumonia | P. aeruginosa | Serretia spp | Sphingimonas spp | Other* | Total (%) |
| **Specimen** | | | | | | | | | |
| Asctic fluid | – | – | – | – | – | – | – | 1 | 1 (0.5) |
| Aspirate | – | 2 | 1 | 1 | – | – | – | – | 4 (2.0) |
| Blood | – | 1 | 2 | 2 | – | – | – | 6 | 11 (5.5) |
| Bronchial Lavage | – | – | 1 | – | – | – | – | – | 1 (0.5) |
| Ear Swab | – | 1 | – | 1 | 1 | 1 | – | 2 | 6 (3.0) |
| Gastric Lavage | – | – | – | 1 | 1 | – | – | 2 | 4 (2.0) |
| Nasal Swab | – | – | – | – | 1 | – | – | – | 1 (0.5) |
| Pleural Fluid | – | – | – | 1 | – | – | 1 | – | 2 (1.0) |
| Pus | – | 3 | – | – | – | – | 1 | 1 | 5 (2.5) |
| Sputum | – | 3 | 3 | 3 | 8 | 3 | 2 | 2 | 24 (12.0) |
| Urethral Swab | 2 | – | – | – | – | – | – | – | 2 (1.0) |
| Urine | 6 | 35 | 5 | 23 | 12 | 4 | 4 | 5 | 94 (47.0) |
| Wound Swab | – | 4 | | 6 | 16 | – | 3 | 16 | 45 (22.5) |
| **WARD/DEPT** | | | | | | | | | |
| A &E | 1 | 2 | – | 2 | 2 | 1 | 1 | 1 | 10 (5.0) |
| Child Health | 1 | 12 | 3 | 11 | 3 | – | 1 | 8 | 39 (19.5) |
| Medical ICU | 2 | 14 | 6 | 10 | 21 | 5 | 4 | 16 | 78 (39.0) |
| OBS &GYN | 2 | 3 | 2 | 4 | 2 | 1 | 1 | 2 | 17 (8.5) |
| OPD | 2 | 12 | 1 | 9 | 5 | 1 | 3 | 6 | 39 (19.5) |
| Surgery | – | 6 | – | 2 | 6 | – | – | 3 | 17 (8.5) |
| **Diagnosis** | | | | | | | | | |
| Abscess | – | 1 | 1 | 1 | 1 | 1 | – | 2 | 7 (3.5) |
| Appendicitis | – | 1 | – | – | – | – | – | – | 1 (0.5) |
| Bacteremia | – | 1 | – | – | – | – | – | – | 1 (0.5) |
| Bronchitis | – | – | – | 1 | 1 | – | – | – | 2 (1.0) |
| Cellulitis | – | – | – | – | – | – | – | 1 | 1 (0.5) |
| Cirrhosis | – | 1 | 1 | – | – | – | – | – | 2 (1.0) |
| Cystitis | – | – | – | 1 | – | – | – | – | 1 (0.5) |
| Diabetic foot ulcer | – | 1 | 1 | – | 4 | – | 1 | 3 | 10 (5.0) |
| Gastroenteritis | – | 4 | – | 1 | – | – | – | – | 5 (2.5) |
| Nephritis | – | 6 | – | 3 | – | 1 | – | 1 | 11 (5.5) |
| Otitis | – | 1 | – | – | – | – | – | 1 | 2 (1.0) |
| Pericarditis | – | 1 | – | – | 2 | – | – | – | 3 (1.5) |
| Peritonitis | – | 1 | – | – | 1 | – | – | – | 2 (1.0) |
| Pneumoniae | – | – | – | 1 | – | 2 | 1 | – | 4 (2.0) |
| Prostitis | – | – | – | – | – | 1 | – | – | 1 (0.5) |
| RTI | – | – | – | 1 | 1 | – | 2 | 1 | 5 (2.5) |
| Sepsis | 1 | 6 | 1 | 4 | 4 | 2 | 3 | 8 | 29 (14.5) |
| Surg. site infection | – | 1 | – | 4 | 4 | – | – | 1 | 10 (5.0) |
| Tuberculosis | – | 1 | 4 | 2 | **7** | 1 | 1 | 2 | 18 (9.0) |

**Table 1** Distribution of isolates among clinical specimen, wards and diagnosis *(Continued)*

| | Isolates (N) | | | | | | | | |
| | Acinetobacter spp | E. coli | Enterobacter spp | K. pneumonia | P. aeruginosa | Serretia spp | Sphingimonas spp | Other* | Total (%) |
|---|---|---|---|---|---|---|---|---|---|
| UTI | 7 | 24 | 4 | 17 | 9 | – | 2 | 6 | 69 (34.5) |
| Ulcer | – | – | – | – | 1 | – | – | 1 | 2 (1.0) |
| Wound infection | – | – | – | 1 | 4 | – | – | 7 | 12 (6.0) |
| Frequency (%) | **8 (4.0)** | **49 (24.5)** | **12 (6.0)** | **38 (19.0)** | **39 (19.5)** | **8 (4.0)** | **10 (5.0)** | **36 (18.0)** | **200 (100)** |

*Abbreviation: A&E Accident and Emergency, OPD Out-Patient Department, OBS&GYN Obstetrics and Gynecology, Other\* Other Gram-negative bacteria. The In-- Patient Department comprises of A&E, Medical ICU, OBS&GYN and Surgical ward, –: Non-detected*

**Table 2** Distribution of infections among gender and patients' age groups

| | Age (Years) Number of Cases (N) | | | | | | | |
| | < 10 | 10–19 | 20–29 | 30–39 | 40–49 | 50–59 | ≥60 | Total (%) |
|---|---|---|---|---|---|---|---|---|
| Gender | | | | | | | | |
| Female | 21 | 8 | 20 | 13 | 11 | 9 | 17 | 99 (49.5) |
| Male | 27 | 11 | 6 | 8 | 9 | 8 | 32 | 101 (50.1) |
| Infections | | | | | | | | |
| Abscess | 2 | 1 | 2 | 1 | – | 1 | – | 7 (3.5) |
| Appendicitis | – | 1 | – | – | – | – | – | 1 (0.5) |
| Bacteremia | 1 | – | – | – | – | – | – | 1 (0.5) |
| Bronchitis | 1 | – | – | – | – | – | 1 | 2 (1.0) |
| Cellulitis | – | – | – | – | – | – | 1 | 1 (0.5) |
| Cirrhosis | – | 1 | 1 | – | – | – | – | 21.0) |
| Cystitis | 1 | – | – | – | – | – | – | 1 (0.5) |
| Diabetic foot ulcer | – | – | 1 | – | 1 | 1 | 7 | 10 (5.0) |
| Gastroenteritis | 4 | 3 | – | – | – | – | – | 7 (3.5) |
| Nephritis | – | 1 | 1 | 1 | 1 | 1 | 6 | 11 (3.5) |
| Otitis | 1 | – | 1 | – | – | – | – | 2 (1.0) |
| Pericarditis | – | – | – | – | 2 | – | 1 | 3 (1.5) |
| Peritonitis | 2 | – | – | – | – | – | – | 2 (1.0) |
| Pneumoniae | – | 1 | – | – | – | – | 3 | 4 (2.0) |
| Prostitis | – | – | – | – | – | – | 1 | 1 (1.0) |
| RTI | 2 | 1 | – | 1 | 1 | – | – | 5 (2.5) |
| Sepsis | 8 | 3 | 1 | – | 1 | 2 | 5 | 20 (10.0) |
| Surgical wound infection | 1 | 1 | 2 | 2 | – | 2 | 2 | 10 (5.0) |
| Tuberculosis | 1 | 1 | 3 | – | 6 | 3 | 4 | 18 (9.0) |
| UTI | 23 | 4 | 10 | 12 | 7 | 4 | 9 | 69 (34.5) |
| Ulcer | – | 1 | – | – | 1 | – | – | 2 (1.0) |
| Wound infection | 1 | – | 2 | 2 | 1 | 2 | 2 | 10 (5.0) |
| Frequency (%) | **48 (24.0)** | **19 (9.5)** | **26 (13.0)** | **21 (10.5)** | **20 (10.0)** | **17 (8.5)** | **49 (24.4)** | **200 (100)** |

*Abbreviation: UTI Urinary tract infection, RTI Respiratory tract infection, –: Non-detected*

## Susceptibility profile

The antibiotic susceptibility profile showed that the isolates were most resistant to ampicillin (94.4%), trimethoprim/sulfamethoxazole (84.5%), cefuroxime/Axetil (80.0%), cefuroxime (79.0%), cefotaxime (71.3%), cefoxitin (57.5%) and were least resistant to ertapenem (1.5%) (Table 3).

### Multi-drug resistance

Multidrug resistance was observed in 89.5% of the bacterial isolates, ranging from 53.8% in *Enterobacter* spp. to 100.0% in *Acinetobacter* spp. and *P. aeruginosa* (Table 4).

## Discussion

Epidemiological surveillance of bacterial infection and resistance to antibiotics are essential for awareness creation, implementation of control measures and effective management of infections. This is important in developing countries particularly in sub-Saharan Africa where studies have indicated that many hospitals have rudimentary and poor enforcement of infection control measures and marginal awareness on the extent of infections caused by multi-drug resistant bacteria which have resulted in increased morbidity and mortality [10, 11].

Our study observed higher prevalence of infections among in-patients (80.5%) compared to the out-patients (19.5%), with ICU accounted for highest incidence. The frequency of bacterial pathogens isolated from male (50.5%) and female (49.5%) patients, showed no appreciable

difference. The high infections of in-patients is consistent with the finding from nationwide surveillance on antimicrobial resistant pathogens from patients' blood cultures, which recorded prevalence of >70% of bacterial infections among in-patients in Ghanaian hospitals [12]. Several predisposing factors are associated with the higher infection rates among hospitalized patients such as the use of invasive procedures like catheterization, central lines and mechanical ventilation [13]. A number of risk factors account for the high ICU infections including non-compliance of care professionals (physicians and nurses) to hand-hygiene practices which has been identified in a study conducted in a neonatal ICU in a Ghanaian tertiary care hospital as a major factor contributing to healthcare infections in ICU [14]. The ICU houses critically ill patients and are often exposed to extensive use of antibiotics causing selection pressure for the emergence of resistance. These factors coupled with interventional instrumentations such as mechanical ventilation and invasive procedures, commonly used in ICU [15], exposes the patients to high risk of infections. KATH is the only tertiary and referral facility receiving patients into the ICU from many healthcare facilities within the region and other parts of the country, often resulting in congestion or overcrowding, thus increasing chances of transmitting infections among patients.

This study indicated high infections among advancing and infant age-groups with UTI and sepsis recorded as most frequent. The geriatric and pediatric patients are

**Table 3** Antibiotic susceptibility profile of isolates

| Antibiotics | Total number of isolates (N) | Susceptible N (%) | Intermediate N (%) | Resistant N (%) |
|---|---|---|---|---|
| Ampicillin | 162 | 7 (4.3) | 2 (1.2) | 153 (94.4) |
| Amox/clav | 200 | 51 (25.5) | 47 (23.5) | 102 (51.5) |
| Piperacillin-tazobactam | 198 | 109 (54.5) | 62 (31.0) | 27 (13.5) |
| Cefuroxime | 200 | 35 (17.5) | 7 (3.5) | 158 (79.0) |
| Cefoxitin | 200 | 74 (37.0) | 11 (5.5) | 115 (57.5) |
| Cefotaxime | 199 | 44 (22.1) | 12 (6.0) | 143 (71.3) |
| Ceftazidime | 200 | 104 (52.0) | 15 (7.5) | 81 (40.5) |
| Cefepime | 200 | 119 (59.5) | 64 (32.0) | 17 (8.5) |
| Ertapenam | 132 | 130 (98.5) | 1 (0.8) | 1 (0.8) |
| Imipenem | 199 | 191 (95.5) | 0 (0.0) | 8 (4.0) |
| Meropenem | 198 | 192 (97.0) | 1 (0.5) | 5 (2.5) |
| Amikacin | 199 | 178 (89.4) | 14 (7.0) | 7 (3.5) |
| Gentamicin | 198 | 105 (53.0) | 5 (2.5) | 88 (44.4) |
| Ciprofloxacin | 200 | 116 (58.0) | 2 (1.0) | 82 (41.0) |
| Tetracycline | 199 | 124 (62.3) | 14 (7.0) | 61 (30.7) |
| Nitrofuratoin | 200 | 84 (42.0) | 17 (8.5) | 99 (49.5) |
| Collistin | 198 | 164 (82.8) | 2 (1.0) | 32 (16.2) |
| Trim/Sulfamethoxazole | 200 | 31 (15.5) | 0 (0.0) | 169 (84.5) |

Not all the antibiotics were tested for all 200 isolates and not all N-values added up to 200

*Abbreviation*: *amox/clav* amoxicillin-clavulanate, *trim/sulfamethoxazole* trimethoprim-sulfamethoxazole

**Table 4** MDR among Isolates

| Bacterial Isolates | Number of Isolates (N) | MDR N (%) |
| --- | --- | --- |
| Acinetobacter spp | 8 | 8 (100.0) |
| E. coli | 49 | 44 (89.9) |
| Enterobacter spp | 12 | 7 (53.8) |
| K. pneumoniae | 38 | 36 (94.7) |
| P. aeruginosa | 39 | 39 (100.0) |
| Serratia spp | 8 | 7 (87.5) |
| Sphingomonas paucimobilis | 10 | 9 (90.0) |
| Other Gram negative | 36 | 29 (80.6) |
| Frequency | **200** | **179 (89.5)** |

usually more disposed to infections due to their immune status. The advancing age are commonly associated with risk factors including reduced immunity, co-morbid diseases such as diabetes mellitus, chronic heart diseases, neurogenic bladder [13, 16] whilst in infants, lack of fully developed immunity, malnutrition as well as inadequate hygiene [17] put them at greater risk of infections. Urinary tract infection (34.5%) was most prevalent within the period of our study, and is comparable to 31.5% reported from a study on prevalence and antibiotic susceptibility pattern of uropathogens conducted in secondary hospital in Ghana [18]. Our study found, E. coli and K. pneumoniae as most predominant pathogens implicated in UTI. Several studies conducted in the region and other parts of the country have reported UTI as most common infections frequently caused by E.coli and K. pneumoniae with high resistance to broad spectrum antibiotics, that remains a major clinical problem in health care system in Ghana [19, 20]. Among the isolates, E. coli, K. pneumoniae Proteus mirabilis, P. aeruginosa, Enterobacter, Acinetobacter and Serratia spp. in the present study have been reported as clinically important urine pathogens [18, 21], associated with about 90% of both community and hospital acquired UTIs [22, 23]. Urinary tract infection prevalence was high among infants and the middle aged with incidence higher in females (10.8%) than the males (6.6%) in the middle age group. In infants predisposing factors such as lack of personal hygiene, incomplete emptying of the bladder with residual urine and severe acute malnutrition have been reported [24], whilst the middle aged, in particular females, high parity coupled with increased frequency of sexual activities have been identified, contributing to the high incidence [25]. The prevalence of sepsis among infants, 40.0% (Table 2), was higher compared to the 25.9% previously reported in the country [26]. The higher prevalence is attributed to higher patients' intake in the study site and also situated in most populous region, thus receiving higher numbers of patients (infants) with complications compared to other regions of Ghana. This study is however limited in its representativeness of the entire hospital because we did not systematically collect data on how much of each specimen type was sent to the lab and which types of isolates were obtained from each specimen type.

Among the isolates, E. coli, P. aeruginosa and K. pneumoniae were most prevalent pathogens implicated in 63.0% (Table 1) of the infections with high resistance to antibiotics commonly used in Ghana. The finding that E coli, P. aeruginosa and K. pneumoniae were most prevalent Gram-negative pathogens is consistent with previous studies conducted in Ashanti region of Ghana [20] and other parts of the country [26, 27]. A nationwide surveillance on antimicrobial resistant pathogens study, conducted by Opintan et al. also indicated E.coli and P. aeruginosa, Enterobacter, Citrobacter spp. and K. pneumoniae as most common gram-negative bacterial pathogens in Ghana [28]. The current prioritized lists of bacterial pathogens by World Health Organization (WHO), categorized E. coli, P. aeruginosa, K. pneumoniae, Acinetobacter, Enterobacter, Serratia, Proteus and Providencia spp. identified in our study, as critical or most life-threatening Gram-negative pathogens under surveillance due to their high antibiotic resistance especially to carbapenems and third generation cephalosporins, associated with attributable mortality [29]. In particular, K. pneumoniae, P. aeruginosa, Acinetobacter and Enterobacter spp. have further been described by the Infectious Diseases Society of America as Gram-negative ESKAPE (Enterococcus faecium, Staphylococcus aureus, Klebsiella pneumoniae, Acinetobacter baumannii, Pseudomonas aeruginosa and Enterobacter spp) pathogens, frequently associated with multidrug resistance [30, 31]. These ESKAPE Gram-negative pathogens were implicated in 48.5% (Table 1) of the infections which is higher than 35.6% previously reported [27]. The pathogens were also implicated in 50% (Table 1) of the ICU infections, and therefore posing a major threat to public healthcare in Ghana.

The susceptibility profile of the isolates displayed high level multidrug resistance of 89.5% with high resistance to ampicillin (94.4%), trimethoprim sulfamethoxazole (84.5%), cefuroxime (79.0%) cefotaxime (71.3%), cefoxitin (57.5%) and amoxacillin-clavulanate (51.5%) observed, was consistent with other studies conducted in Ghana [27, 32]. The degree of resistance among the isolates to ampicillin, trimethoprim/sulfamethoxazole and amoxacillin-clavulanate showed in the study, also agreed with other studies conducted in the sub-Sahara African countries such as Tanzania [7], Nigeria [33], Ethiopia [34], Zimbabwe [35] and Rwanda [6]. The high resistance trend in the sub region is indicative of high antibiotic selection pressure largely due to relatively cheap and easy availability of these agents, mostly used as first line or common choice of treatment in many healthcare settings in the sub region [36–38].

The decreased susceptibility of isolates to the beta-lactam/beta-lactamases inhibitor combination antibiotic therapy and fluoroquinolones (ciprofloxacin) is comparable to other studies in Ghana [20, 27], which poses a challenge to treatment of common infections as these agents are readily available therapeutic options [39]. The high resistance to second and third-generation cephalosporins (cefuroxime [79.0%], cefoxitin [57.5%] and cefotaxime [71.3%]), may suggest high expression or production of extended spectrum beta-lactamases among Gram-negative bacteria as previously reported in Ghana [40]. The carbapenems (imipenem, ertapenem and meropenem), amikacin and colistin were sensitive, as these antibiotics are used as last resort in treatment of serious infections. In addition the carbapenems have been introduced into Ghanaian market for relatively short span of time and is comparatively more expensive than the mainstay antibiotics and therefore, not commonly used.

This has possibly led to relatively low natural selection and hence low development of antibiotic resistance among the isolates.

## Conclusion

The study demonstrated high multidrug resistant Gram-negative bacteria implicated in the infections, with UTI as most frequently diagnosed among patients. Infections were common among the elderly and infants, and predominantly caused by *E. coli*, *K. pneumoniae* and *P. aeruginosa* during the period of our study. These results should inform the empirical treatment of infections in Komfo Anokye Teaching Hospital of Ghana as appropriate.

### Acknowledgements

We would like to thank the Komfo Anokye Teaching Hospital staff, especially the technical staff in the Microbiology laboratory for their support during sample collection and preliminary identification, the Physicians and Nursing staff in various wards for their assistance. We also thank the staff of National Health Laboratory Services (NHLS), Albert Luthuli Hospital in South Africa for further bacteria identification and the antibiotics susceptibility profile testing.

### Funding

This study was supported by the National Research Foundation Incentive Funding for Rated Researchers Grant No.: 85595 awarded to Professor S.Y. Essack and a PhD Scholarship awarded to N Agyepong by the College of Health Sciences, University of KwaZulu-Natal.

### Authors' contributions

The study was co-conceptualized and jointly designed by NA, AO and SE. NA collected the data and undertook laboratory analysis with the help from UG. NA analyzed and interpreted the data with assistance from AO & SE. All the authors contributed in preparation and submission of manuscript. All authors read and approved the final manuscript.

### Competing interests

Professor Essack is a member of the Global Respiratory Infection Partnership sponsored by an unrestricted educational grant from Reckitt and Benckiser, UK. The other authors have no competing interest to declare.

### Author details

[1]Antimicrobial Research Unit, Discipline of Pharmaceutical Sciences, University of Kwa-Zulu Natal, Durban, South Africa. [2]School of Medical Sciences, Kwame Nkrumah University of Science and Technology, Kumasi, Ghana.

### References

1. Singh N, Manchanda V. Control of multidrug-resistant gram-negative bacteria in low-and middle-income countries—high impact interventions without much resources. Clin Microbiol Infect. 2017;23:216–8.
2. De Angelis G, D'Inzeo T, Fiori B, Spanu T, Sganga G. Burden of antibiotic resistant gram negative bacterial infections: evidence and limits. J Med Microbiol Diagn. 2014;3:132–8.
3. Rossolini GM, Mantengoli E, Docquier J, Musmanno RA, Coratza G. Epidemiology of infections caused by multiresistant gram-negatives: ESBLs, MBLs, panresistant strains. New Microbiol. 2007;30:332.
4. Oduro-Mensah D, Obeng-Nkrumah N, Bonney EY, Oduro-Mensah E, Twum-Danso K, Osei YD, Sackey ST. Genetic characterization of TEM-type ESBL-associated antibacterial resistance in Enterobacteriaceae in a tertiary hospital in Ghana. Ann Clin Microbiol Antimicrob. 2016;15:29–38.
5. Le Doare K, Bielicki J, Heath PT, Sharland M. Systematic review of antibiotic resistance rates among gram-negative bacteria in children with sepsis in resource-limited countries. J Pediatric Infect Dis Soc. 2015;4:11–20.
6. Carroll M, Rangaiahagari A, Musabeyezu E, Singer D, Ogbuagu O. Five-year antimicrobial susceptibility trends among bacterial isolates from a tertiary health-care facility in Kigali, Rwanda. Am J Trop Med Hyg. 2016;95:1277–83.
7. Kumburu HH, Sonda T, Mmbaga BT, Alifrangis M, Lund O, Kibiki G, Aarestrup FM. Patterns of infections, aetiological agents, and antimicrobial resistance at a tertiary care hospital in northern Tanzania. Tropical Med Int Health. 2017;22:454–64.
8. Allegranzi B, Nejad SB, Combescure C, Graafmans W, Attar H, Donaldson L, Pittet D. Burden of endemic health-care-associated infection in developing countries: systematic review and meta-analysis. Lancet. 2011;377:228–41.
9. Owusu G, Oteng-Ababio M. Moving unruly contemporary urbanism toward sustainable urban development in Ghana by 2030. Am Behav Sci. 2015;59: 311–27.
10. Huttner A, Harbarth S, Carlet J, Cosgrove S, Goossens H, Holmes A, Jarlier V, Voss A, Pittet D. Antimicrobial resistance: a global view from the 2013 World Healthcare-Associated Infections Forum. Antimicrob Resist Infect Control. 2013;2:2–31.
11. Samuel S, Kayode O, Musa O, Nwigwe G, Aboderin A, Salami T, Taiwo S. Nosocomial infections and the challenges of control in developing countries. Afr J Clin Exp Microbiol. 2010;11:102–9.
12. Opintan JA, Newman MJ. Prevalence of antimicrobial resistant pathogens from blood cultures: results from a laboratory based nationwide surveillance in Ghana. Antimicrob Resist Infect Control. 2017;6:64–70.
13. Chang YJ, Yeh ML, Li YC, Hsu CY, Lin CC, Hsu M-S, Chiu WT. Predicting hospital-acquired infections by scoring system with simple parameters. PLoS One. 2011;6:1–11.
14. Asare A, Enweronu-Laryea CC, Newman MJ. Hand hygiene practices in a neonatal intensive care unit in Ghana. J Infect Dev Ctries. 2009;3:352–6.
15. Ulu-Kilic A, Ahmed S, Alp E, Doğanay M. Challenge of intensive care unit-acquired infections and Acinetobacter baumannii in developing countries. Crit Care. 2013;1:2–7.
16. Simonetti AF, Viasus D, Garcia-Vidal C, Carratalà J. Management of community-acquired pneumonia in older adults. Ther Adv Infect Dis. 2014;2:3–16.
17. Hill R, Paulus S, Dey P, Hurley MA, Carter B. Is undernutrition prognostic of infection complications in children undergoing surgery? A systematic review. J Hosp Infect. 2016;93:12–21.
18. Gyansa-Lutterodt M, Afriyie D, Asare G, Amponsah S, Abutiate H, Darko D. Antimicrobial use and susceptibility pattern of uropathogens associated with urinary tract infections at the Ghana Police Hospital. Glob J Pharmacol. 2014;8:306–15.
19. Obirikorang C, Quaye L, Bio F, Amidu N, Acheampong I, Addo K. Asymptomatic bacteriuria among pregnant women attending antenatal clinic at the University Hospital, Kumasi, Ghana. J Med Biomed Sci. 2012;1:38–44.
20. Gyasi-Sarpong CK, Nkrumah B, Yenli EMT-A, Appiah AA, Aboah K, Azorliade R, Kolekang AS, Ali I. Resistance pattern of uropathogenic bacteria in males with lower urinary tract obstruction in Kumasi, Ghana. Afr J Microbiol Res. 2014;8:3324–9.

21. Wireko S, Abubakari A, Opoku B. In vitro activities of antimicrobial agents against uropathogenic isolates at Brong Ahafo regional hospital, Ghana. Int J Curr Microbiol App Sci. 2017;6:193–201.

22. Linhares I, Raposo T, Rodrigues A, Almeida A. Frequency and antimicrobial resistance patterns of bacteria implicated in community urinary tract infections: a ten-year surveillance study (2000–2009). BMC Infect Dis. 2013; 13:19–33.

23. Farajnia S, Alikhani MY, Ghotaslou R, Naghili B, Nakhlband A. Causative agents and antimicrobial susceptibilities of urinary tract infections in the northwest of Iran. Int J Infect Dis. 2009;13:140–4.

24. Uwaezuoke SN. The prevalence of urinary tract infection in children with severe acute malnutrition: a narrative review. Pediatric Health Med Ther. 2016;7:121–7.

25. Komala M, Kumar KS. Urinary tract infection: causes, symptoms, diagnosis and it's management. Indian J Res Pharm Biotechnol. 2013;1:226–33.

26. Acquah SE, Quaye L, Sagoe K, Ziem JB, Bromberger PI, Amponsem AA. Susceptibility of bacterial etiological agents to commonly-used antimicrobial agents in children with sepsis at the Tamale Teaching Hospital. BMC Infect Dis. 2013;13:1–14.

27. Newman MJ, Frimpong E, Donkor ES, Opintan JA, Asamoah-Adu A. Resistance to antimicrobial drugs in Ghana. Infect Drug Resist. 2011;4:215–20.

28. Opintan JA, Newman MJ, Arhin RE, Donkor ES, Gyansa-Lutterodt M, Mills-Pappoe W. Laboratory-based nationwide surveillance of antimicrobial resistance in Ghana. Infect Drug Resist. 2015;8:379–85.

29. WHO. Global priority list of antibiotic-resistant bacteria to guide research, discovery, and development of new antibiotics. Geneva: World Health Organization; 2017.

30. Navidinia M. The clinical importance of emerging ESKAPE pathogens in nosocomial infections. J Paramed Sci. 2016;7:43–57.

31. Cerceo E, Deitelzweig SB, Sherman BM, Amin AN. Multidrug-resistant gram-negative bacterial infections in the hospital setting: overview, implications for clinical practice, and emerging treatment options. Microb Drug Resist. 2016;22:412–31.

32. Obeng-Nkrumah N, Twum-Danso K, Krogfelt KA, Newman MJ. High levels of extended-spectrum beta-lactamases in a major teaching hospital in Ghana: the need for regular monitoring and evaluation of antibiotic resistance. Am J Trop Med Hyg. 2013;89:960–4.

33. Ogbolu D, Daini O, Ogunledun A, Alli A, Webber M. High levels of multidrug resistance in clinical isolates of gram-negative pathogens from Nigeria. Int J Antimicrob Agents. 2011;37:62–6.

34. Muluye D, Wondimeneh Y, Ferede G, Nega T, Adane K, Biadgo B, Tesfa H, Moges F. Bacterial isolates and their antibiotic susceptibility patterns among patients with pus and/or wound discharge at Gondar university hospital. BMC Res Notes. 2014;7:619–24.

35. Mbanga J, Dube S, Munyanduki H. Prevalence and drug resistance in bacteria of the urinary tract infections in Bulawayo province, Zimbabwe. East Afr J Public Health. 2010;7:229–32.

36. Mshana SE, Matee M, Rweyemamu M. Antimicrobial resistance in human and animal pathogens in Zambia, Democratic Republic of Congo, Mozambique and Tanzania: an urgent need of a sustainable surveillance system. Ann Clin Microbiol Antimicrob. 2013;12:28–38.

37. Ocan M, Bwanga F, Bbosa GS, Bagenda D, Waako P, Ogwal-Okeng J, Obua C. Patterns and predictors of self-medication in northern Uganda. PLoS One. 2014;9:92323–30.

38. Donkor ES, Tetteh-Quarcoo PB, Nartey P, Agyeman IO. Self-medication practices with antibiotics among tertiary level students in Accra, Ghana: a cross-sectional study. Int J Env Res Public Health. 2012;9:3519–29.

39. Hackman HK, Osei-Adjei G, Ameko E, Kutsanedzie F, Gordon A, Laryea E, Quaye S, Anison L, Brown CA, Twum-Danso K. Phenotypic determination and antimicrobial resistance profile of extended spectrum beta-lactamases in Escherichia coli and Klebsiella pneumoniae in Accra, Ghana. J Nat Sci. 2013;3:75–83.

40. Feglo P, Adu-Sarkodie Y. Antimicrobial resistance patterns of extended spectrum B-lactamase producing Klebsiellae and E. coli isolates from a tertiary hospital in Ghana. Eur Sci J. 2016;12:174–87.

# 16

# Extended spectrum and metalo beta-lactamase producing airborne *Pseudomonas aeruginosa* and *Acinetobacter baumanii* in restricted settings of a referral hospital: a neglected condition

Fithamlak Bisetegen Solomon[1*], Fiseha Wadilo[2], Efrata Girma Tufa[3] and Meseret Mitiku[4]

## Abstract

**Background:** Frequently encountered multidrug-resistant bacterial isolates of *P. aeruginosa* and *A. baumannii* are common and prevalent in a hospital environment. The aim of this study was to determine the prevalence and pattern of antibiotic resistance, extended spectrum and metallo beta-lactamase producing *P. aeruginosa* and *A. baumannii* isolates from restricted settings of indoor air hospital environment.

**Methods:** A hospital-based cross-sectional study was conducted in Wolaita Sodo University Teaching and referral Hospital, Ethiopia from December 1/2015 to April 30/2015. The Air samples were collected from delivery room, intensive care unit and operation theatre of the hospital by active, Anderson six slate sampler technique during the first week of the months, twice a week during Monday's and Friday's. Standard microbiological procedures were followed to isolate *P. aeruginosa* and *A. baumannii*. Susceptibility testing was performed on isolates using the Kirby-Bauer disk diffusion technique. Extended spectrum beta lactamase production was detected by double disc synergy test and Imipenem-resistant isolates were screened for producing Metallo-beta lactamase.

**Results:** A total number of 216 indoor air samples were collected from the delivery room, intensive care unit, and operation room. Correspondingly, 43 *A. baumannii* isolates were identified (13 from delivery room, 21 from intensive care unit and 9 from operation room). Likewise 24 *P. aeruginosa* isolates were obtained (4 from delivery room, 13 from intensive care unit and 7 from operation room). Extended spectrum beta lactamase and metalo-beta lactamase production were observed in 24 (55.8%) and 13 (30.2%) isolates of *A. baumannii* respectively, whereas *P. aeruginosa* showed 15 (62.5%) extended spectrum beta lactamase and 9 (37.5%) metallo-beta lactamase production.

**Conclusions:** Extended spectrum beta lactamase and metalo-beta lactamase producing bacteria in hospital air is a new dimension for specific setting of the study area where antimicrobial resistance is increasing and surgical site infection is prevalent. So, identification of these microorganisms has a great role in reducing the burden of antibiotic resistance and could also provide a significant input for framing hospital infection control policies.

**Keywords:** Antibiotic resistance, ESBL, MBL, *P. aeruginosa*, *A. Baumannii*, MDR, Airborne

* Correspondence: fitha2007@yahoo.com
[1]School of Medicine, Wolaita Sodo University, PO box 138, Sodo, Ethiopia
Full list of author information is available at the end of the article

Extended spectrum and metalo beta-lactamase producing airborne Pseudomonas aeruginosa...

111

## Background

Airborne microorganisms could cause respiratory disorders, severe infections, hypersensitivity pneumonitis and toxic reactions [1]. Frequently encountered multidrug-resistant (MDR) bacterial isolates like Ceftazidime-resistant *Pseudomonas aeruginosa* and Imipenem-resistant *Acinetobacter baumannii* are common and prevalent in a hospital environment [2–5].

Multidrug-resistant *P. aeruginosa* is inherently resistant to many drug classes and is able to acquire resistance to all effective antimicrobial drugs [6]. MDR *P. aeruginosa* elaborates inactivating enzymes that make beta-lactams and carbapenems ineffective, such as extended spectrum beta lactamases (ESBLs) and metallo-β-lactamases (MBLs) [7].

*A. baumannii* also remain problematic because of its high intrinsic resistance to a wide variety of antimicrobial agents. Moreover, the ability of resistant strains of *A. baumannii* to survive for prolonged periods in the hospital environment contributes significantly to antimicrobial resistance, thereby posing a difficult challenge for infection control [8, 9]. Carbapenems used to be the drugs of choice for treating burn infections caused by *A. baumannii* strains. Consequently, due to selective pressure on carbapenems and the increased use of this antibiotic, carbapenem-resistant *A. baumannii* has emerged. This problem worsens in cases of MBL production when the drug of last choice, carbapenems, is inactive [10].

The uncontrolled movement of air in and out of the hospital environment makes the bacterial persistence worse since these infectious microorganisms may spread easily into the environment through sneezing, coughing, talking and contact with hospital materials. It can affect patients admitted to rooms in which the prior occupants tested positive for a pathogen and also other patients in the facility [11, 12].

Therefore, the main objective of this study was to determine the prevalence and pattern of ESBL and MBL producing *P. aeruginosa* and *A. baumannii* from hospital indoor air of Wolaita Sodo University Teaching and Referral Hospital (WSUTRH).

## Methods

### Study area

The study was conducted at Wolaita Sodo University Teaching and Referral Hospital (WSUTRH), Sodo, located South Central Ethiopia. It is serving people in catchment's area of 2 million people. The hospital has 320 beds for inpatient service which are on medical, pediatrics, surgical, intensive care unit, gynecology and obstetrics wards.

### Study design and period

A hospital based cross sectional study was conducted to determine the prevalence and pattern of antibiotic resistance, extended spectrum and metallo beta-lactamase producing *P. aeruginosa* and *A. baumannii* isolates from restricted settings of indoor air hospital environment. The study was undertaken from December 1, 2015 to April 30, 2016 in WSUTRH.

### Sampling techniques

The Air samples were collected during the first week of the months, twice a week during Monday's and Friday's. All microbiological procedures were conducted in Wolaita Sodo University microbiology laboratory which is an accredited laboratory with bio-safety cabinet two and vitek 2 microbiology apparatus. The laboratory built independently 5 km far from the clinical departments where air samples were conducted.

### Active air sampling

Active air sampler, Anderson six state cascade impactor, which sucks 28.3 l of air per minute, was used and the Petridish was placed in the impactor for 5 minutes [13]. After that the Petridish was shipped to Wolaita Sodo university microbiology laboratory. Petri dishes were labeled with sample number, hospital ward, date and time (hour, minute and second) of sample collection.

Three agar plates were placed at various distances in each of the selected wards with five meter apart. Self-contamination was prevented by wearing sterile surgical gloves, mouth masks, and protective gown.

### Processing of specimens and preliminary identification

Following collection, colonies on tryptic soya agar were inoculated into MacConkey agar, and blood agar plates. The inoculated plates were incubated at 35 °C for 24–48 h. Then the growth was inspected to identify the bacteria.

*P. aeruginosa* isolates were presumptively identified by gram staining, colony morphology, pigment formation, mucoid, haemolysis on blood agar, positive oxidase test, grape-like odour, growth at 42 °C on nutrient agar, and positive motility [14].

Genus *Acinetobacter* was identified by Gram staining, cell and colony morphology, positive catalase test, negative oxidase test and absence of motility. Suspected *A. baumanii* isolates were confirmed by API-20 NE kit (biomerieux, France) system.

### Antibiotic susceptibility testing

The drug susceptibility testing of the isolates was done by Kirby-Bauer disc diffusion method [15] following Clinical Laboratory Standards Institute (CLSI) guide lines. The grades of susceptibility pattern were recognized as sensitive, intermediate and resistant by comparison of the zone of inhibition as indicated by CLSI, 2014 [16]. Intermediate isolates were taken as sensitive for the purpose of this study. The antibiotic discs were obtained from Oxoid, England, with the following concentrations: amikacin (30 µg), cefotaxime (30 µg), cefepime (30 µg), azetronam (30 µg) amoxicillin-clavulanic acid (30 µg), ceftazidime (30 µg), ceftriaxone (30 µg), ciprofloxacin (10 µg), meropenem (10 µg), gentamicin (10 µg), imipenem (10 µg), trimethoprim-sulphamethoxazole (25/1.25 µg). Antibiotics were selected based on local availability, their effectiveness, guideline provided by CLSI and from literatures.

### Phenotypic detection of extended spectrum beta-lactamase producing bacteria

Extended spectrum beta-lactamase (ESBL) production was detected by double disc synergy test (DDST) [17]. Accordingly, 3–5 selected colonies were taken from a pure culture and transferred to a tube containing 5 ml sterile nutrient broth and mixed gently until a homogenous suspension was formed. The suspension was incubated for 4–6 h at 37 °C until the turbidity was matched with the 0.5 McFarland standards. A sterile cotton swab was then used to distribute the bacteria evenly over the entire surface of Mueller Hinton agar (Oxoid, England).

Amoxicillin-clavulanic acid disc was placed in the center of the plate whereas ceftriaxone, ceftazidime and cefotaxime (30 µg each) discs were placed at a distance of 20 mm (center to center) from the amoxicillin-clavulanic acid disk. The plates were then incubated at 37 °C for 24 h and results were read. Enhancement of zone of inhibition of the cephalosporin disc towards clavulanic acid containing disc was inferred as synergy and the strain considered as ESBL producer.

### Phenotypic detection of metalo-beta lactamase producing bacteria

Imipenem-resistant isolates were screened for producing MBL. The double disk method was used to detect this enzyme. Colonies from overnight cultures on blood agar plates were suspended in Mueller-Hinton broth and the turbidity standardized to equal that of a bacterial concentration of 1:100 suspensions of the 0.5 McFarland standards. Then the suspension was streaked onto Mueller-Hinton agar plates (Hi Media, Mumbai, India). A disc of Imipenem alone (10 µg) and Imipenem (10 µg) in combination with EDTA (750 µg/disc) was placed at the distance of 20 mm (centre to centre). After overnight incubation at 35 °C, a ≥ 7 mm increase in the inhibition zone of diameter around Imipenem-EDTA discs, as compared to imipenem discs alone, interpreted as indicative of MBL production [18].

### Operational definitions

**MDR** was defined as acquired non-susceptibility to at least one agent in three or more antimicrobial categories.

**Pan resistance**-resistance for all antibiotics tested.

**High MDR**: resistance rate of the isolates for more than 60% of the antibiotics.

### Quality controls

Standard operating procedures were prepared and followed from sample collection to reporting. Culture medias were prepared based on the manufacturers' instruction then the sterility was checked by incubating 5% of the batch at 35-37 °C for overnight and observing bacterial growth. Those Media which showed growth were discarded. Anderson air sampler was handled by environmental microbiologist and as per the manufacturer's instruction.

*Escherichia coli* ATCC 25922 and *Pseudomonas aeruginosa* ATCC 27853 were used as control strains.

### Data analysis

Statistical analysis was performed by using SPSS version 20 software program and descriptive statistics were used.

## Results

### Microbial load of hospital wards

A total of 216 indoor samples were collected from intensive care unit (ICU), delivery room (DR) and operation room (OR). Correspondingly, 67 isolates (43 *A. baumannii* and 24 *P. aeruginosa*) were obtained with an overall isolation rate of 31% (67/216). Of those isolates, the highest rate (50.7%) was identified from ICU, whereas the lowest rate (23.9%) was from OR (Table 1).

### Antibiotic resistance profile of air-borne bacterial pathogens

*A. baumannii* showed a high level of resistance, i.e. >80%, for each of trimethoprim-sulfamethoxazole, cefepime, ciprofloxacin and ceftriaxone antibiotics whereas *P.aeruginosa* showed a high resistance percentage for trimethoprim-sulfamethoxazole, ciprofloxacin and ceftriaxone antibiotics with the rate of 88.2%, 83.3, and 79.1% respectively (Table 2).

### ESBL and MBL production by *A. baumannii*

From the total isolates of *A. baumannii*, 38 (88.4%) of them showed resistance to at least one of the third generation cephalosporins (3GC). ESBL and MBL production were observed in 24(55.8%) and 13 (30.2%) of the

**Table 1** Distribution of airway *A. baumannii* and *P. aeruginosa* isolates in wards of WSUTRH

| Wards | *A. baumannii* n = 43 | *P. aeruginosa* n = 24 | Total isolates n = 67 |
|---|---|---|---|
| Delivery room | 13 | 4 | 17 |
| Intensive care unit | 21 | 13 | 34 |
| Operation room | 9 | 7 | 16 |

**Table 2** Antibiotic resistance profile of air-borne *A. baumannii* and *P. aeruginosa*

| Antibiotics | *A. baumannii* (n = 43) No (%) | *P.aeruginosa* (n = 24) No (%) |
|---|---|---|
| Amikacin | 30 (69.8) | 6 (25) |
| Cefotaxime | 32 (74.4%) | 17 (70.8) |
| Cefepime | 38 (88.4%) | 14 (58.3) |
| Ceftazidime | 28 (65.1) | 7 (29.1) |
| Ciprofloxacin | 38 (88.4%) | 20 (83.3) |
| Gentamicine | 33 (76.7) | 19 (79.1) |
| Ceftriaxone | 36 (83.7) | 19 (79.1) |
| Aztreonam | 19 (44.2) | 14 (58.3) |
| Meropenem | 13 (30.2) | 10 (41.7) |
| Imipenem | 16 (37.2) | 10 (41.7) |
| Trimethoprim-Sulfamethoxazole | 40 (93.0) | 21(87.5) |

isolates respectively. Coexistence of both ESBL and MBL producers was seen in 5(11.6%) isolates of *A. baumannii* (Table 3).

**ESBL and MBL production by *P. aeruginosa***

Out of 24 isolates of *P. aeruginosa,* 15 (62.5%) were found to become ESBL producers. Metalo-beta-lactamase production was observed in 9 (37.5%) of *P. aeruginosa* isolates. Co-occurrence of both ESBL and MBL producers were seen in 5 (20.8%) isolates (Table 4).

**MDR patterns of aerosol *A. baumannii* and *P.aeruginosa***

A total of 35 (81.4%) *A. baumannii* isolates were found out to be multi-drug resistant. Moreover, 7 (16.3%) of the isolates were pan-drug resistant. Likewise about 20 (83.3%) *P. aeruginosa* isolates were multi-drug resistant with 5 (20.8%) of them pan-drug resistant isolates (Table 5).

**Discussion**

Several studies have documented extensive contamination by *Acinetobacter spp.* of the environment,

**Table 3** ESBL and MBL producing airway *A.baumannii* isolates in restricted settings of the Hospital

Number of resistance isolates (%)

| Antibiotics | Total isolates n = 43 | ESBL producer n = 24 | MBL producer n = 13 |
|---|---|---|---|
| Ceftazidime | 28 (65.1) | 19 (79.2) | 8 (61.5) |
| Ceftriaxone | 36 (83.7) | 22 (91.7) | 10 (76.9) |
| Cefepime | 38 (88.4) | 23 (95.8) | 11 (84.6) |
| Cefotaxime | 32 (74.4) | 20 (83.3) | 9 (69.2) |
| Aztreonam | 19 (44.2) | 21 (87.5) | 12 (92.3) |
| Impeniem | 16 (37.2) | 5 (20.8) | 13 (100) |
| Meropenem | 13 (30.2) | 3 (12.5) | 13 (100) |

**Table 4** ESBL and MBL producing airway *P. aeruginosa* isolates in intensive care unit of the hospital

Number of resistance isolates (%)

| Antibiotics | Total isolates n = 24 | ESBL producer n = 15 | MBL producer n = 9 |
|---|---|---|---|
| Ceftazidime | 7 (29.1) | 11 (73.3) | 7 (77.8) |
| Ceftriaxone | 19 (79.1) | 13 (86.7) | 8 (88.9) |
| Cefipime | 14 (58.3) | 10 (66.7) | 5 (55.6) |
| Cefotaxime | 17 (70.8) | 11 (73.3) | 8 (77.8) |
| Aztreonam | 14 (58.3) | 10 (66.7) | 9 (100) |
| Impenem | 10 (41.7) | 5 (50.0) | 9 (100) |
| Meropenem | 10 (41.7) | 3 (20.0) | 9 (100) |

including respirators and air samples, in the vicinity of infected or colonized patients [19]. In an outbreak of infection with Multi-resistant *Acinetobacter spp.* extensive contamination of the environment, including air was found [19].

The presence of *A.baumannii* as bioaerosols in this study could be supported by its higher survival ability (3 days to 11 months) in the environment and its disinfectant resistance. As the best of the investigators knowledge, this is the first finding of *A.baumannii* in Hospital air in Ethiopian setup. But our finding was corroborated with previous reports in Taiwan [20], Iran [21] and Nepal [22].

High percentage of antibiotic resistance, more than 80%, *A. baumannii* isolates were detected for trimethoprim-sulfamethoxazole, ciprofloxacin, cefepime and ceftriaxone in this study which is corroborated with findings of previous reports in Iran [23, 24], Turkey [25] and Italy hospital intensive care units [26]. A study in Romania reported highly resistant *A. baumannii* isolates with 75% resistance for ceftriaxone, ceftazidime, gentamicin and kanamycin antibiotics each [27] and a study conducted in Ethiopia also revealed 100% and 88% resistant Ciprofloxacin and Gentamicin *A.baumannii* from environmental isolates respectively [28]. Ciprofloxacin resistant, 86.5% *A.baumannii* isolates were also detected in clinical and environmental isolates in Brazil [29] and 92.2% TMP-SXT resistant isolates were also identified in hospital waste effluent in Denmark [30]. Similarly, high antibiotic resistance percentage were also found in Bangladesh from isolates collected from endotracheal tube with 100% resistance for ceftriaxone and gentamicin, and 66.7% for amikacin and impenem 66.7% [31].

Meropenem and imipenem depicted 30.2% and 37.2% resistance *A. baumannii* in the current study which is in harmony with previous findings of 30.2% Meropenem resistance in India [32], 33.3% and 28.1% imipenem resistance in Egypt [33] and Brazil [29] respectively but much lower than 87.7% and 95% resistance reported for both antibiotics in Turkey [34] respectively which could

**Table 5** Antibiogram of air-borne *A. baumannii* and *P. aeruginosa* isolates

| Bacteria | Quantity | Resistance pattern | Frequency | Class |
|---|---|---|---|---|
| *P.aeruginosa* n = 24 | Max | TMP-SXT, CIP, GEN, CRO, CTX, ATM, FEP, IMP, MEM, CAZ, AMK | 5 | 6 |
| | | TMP-SXT, CIP, GEN, CRO, CTX, ATM, FEP, IMP, MEM, CAZ | 2 | 6 |
| | | TMP-SXT, CIP, GEN, CRO, CTX, ATM, FEP, IMP, MEM | 2 | 6 |
| | | TMP-SXT,CIP, GEN, CRO, CTX, FEP, IMP, MEM,AMK | 1 | 5 |
| | | TMP-SXT, CIP, GEN, CRO, CTX, ATM, FEP | 4 | 5 |
| | | TMP-SXT, CIP, GEN, CRO, CTX | 3 | 4 |
| | | TMP-SXT, CIP, GEN, CRO, ATM | 1 | 4 |
| | | TMP-SXT, CIP, GEN | 1 | 3 |
| | Min | TMP-SXT, CIP, CRO | 1 | 3 |
| *A. baumannii* n = 43 | Max | TMP-SXT, CIP, FEP, CRO, GEN, CTX, AMK, CAZ, ATM, IMP, MEM | 7 | 6 |
| | | TMP-SXT, CIP, FEP, CRO, GEN, CTX, AMK, CAZ, ATM, IMP | 3 | 6 |
| | | TMP-SXT, CIP, FEP, CRO, GEN, CTX, AMK, CAZ, IMP, MEM | 3 | 5 |
| | | TMP-SXT, CIP, FEP, CRO, GEN, CTX, AMK, CAZ, ATM | 6 | 5 |
| | | TMP-SXT, CIP, FEP, CRO, GEN, CTX, AMK, CAZ | 6 | 4 |
| | | TMP-SXT, CIP, FEP, CRO, GEN, CTX, AMK | 2 | 4 |
| | | TMP-SXT, CIP, FEP, CRO, GEN, CTX | 2 | 4 |
| | | TMP-SXT, CIP, FEP, CRO | 4 | 3 |
| | Min | TMP-SXT, CIP, FEP | 2 | 3 |

Key: AMK-Amikacin, CTX-Cefotaxime, FEP-cefepime CAZ-Ceftazidime, CIP-Ciprofloxacin GEN-Gentamicine CRO-Ceftriaxone, ATM-Aztreonam, MEM-Meropenem, IMP-Imipenem, TMP-SXT-Trimethoprime-Sulphamethoxazole

be due to difference in availability and prescribing pattern of antibiotics where these antibiotics were introduced in our country recently.

ESBLs were reported in the species belonging to the genera of *Enterobacter* and *Klebsiella* isolated from the air of hospital associated environment. 55.8% of *A. baumannii* isolates were ESBL producing. This finding is higher than 21% ESBL production rate reported in Tehran [35] and 28% in India [36].

MBL producer *A. baumannii* rate identified in this study (30.2%) was lower than 48% reported in India [37] and 81.48% reported in environmental isolates in Egypt [38], which could be explained by difference in samples, and reduced selective pressure of *Acinetobacter* for impenem and meropenem antibiotics in our country setups.

Generally *A.baumannii* showed the highest percentage of resistance for most antibiotics tested, this could possibly be due to the bacterial ability to resist many antibiotics and disinfectant or could possibly be due to selective pressure or abusing of the drugs in the hospital.

*P. aeruginosa* associated infection is a recognized public health threat often acquired from the hospital environment. It is not only an important cause of morbidity but also increases the stay of the patient in the hospital and increases the cost of treatment [39]. The isolation of epidemic *P. aeruginosa* from room air in the presence of patients increases the possibility that there may be airborne spread of epidemic *P. aeruginosa* strains between patients [40].

The antibiotic susceptibility pattern of environmental isolates of *P. aeruginosa* is mostly overlooked and rarely reported. A few reports available on susceptibility pattern of *P. aeruginosa* suggest significant resistance to a variety of antibacterial agents. In this study, high rate (> 60%) of antibiotic resistant *P.aeruginosa* isolates were observed for amikacin, cefotaxime, cefepime, ceftazidime, ciprofloxacin, gentamicin and trimethoprim-sulphamethoxazole. This finding is corroborated with previous study from environmental isolates in Egypt where isolates from the hospital environment have showed more antibiotic resistance than the clinical isolates with rate of resistance 100% for cefotaxime, 92% for ceftriaxone, 85% for gentamicin, 85%, and 62% for ciprofloxacin [41].

A previous study conducted in Ethiopia revealed high antibiotic resistant *P.aeruginosa* isolates in hospital environment. Indoor air pseudomonas species were also showed significant percentage of resistance for Gentamicin (73.7%) and Ciprofloxacin (78.9%) [42]. Higher levels of *P.aeruginosa* resistance to trimethoprim-sulfamethoxazole, gentamicin and ceftriaxone in the present study is comparable with the study conducted in Ethiopia where 95.1% to trimethoprim-sulphametoxazole, 62% to gentamicin, and 58% to ceftriaxone resistance revealed [43].

The rate (41.7%) of resistance of the *P.aeruginosa* isolates to imipenem seen in this study is higher than 18and 18.9% reported in India [44, 45]. Ceftazidime resistance (29.1%), *P.aeruginosa* isolates in this study is different from the previous reported findings in Nigeria 34.6% [46] and India 36% [44]. Variation of resistance across different studies could be due to availability of antibiotics at the hospital as well as community level, type of patients, number of samples, and genotypic resistance mechanisms.

ESBL producing *P.aeruginosa* isolates were mostly detected in clinical isolates in hospital setup according to the university hospital microbiology report. ESBL producing *P.aeruginosa* isolates detected in this study corroborated with a study in Egypt where 95% of *P.aeruginosa* isolates were beta-lactamase producers [6] and all isolates from surface water were ESBL producer in study conducted by Nasereen et al. [47].

In our finding, 37.5% MBL production by *P. aeruginosa* was observed. A study conducted in India, Brazil and Iran revealed 32.9%, 30%, 48.3% MBL production respectively [48–50]; however those studies used clinical specimen. These *P. aeruginosa* isolates could be causes for several nosocomial infections, illustrating the need for proper infection control practices [51].

## Conclusions

Higher rate of MDR, ESBL and, MBL producing antibiotic resistant *P.aeruginosa* and *A.baumannii* isolates were found in indoor air. Though the current isolates were not identified from patients in this study, the role of contaminated indoor air for the production of ESBL and MBL isolates could play a major role if contact is established. So it is pertinent that their presence should be controlled and antimicrobial stewardship programs should be designed to prevent the further spread of these isolates. ESBL and MBL strains as airborne microbiota are the first finding in Ethiopian that could provide a new insight for antimicrobial stewardship programs and future studies.

## Strength

These bacteria especially *A.baumannii* is the first finding as airborne organism in Ethiopia. Many antibiotics as per the guidelines were tested for these findings and post intervention phase is started after fumigation.

## Weakness

The study didn't have a plan of post intervention phase by the investigators due to budget limitation even though now the budget was approved for it. The cross sectional nature of this study may increase and decrease the prevalence of the bacteria since patient trafficking, type of patients and other environmental factors like humidity and others may differ in a given day.

## Abbreviations
ATCC: American Type Culture Collection; BAP: Blood agar plates; DR: Delivery room; ESBLs: Extended spectrum beta lactamases; HAI: Health care associated infections; ICU: Intensive care unit; MBLs: Metallo-β-lactamases; MDR: Multidrug-resistant; OR: Operation room; TSA: Tryptic soya agar; WSUTRH: Wolaita Sodo University Teaching and Referral Hospital

## Acknowledgements
We acknowledge all the nurses and midwives, Laboratory technologists of WSUTRH, Wolaita Sodo University ethical review committee for the ethical clearance, and WSU for Financial support.

## Funding
The research budget is funded by Wolaita Sodo University. Grant number 239/2015WSU.

## Author's contributions
FS: Conceived the study, FS, FW: Participated in the design of the study and performed the statistical analysis, FS, FW: Interpreted the data: FS, EG: Obtained ethical clearance and permission for study: FW: Supervised data collectors: FS, FW, MM: Drafting the article or revisiting it critically for important intellectual content. All authors read and approved the final manuscript.

## Consent for publication
Not applicable.

## Competing interest
All authors declare that they have no competing interest.

## Author details
[1]School of Medicine, Wolaita Sodo University, PO box 138, Sodo, Ethiopia. [2]Wolaita Sodo University, School of Medicine, Sodo, Ethiopia. [3]Department of medical laboratory, Wolaita Sodo University, Sodo, Ethiopia. [4]College of health science and medicine, school of medicine, MaddaWalabu University, Bale Goba, Ethiopia.

## References
1. Gorny R. Filamentous microorganisms and their fragments in indoor air: a review. Ann Agric EnvironMed. 2004;11:185–97.
2. Asghar AH, Faidah HS. Frequency and antimicrobial susceptibility of gram- negative bacteria isolated from 2 hospitals in Makkah. Saudi Arabia Saudi Med J. 2009;30:1017–23.
3. WHO. The evolving threats of antimicrobial resistance, option for action ISSN 9789241503181. 2012.
4. CDC. Antibiotic resistance threats in the United States. 2013.
5. Lee TB, Baker OG, Lee JT, Scheckler WE. Recommended practices for surveillance. Am J Infect Contr. 1998;26:277–88.
6. Gad G, Eldomany E, Zaki S, Ashour H. Characterization of *Pseudomonas Aeruginosa* isolated from clinical and environmental samples in Minia, Egypt: prevalence, Antibiogram and resistance mechanisms. J Antimicrob Chemother. 2007;60:1010–7.
7. Vahdani M, Azimi L, Asghari B, Bazmi F, Rastegar LA. Phenotypic screening of extended-spectrum ß-lactamase and metallo-ß-lactamase in multidrug-resistant Pseudomonas Aeruginosa from infected burns. Ann Burns Fire Disasters. 2012;25(2):78–81.
8. Manchanda V, Sanchaita S, Singh NP. Multidrug Resistant Acinetobacter. J Glob Infect Dis. 2010;2(3):291–304.
9. Vila J, Pachón J. Therapeutic options for Acinetobacterbaumannii infections. Expert OpinPharmacother. 2008;9:587–99.
10. Owlia P, Azimi L, Gholami A, Asghari B, Lari AR. ESBL and MBL mediated resistance in *Acinetobacterbaumannii*: a global threat to burnt patients. Infez Med. 2012;20(3):182–7.
11. Roy FC, Sarah S, Charles D. The role of the healthcare environment in the spread of multidrug-resistant organisms: update on current best practices for containment. TherAdv Infect Dis. 2014;2:79–90.

12. Pasquarella C, Pitzurra O, Savino A. The index of microbial air contamination (review). J Hosp Infect. 2000;46:241–56.

13. Anderson AA. New sampler for the collection, sizing and enumeration of viable airborne particles. J Bacteriol. 1958;76(5):471–84.

14. Govan JR. Pseudomonas aeruginosa. In: Collee G, Barrie PM, Andrew PF, Anthony S, editors. Mackie and McCartney practical medical microbiology. 14th ed. New York: Churchill Livingstone; 2006. p. 413–24.

15. Bauer A, Kirby W, Sherris J, Turck M. Antibiotic susceptibility testing by a standardized single disk method. Am J ClinPathol. 1966;45:493–6.

16. Clinical and Laboratory Standards Institute. Performance Standards for Antimicrobial Susceptibility Testing; Twenty-Fourth Informational Supplement, M100-S24, 2014.

17. Clinical Laboratory Standards Institute. Performance standards for antimicrobial susceptibility testing. Sixteenth informational supplement. Approved standards, M100 -S16, Wayne, PA. 2007.

18. Yong D, Lee K, Yum J, Shin H, Rossolini G, Chong Y. Imipenem-EDTA disk method for differentiation of metallo-betalactamase- producing clinical isolates of pseudomonas spp. and Acinetobacter spp. J ClinMicrobiol. 2002;40:3798–801.

19. Bergogne E and Towner K. *Acinetobacter spp.* as Nosocomial Pathogens: Microbiological, Clinical, and Epidemiological Features. Clinical microbiology reviews. 1996;9(2):148–65.

20. Huang PY, Shi ZY, Chen CH, Den W. Airborne and surface-bound microbial contamination in two intensive care units of a medical Center in Central Taiwan. Aerosol Air Qual Res. 2013;13:1060–9.

21. Alireza A, Sanam M. Microbial profile of air contamination in hospital Ward. Iranian J Pathol. 2012;7:168–74.

22. Kritu P, Prakash G, Shiba K, Reena K, Mukhiya RN, Ganesh R. Screening of Antibiotype among environmental isolates of Acinetobacter spp.in hospital setting. Nepal J Sci Technol. 2012;13(2):203–8.

23. HakemiVala M, Hallajzadeh M, Fallah F, Hashemi A, Goudarzi H. Characterization of theextended-spectrum beta-lactamase producers among non-fermenting gram-negative bacteria isolated from burnt patients. Arch Hyg Sci. 2013;2(1):1–6.

24. Mirnejad R, Vafaei S. Antibiotic resistance patterns and the prevalence of ESBLs amongstrains of *A. baumannii* isolated from clinical specimens. JGMI. 2013;2:1–8.

25. Aktas O, Ozbek A. Prevalence and *In-vitro* antimicrobial susceptibility patterns of *Acinetobacter* strains isolated from patients in intensive care units. J Int Med Res. 2003;31:272–80.

26. Parviz O, Leila A, Abbas G, Abdolaziz R. L. ESBL- and MBL-mediated resistance in *Acinetobacter baumannii*: a global threat to burn patients. Infez Med. 2012;3:182–7.

27. Sofia C, Angela R, Luminiţa S, Raluca F, Iuliana T. Cultural and biochemical characteristics of acinetobacter spp. strains isolated from hospital units. J Prev Med. 2004;12(3–4):35–42.

28. Agersew A, Degisew M, Yitayih W. Bacterial profile and their antimicrobial susceptibility patterns of computer keyboards and mice at Gondar University hospital, Northwest Ethiopia. Biomedicine Biotechnology. 2015;3(1):1–7.

29. Medeiros M, Lincopan N. Oxacillinase (OXA)-producing *Acinetobacter baumannii*in Brazil: clinical and environmental impact and therapeutic options. J Bras Patol Med Lab. 2013;49(6):391–405.

30. Luca G, Andreas P, John E, Anders D. Antibiotic resistance in *Acinetobacter* spp. isolated from sewers receiving waste effluent from a hospital and a pharmaceutical plant. Appl Environ Microbiol. 1998;64(9):3499–502.

31. Azizun N, Shasheda A, Ruhulu AM AAS. Isolation of and their antimicrobial resistance pattern in an intensive care unit (ICU) of a tertiary care hospital in Dhaka, Bangladesh. Bangladesh J Med Microbiol. 2012;06(01):03–6.

32. Mahua S, Srinivasa H, Macaden R. Antibiotic resistance profile & extended spectrum beta-lactamase (ESBL) production in *Acinetobacter*species. Indian J Med Res. 2007;63–7.

33. Enas A, Ismael S, Ahmad S, Sherein G, Entsar H, Ibrahim M. Relationship between clinical and environmental isolates of *Acinetobacter baumannii*in Assiut university hospitals. J Am Sci. 2013;9(11):67–73.

34. Aktas O, Ozbek A. Prevalence and in-vitro antimicrobial susceptibility patterns of Acinetobacter strains isolated from patients in intensive care units. J Int Med Res. 2003;31:272–80.

35. Ava B, Mohammad R, Jalil V. Frequency of extended spectrum beta-lactamase (ESBLs) producing *Escherichia coli* and *klebseilla pneumonia* isolated from urine in an Iranian 1000-bed tertiary care hospital. Afr J Microbiol Res. 2010;4(9):881–4.

36. Sinha M, Srinivasa H, Macaden R. Antibiotic resistance profile & extended spectrum beta-lactamase (ESBL) production in Acinetobacter species. Indian J Med Res. 2007;126(1):63–7.

37. Goel V, Hogade SA, Karadesai SG. Prevalence of extended spectrum beta lactamases, AmpC beta lactamase, and metallo beta lactamase producing Pseudomonas Aeruginosa and Acinetobacterbaumannii in an intensive care unit in a tertiary care hospital. J Sci Soc. 2013;40(1):28–31.

38. Enas A, Ismael S, Ahmad S, et al. Relationship between Clinical and Environmental Isolates of *Acinetobacter baumannii* in Assiut University Hospitals Journal of American Science 2013;9(11):67-73.

39. Elizabeth B, Vincent HT. Impact of multidrug-resistant *Pseudomonas aeruginosa* infection on patient outcomes. Expert Rev Pharmacoecon Outcomes Res. 2010;10(4):441–51.

40. Jones AM, Govan JR, Doherty CJ, et al. Identification of airborne dissemination of epidemic multiresistant strains of Pseudomonas Aeruginosa at a CF Centre during a cross infection outbreak. Thorax. 2003;58:525–7.

41. Gamal F, Ramadan A, Sahar Z, Hossam M. Characterization of *Pseudomonas aeruginosa* isolated from clinical and environmental samples in Minia, Egypt: prevalence, antibiogram and resistance mechanisms. J Antimicrob Chemother. 2007 Nov;60(5):1010–7.

42. Teklu S, Lakew G, Girma M, Adinew Z, Feleke B, Daba M, Endalew Z. Bacterial indoor-air load and its implications for healthcare-acquired infections in a teaching hospital in Ethiopia. Int J Infect Control. 2016;12:1–9.

43. Meseret M, Solomon A, Gebre K. Antimicrobial drug resistance and disinfectants susceptibility of *Pseudomonas aeruginosa* isolates from clinical and environmental samples in Jimma University specialized hospital, Southwest Ethiopia. Am J Biomedical Life Sci. 2014; 2 (2). 40-45. doi:10.11648/j.ajbls.20140202.12.

44. Sivaraj S, Murugesan S. Muthuvelu S, et al. Comparative study of Pseudomonas aeruginosaisolate recovered from clinical and environmental samples against antibiotics. Int J Pharm PharmSci. 2012;4:103–107.

45. Indu B, BalvInder S, Imple K. Incidence of multidrug resistant *Pseudomonas aeruginosa* isolated from burn patients and environment of teaching institution. J Clin Diagnostic Research. 2014;8(5):26–9.

46. Eyo AA, Ibeneme BD, Thumamo AE. Antibiotic resistance profiles of clinical and environmentalisolates of *Pseudomonas aeruginosa*in Calabar, Nigeria. J Pharm Biol Sci. 2015;10(4):09–15.

47. Nasreen M, Sarker A, Malek MA, Ansaruzzaman Md, Rahman M. Prevalence and resistance pattern of *Pseudomonas aeruginosa*solated from surface water. Adv Microbiol. 2015;5:74-81. doi:10.4236/aim.2015.51008.

48. Gaikwad V., Bharadwaj R., Dohe V. Study the Prevalence and Risk Factors of Metallo- Betalactamase Producing *Pseudomonas aeruginosa* from Teriary Care Centre. 2015;4(5):3126–32.

49. Inacio H, Bomfim M, França R, Farias LM, Carvalho M, Serufo J, Santos S. Phenotypic and Genotypic Diversity of Multidrug-Resistant Pseudomonas aeruginosa Isolates from Bloodstream Infections Recovered in the Hospitals of Belo Horizonte, Brazil. Chemotherapy. 2014;60:54-62.

50. Alisha A, Afsaneh S, Bizhan N, Kamal A. Prevalence and Clonal dissemination of Metallo-Beta-Lactamase-producing Pseudomonas Aeruginosa in Kermanshah. Jundishapur J Microbiol. 2015 Jul;8(7):e20980.

51. Arunava K, Sreenivasan S, Shailesh K, Hema A, Akhila K, Sivaraman U. Incidence of metallo beta lactamase producing *Pseudomonas aeruginosa* in ICU patients. Indian J Med Res. 2008 Apr;127(4):398–402.

# 17

# Risk factors for hospitalized patients with resistant or multidrug-resistant *Pseudomonas aeruginosa* infections

Gowri Raman[1]*(iD), Esther E. Avendano[1], Jeffrey Chan[1], Sanjay Merchant[2] and Laura Puzniak[2]

## Abstract

**Background:** Identifying risk factors predicting acquisition of resistant *Pseudomonas aeruginosa* will aid surveillance and diagnostic initiatives and can be crucial in early and appropriate antibiotic therapy. We conducted a systematic review examining risk factors of acquisition of resistant *P. aeruginosa* among hospitalized patients.

**Methods:** MEDLINE®, EMBASE®, and Cochrane Central were searched between 2000 and 2016 for studies examining independent risk factors associated with acquisition of resistant *P. aeruginosa*, among hospitalized patients. Random effects model meta-analysis was conducted when at least three or more studies were sufficiently similar.

**Results:** Of the 54 eligible articles, 28 publications (31studies) examined multi-drug resistant (MDR) or extensively drug resistant (XDR) *P. aeruginosa* and 26 publications (29 studies) examined resistant *P. aeruginosa*. The acquisition of MDR *P. aeruginosa*, as compared with non-MDR *P. aeruginosa*, was significantly associated with intensive care unit (ICU) admission (3 studies: summary adjusted odds ratio [OR] 2.2) or use of quinolones (4 studies: summary adjusted OR 3.59). Acquisition of MDR or XDR compared with susceptible *P. aeruginosa* was significantly associated with prior hospital stay (4 studies: summary adjusted OR 1.90), use of quinolones (3 studies: summary adjusted OR 4.34), or use of carbapenems (3 studies: summary adjusted OR 13.68). The acquisition of MDR *P. aeruginosa* compared with non-*P. aeruginosa* was significantly associated with prior use of cephalosporins (3 studies: summary adjusted OR 3.96), quinolones (4 studies: summary adjusted OR 2.96), carbapenems (6 studies: summary adjusted OR 2.61), and prior hospital stay (4 studies: summary adjusted OR 1.74). The acquisition of carbapenem-resistant *P. aeruginosa* compared with susceptible *P. aeruginosa*, was statistically significantly associated with prior use of piperacillin-tazobactam (3 studies: summary adjusted OR 2.64), vancomycin (3 studies: summary adjusted OR 1.76), and carbapenems (7 studies: summary adjusted OR 4.36).

**Conclusions:** Prior use of antibiotics and prior hospital or ICU stay was the most significant risk factors for acquisition of resistant *P. aeruginosa*. These findings provide guidance in identifying patients that may be at an elevated risk for a resistant infection and emphasize the importance of antimicrobial stewardship and infection control in hospitals.

**Keywords:** Resistant, Multi-drug resistant, Pseudomonas aeruginosa, Risk factors, Acquisition

* Correspondence: graman@tuftsmedicalcenter.org
[1]Center for Clinical Evidence Synthesis, Tufts Medical Center, 800 Washington Street, Box 63, Boston, MA 02111, USA
Full list of author information is available at the end of the article

# Background

There is an alarming increase in antibiotic-resistant Gram-negative infections [1–3]. Among Gram-negative infections, *Pseudomonas aeruginosa*is is one of the most common gram-negative bacteria causing nosocomial and healthcare-associated infections (HAIs) in hospitalized patients [4]. The World Health Organization places carbapenem-resistant *P. aeruginosa* as a critical priority pathogen that desperately requires new treatment options [5]. Increasing rates of multidrug-resistant (MDR) *P. aeruginosa* in HAIs and among hospitalized patients is a major public health problem [6]. MDR *P. aeruginosa* infections in the hospital setting are associated with poor outcomes including increased resource utilization and costs, morbidity, and mortality [7].

MDR *P. aeruginosa* account for 13–19% of HAIs each year in the US. The increasing level of resistance in MDR *P. aeruginosa* is often attributed to patient-to-patient transmission of resistant strains as well as newly acquired resistance owing to previous antibiotic exposure. As per standardized international terminology, MDR is defined as non-susceptibility to at least one agent in three or more antimicrobial categories and XDR is defined as non-susceptibility to at least one agent in all but two or fewer antimicrobial categories (i.e. bacterial isolates remain susceptible to only one or two categories) [8]. In severe systemic infections, consideration of MDR/XDR *P. aeruginosa* when selecting treatment is warranted to ensure timely and appropriate initial therapy. Lack of effective antibacterial therapies against *P. aeruginosa* infections severely limit effective therapeutic options and consequently, lead to inappropriate initial therapy that adversely impacts health outcomes [9]. Typically it takes 48 h to definitively identify MDR *P. aeruginosa*, which can be a detrimental delay for these patients.

There are considerable gaps and inconsistencies in knowledge regarding risk factors associated with the occurrence of MDR *P. aeruginosa* in nosocomial infections and HAIs. Identifying risk factors predicting acquisition of MDR *P. aeruginosa* or identifying subgroups of patients who are at an increased risk for acquisition of MDR *P. aeruginosa* in the hospital setting will assist in providing timely and appropriate treatment. While a recent review examined the risk factors independently associated with extensively drug-resistant (XDR) *P. aeruginosa*, there has not been a comprehensive analysis of contemporary literature reporting all levels of resistance (MDR or XDR or resistant) of *P. aeruginosa* infections [6]. This systematic review of recent published literature evaluates risk factors that are independently associated with acquisition of microbiologically identified MDR or XDR, or resistant (single drug class) *P. aeruginosa* from various sites among inpatients, hospitalized in any of the following setting including wards, intensive care units, and other types of inpatient settings.

# Methods

We performed a systematic search in the MEDLINE, Cochrane Library, and EMBASE databases for citations indexed from January 01, 2000 through December 31, 2016. The initial search strategy (Additional file 1: Table S1) includes terms related to the pathogen (*P. aeruginosa*), mode of infection (nosocomial, hospital-acquired, healthcare-acquired, hospital-associated, healthcare-associated), and risk factor assessment (risk factors, predict, risk score, risk assessment, and multivariate analysis). Additionally, search terms for Gram-negative infections, beta-lactamases, and metallo-beta-lactamases attributed to carbapenem resistance were included to increase the yield of studies with resistant (single drug class) *P. aeruginosa*. These three databases were searched because they index most of the published citations. To supplement this search, we reviewed reference lists of eligible studies using an iterative process to maximize inclusion of relevant data. We did not perform grey literature searches or systematically search for unpublished data. We reviewed abstracts from conference proceedings if they were indexed in the three aforementioned databases.

## Study definitions

Our primary objective was to examine studies evaluating risk factors associated with acquisition of MDR or XDR, or resistant *P. aeruginosa* among inpatient adult patients evaluated in the hospital setting. In this review, the hospital setting comprises all types of units, including intensive care units, emergency room/casualty, or other wards where patients were located at the time of collection of the resistant *P. aeruginosa* microbiological specimen and underwent further treatment in the hospital setting. The acquisition of resistant *P. aeruginosa* could have been either community- or hospital-acquired, but all patients must have been evaluated and treated in the hospital setting. We accepted MDR and XDR *P. aeruginosa* as defined by individual studies, although we noted considerable heterogeneity in the definitions. Non-MDR *P. aeruginosa* was also defined by the individual studies and varied in definition to include *P. aeruginosa* infections other than MDR such as susceptible *P. aeruginosa* (susceptible to all antipseudomonal agents) or resistant to any one class of drug. Non- *P. aeruginosa* was also defined by the individual studies and varied in definition to include pathogens other than *P. aeruginosa*.

## Eligibility criteria

Studies evaluating patients hospitalized in a ward, intensive or critical care unit, or any other inpatient healthcare setting (including chronic care facilities), were eligible for inclusion. Studies examining patients with either hospital-acquired or community-acquired were included, provided that they were evaluated in a hospital /inpatient setting. Risk factors that predict acquisition of MDR or XDR, or resistant *P. aeruginosa* were included. Risk factors were categorized into patient characteristics, hospital characteristics, and treatment characteristics.

The exposure and comparators of interest included: MDR or XDR *P. aeruginosa* versus resistant *P. aeruginosa* (to any one class of antibiotic); MDR or XDR *P. aeruginosa* versus susceptible *P. aeruginosa*; MDR or XDR *P. aeruginosa* versus control (any other Gram-negative pathogen or any infection with unspecified pathogen); resistant *P. aeruginosa* versus susceptible *P. aeruginosa*. The outcome of interest was microbiologically confirmed acquisition of MDR or XDR, or resistant *P. aeruginosa*. For studies that reported both the outcome of acquisition of MDR or XDR *P. aeruginosa* and single-drug resistant *P. aeruginosa*, we included the study only once (for the outcome of acquisition of MDR or XDR *P. aeruginosa*) in the analysis. We accepted all study designs except non-comparative studies, case reports, and case series. Studies that reported multivariable results adjusting for any potential confounders were eligible. No minimum study duration or follow-up time was required for inclusion.

We excluded studies of mixed infections that had more than 20% Gram-positive infections (to ensure most (80%) of the evaluated infections in eligible studies were Gram-negative infections) and studies solely examining *P. aeruginosa* resistant due to metallo-beta-lactamases. Studies published in languages other than English were excluded.

All citations identified by literature searches were independently screened by two researchers. Upon the start of citation screening, we implemented a training session where all researchers screened the same articles and conflicts were discussed. We iteratively continued training until we reached consensus regarding the nuances of the eligibility criteria for screening. During double-screening, we resolved conflicts through group discussions.

We assessed the methodological quality of each study based on predefined criteria using the Agency for Healthcare Research and Quality (AHRQ) and the New-Castle Ottawa risk of bias tool, which probes risk of selection, performance, detection, attrition, reporting, and other potential biases. Each study was extracted by one experienced methodologist (GR, EA, and JC). The extraction was reviewed and confirmed by at least one other methodologist. Any disagreements were resolved by discussion amongst the study team. Data were extracted into customized Microsoft Excel™ forms. We tested the data extraction forms on several studies and revised as necessary before full data extraction. Extracted data included variables addressing population characteristics, including severity of illness, description of exposure and comparator groups, sites of infection, outcome

definitions, enrolled and analyzed sample sizes, study design features, and multivariate results. Any missing or unavailable data were deemed as not reported information. We performed random effects model meta-analyses of eligible studies if at least three or more studies were sufficiently similar in population, exposure, and outcomes [10]. If appropriate, we also conducted meta-regression analyses to evaluate study features explaining potential heterogeneity. However, due to the presence of substantial clinical heterogeneity, we also qualitatively compared results across studies (for example, source of infection).

All analyses were performed in Stata version 14 (StataCorp, College Station, Texas) with the metan, metareg, and metabias functions. We tested between study heterogeneity with the Q statistic (significant when $p < 0.10$) and quantified the extent of heterogeneity with the $I^2$ statistic. It is common practice to interpret $I^2 > 50\%$ as representing substantial inconsistency or significant statistical heterogeneity [11].

When applicable, results were also presented in table format. All meta-analyses of adjusted or multivariate results were presented in forest plots. The summary results examining the relationship between risk factors and acquisition of MDR or XDR, or resistant *P. aeruginosa* were presented as adjusted odds ratio or relative risks with 95% confidence intervals.

## Results

The literature search identified 316 citations and an additional 43 citations were identified through bibliographic searches. After removing duplicates, 345 abstracts were eligible for screening. Using a low threshold of eligibility criteria for review of abstracts, 112 full-text articles were retrieved. After full-text review, an additional 58 articles were excluded based on the eligibility criteria (Fig. 1). Of the 54 eligible articles, 28 articles (31 studies) examined MDR or XDR *P. aeruginosa* [12–39] and the remaining 26 articles (29 studies) examined resistant *P. aeruginosa* [41–65].

### Studies of MDR and XDR *P. aeruginosa*

Of the 28 articles ($n = 8935$ subjects) that examined risk factors for acquisition of MDR or XDR *P. aeruginosa* [12–39], nine were prospective studies and 19 were retrospective or unmatched case-control or matched case-control studies. In 31 studies from 28 articles; two articles reported two different control groups [20, 27] and one study reported two different cases [33]. The studies were conducted in Western European countries (16 studies), the USA (3 studies), the USA and Western Europe (2 studies), Asia (6 studies), Turkey (1 study), or Brazil (1 study); 3 studies were conducted in an unclear location (Table 1). Of the 28 articles, three were

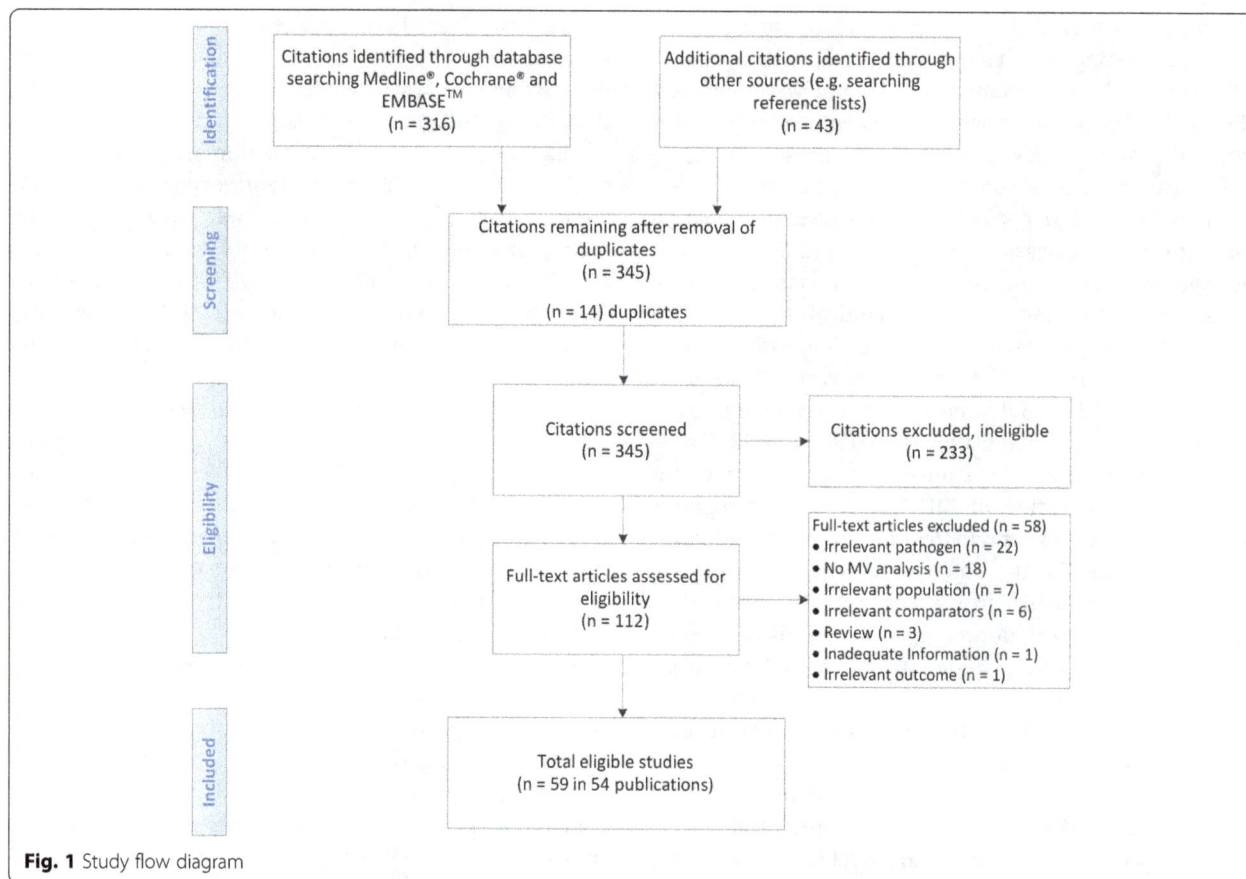

**Fig. 1** Study flow diagram

multi-center studies [26, 32, 35]. Twenty-one were conducted in tertiary care or university hospitals and the other 9 were conducted in any hospital.

Of the included 28 articles, 20 articles (from 22 studies) reported data on MDR*P. aeruginosa* acquisition [12, 14–20, 22, 23, 25–31, 35, 37, 39], six reported on XDR *P. aeruginosa* [13, 24, 32–34, 38], and two included both (MDR acquisition being the most commonly reported) [21, 36]. The most commonly reported definition for MDR was laboratory-confirmed resistance to more than one agent in three or more classes of antibiotics. In five studies, the definitions were similar to the definition of XDR, but they were described as MDR [12, 16, 17, 27, 28]. The most commonly reported definition for XDR was non-susceptibility to at least one agent in all antimicrobial classes, but susceptibility to two or fewer anti-pseudomonal antimicrobials; one study required evidence of resistance to all available anti-pseudomonal antimicrobials [32].

Of 8935 patients, 2446 case patients had MDR or XDR *P. aeruginosa* or both types of resistance and the remaining were control patients. The descriptions of study control groups varied across studies: susceptible *P. aeruginosa* (5 studies [12, 13, 26, 29, 32]); non-MDR *P. aeruginosa* (without MDR phenotype) (14 studies [14, 15,

18–22, 24, 25, 27, 34, 35, 60, 39]); non-XDR *P. aeruginosa* (without XDR phenotype) (2 studies [31, 33]); non-*P. aeruginosa* (any pathogen other than *P. aeruginosa*) (4 studies [16, 23, 26, 30]); non-MDR/non-XDR *P. aeruginosa* plus non-*P. aeruginosa* (2 studies [17, 37]). No data were reported in two studies [11, 19]. The mean age of study subjects ranged from 29.8 years to 73.2 years (cases) and from 37.9 years to 71.1 years (controls). The males included as study subjects ranged from 50 to 91% (cases) and from 46 to 78.3% (controls). Most studies included a mix of patients with respiratory, wound, genitourinary, and bloodstream as the source of infection. Various severity scores were employed across studies including McCabe score, APACHE II, Charlson index, and SAPS II score.

For meta-analysis, we categorized studies based on three control groups: non-MDR *P. aeruginosa* (without MDR phenotype); susceptible *P. aeruginosa*; and any controls (non *P. aeruginosa* or undescribed controls). In analyses of risk for acquisition of MDR *P. aeruginosa*, 21 articles in 23 studies [12, 14–20, 22, 23, 25–31, 33, 35, 37, 39]) reported data on MDR *P. aeruginosa* acquisition and two included both MDR *P. aeruginosa* and XDR *P. aeruginosa* (MDR *P. aeruginosa* acquisition being the most commonly reported) [21, 36].

**Table 1** Baseline characteristics of studies in MDR or XDR *P. aeruginosa*

| Author, Year | Design | Country | Case/Exposure | Control/Comparator | Total N | Age cases (Yr) | Age control (Yr) | Male cases (%) | Male control (%) |
|---|---|---|---|---|---|---|---|---|---|
| Aloush, 2006 [12] | CC, matched | Israel | MDR *P. aeruginosa* | Patients with MDR *P. aeruginosa* | 164 | 65 | 63 | 60 | 50 |
| Bodro, 2015 [13] | P, cohort | Spain | XDR *P. aeruginosa* | Other pathogens | 318 | Median: 59 | Median: 62 | 77.4 | 69.7 |
| Cao, 2004 [14] | CC, unmatched | China | MDR *P. aeruginosa* | *P.aeruginosa* | 112 | 60 | 50 | 59 | 58.8 |
| Cilloniz, 2016 [15] | P, cohort | Spain | MDR *P. aeruginosa* | Non-MDR *P. aeruginosa* (not fully described) | 68 | 72.7 | 71.1 | 90.9 | 78.3 |
| Cobos-Trigueros, 2015 [16] | P, cohort | Spain | MDR *P. aeruginosa* | Susceptible or resistant *P.aeruginosa* and non-*P.aeruginosa* | 850 | NR | NR | NR | NR |
| D'Agata (b), 2006 [17] | CC, matched | USA, Italy | MDR *P. aeruginosa* | Non-*P.aeruginosa* | 302 | 58 | 62 | 62 | 50 |
| Dalfino, 2011 [18] | P, cohort | NR | MDR *P. aeruginosa* | NR | 251 | 63 | 63 | 65 | 61.3 |
| Dantas, 2014 [19] | R, cohort | Brazil | MDR *P. aeruginosa* | Resistant or susceptible *P. aeruginosa* | 120 | 51.5 (total) | 51.5 (total) | 63.3 (total) | 63.3 (total) |
| Defez (a), 2004 [20] | CC, matched | France | MDR *P. aeruginosa*, nosocomial | Hospitalized, non-nosocomial MDR *P. aeruginosa* | 320 | 73.2 | 67 | 56.25 | 52.5 |
| Defez (b), 2004 [20] | CC, unmatched | France | MDR *P. aeruginosa* | Non MDR- *P. aeruginosa* (not described) | 395 (155) | 73.2 | NR | 56.25 | 56 |
| Gomez-Zorilla, 2014 [21] | P, cohort | Spain | MDR *P. aeruginosa* (MDR non-XDR and XDR) | Non-MDR *P. aeruginosa* (not fully described) | 112 | 65.3 (total) | 65.3 (total) | 69 (total) | 69 (total) |
| Johnson, 2009 [22] | R, cohort | USA | MDR *P. aeruginosa* | Non-MDR *P.aeruginosa* (not described) | 503 | median: 59 (total) | median: 59 (total) | 57 (total) | 57 (total) |
| Joo, 2011 [23] | P, cohort | South Korea | MDR *P. aeruginosa* | Resistant or susceptible *P. aeruginosa* | 202 | 55 (total) | 55 (total) | 62.9 (total) | 62.9 (total) |
| Liew, 2013 [24] | CC, matched | Singapore | XDR *P. aeruginosa* | Non-*P. aeruginosa* or other gram-negative | 79 | Median: 47 (total) | NR | 62 (total) | NR |
| Lodise, 2007 [25] | CC, unmatched | USA | MDR *P. aeruginosa* | Non-MDR *P.aeruginosa* (not fully described)[a] | 351 | 60.5 (total) | 60.5 (total) | 61.2 (total) | 61.2 (total) |
| Micek, 2015 [26] | R, cohort | USA, France, Germany, Italy, Spain | MDR *P. aeruginosa* | Non-MDR *P. aeruginosa* (not fully described) | 740 | 53.5 | 62.1 | 62.8 | 70.2 |
| Montero (a), 2010 [27] | CC, unmatched | NR | MDR *P. aeruginosa* | Non-*P. aeruginosa* | 1035 | 67.8 | 67.5 | 72.5 | 54.3 |
| Montero (b), 2010 [27] | CC, unmatched | NR | MDR *P. aeruginosa* | Susceptible *P.aeruginosa* | 877 | 67.8 | 69.1 | 72.5 | 59.4 |
| Nakamura, 2013 [28] | P, cohort | Japan | MDR *P. aeruginosa* | Non MDR *P.aeruginosa* (not fully described)[c] | 435 | NR | NR | NR | NR |
| Nseir, 2011 [29] | P, cohort | France | MDR *P. aeruginosa* | Non MDR *P. aeruginosa* (not fully described) | 511 | 60 | 55 | 65 | 69 |
| Ohmagari, 2005 [30] | CC, unmatched | USA | Patients with cancer with MDR *P. aeruginosa* infection | Patients with cancer with susceptible *P. aeruginosa* infection | 54 | 51.8 | 60.3 | 50 | 58.3 |

**Table 1** Baseline characteristics of studies in MDR or XDR *P.aeruginosa* (Continued)

| Author, Year | Design | Country | Case/Exposure | Control/Comparator | Total N | Age cases (Yr) | Age control (Yr) | Male cases (%) | Male control (%) |
|---|---|---|---|---|---|---|---|---|---|
| Paramythiotou, 2004 [31] | CC, matched | France | MDR *P. aeruginosa* | Non-*P. aeruginosa* | 68 | 59 | 61.5 | 65 | 65 |
| Park, 2011 [32] | CC, matched | South Korea | XDR *P. aeruginosa* | Non-XDR *P.aeruginosa* (not fully described)[b] | 99 | 65 | 56 | 79 | 46 |
| Pena, 2009 [39] | P, cohort | Spain | MDR *P. aeruginosa* | CRPA | 246 | 67 | 65 | 67 | 67 |
| Pena (a), 2012 [33] | R, cohort | Spain | XDR *P. aeruginosa* | Susceptible *P. aeruginosa* | 138 | 64.7 | 65.06 | 86 | 70.5 |
| Pena (b), 2012 [33] | R, cohort | Spain | Non-XDR MDR *P. aeruginosa* | Susceptible *P. aeruginosa* | 108 | 64.85 | 65.06 | 54 | 70.5 |
| Samonis, 2014 [34] | R, cohort | Greece | XDR *P. aeruginosa* | Non-XDR *P. aeruginosa* (MDR and PDR and sensitive) | 89 | 73 | 69 | 81.8 | 57.3 |
| Tumbarello, 2011 [35] | CC, unmatched | Italy | MDR *P. aeruginosa* | Non-*P. aeruginosa* | 252 | 62 | 63 | 57.5 | 57.5 |
| Tuncer, 2012 [36] | CC, unmatched | Turkey | MDR and XDR *P. aeruginosa* | Non-MDR *P.aeruginosa* (not fully described) | 120 | 58.6 | 58.2 | 54.1 | 49.4 |
| Ustun, 2016 [37] | CC, unmatched | Turkey | MDR *P. aeruginosa* | Non-*P. aeruginosa* | 225 | 29.8 | 37.9 | 58.7 | 65.3 |
| Willmann, 2014 [38] | CC, matched | Germany | XDR *P. aeruginosa* | Non-XDR *P. aeruginosa* (not fully described) or non- *P. aeruginosa* | 31 | 56 | 60 | 65 | 78.5 |

*CC* Case-control, *CRPA* carbapenem-resistant *P. aeruginosa*, *MDR* multi-drug resistant, *P* Parallel, *PDR* Pan-Drug-Resistant, *R* Retrospective, *XDR* extremely drug-resistant, *YR* Year
[a]Lodise 2007: Non-MDR *P.aeruginosa* = ≥90% for only amikacin, cefepime, and piperacillin-tazobactam
[b]Park,Y.S 2011:used random selection of controls
[c]Nakamura 2013:Non-MDR defines patients with P. aeruginosa other than the MDR phenotype on the same ward as those with the MDR phenotype within the same month

The risk factors statistically significantly associated with acquisition of MDR *P. aeruginosa* in meta-analysis are described in the following results sections. Additional risk factors that had a statistically significant association with acquisition of MDR *P. aeruginosa* but were not eligible for meta-analysis are listed in Additional file 1: Tables S2-S5.

### MDR P. aeruginosa versus non-MDR P. aeruginosa

Thirteen studies with non-MDR *P. aeruginosa* as a comparator reported risk factors associated with acquisition of MDR *P. aeruginosa* [15, 16, 19–23, 25, 26, 28, 35, 36, 39]. In meta-analysis, prior ICU stay or prior use of quinolones had a statistically significant association with acquisition of MDR *P. aeruginosa*. Two other predictors, surgery and prior use of carbapenems, were not associated with an increased risk of acquisition (Fig. 2).

### MDR P. aeruginosa versus susceptible P. aeruginosa

Four studies with susceptible *P. aeruginosa* as a comparator reported risk factors for acquisition of MDR *P. aeruginosa* [14, 27, 30, 33]. In meta-analysis, prior admission, use of quinolones, and use of carbapenems had a statistically significant association with future acquisition of MDR *P. aeruginosa*. Two other predictors (comorbid

severity scores and chronic obstructive pulmonary disease [COPD]) were not associated with a risk of acquisition of MDR *P. aeruginosa* in meta-analysis (Fig. 3).

Of note, the following factors were not combined in a meta-analysis; but were reported to be not associated with acquisition of MDR *P. aeruginosa*: colonization of *P. aeruginosa* in isolate sources other than blood preceding a diagnosis of bacteremia, isolation of multiple pathogens in culture, and history of previous *P. aeruginosa* infection.

### MDR P. aeruginosa versus non-P. aeruginosa

Seven studies with non-*P. aeruginosa* or any undescribed control as a comparator reported risk factors for acquisition of MDR *P. aeruginosa* [12, 17, 18, 27, 29, 31, 37]. In meta-analysis, penicillins, carbapenems, quinolones, disease severity, and prior admissions predicted a statistically significant increased risk of acquiring MDR *P. aeruginosa*, compared with non-*P. aeruginosa* (Fig. 4).

Both diabetes and sepsis were not associated with the risk of acquiring MDR *P. aeruginosa*, compared with non-*P. aeruginosa*.

### XDR P. aeruginosa studies

Six studies reported risk factors for acquisition of XDR *P. aeruginosa* alone, compared with different controls

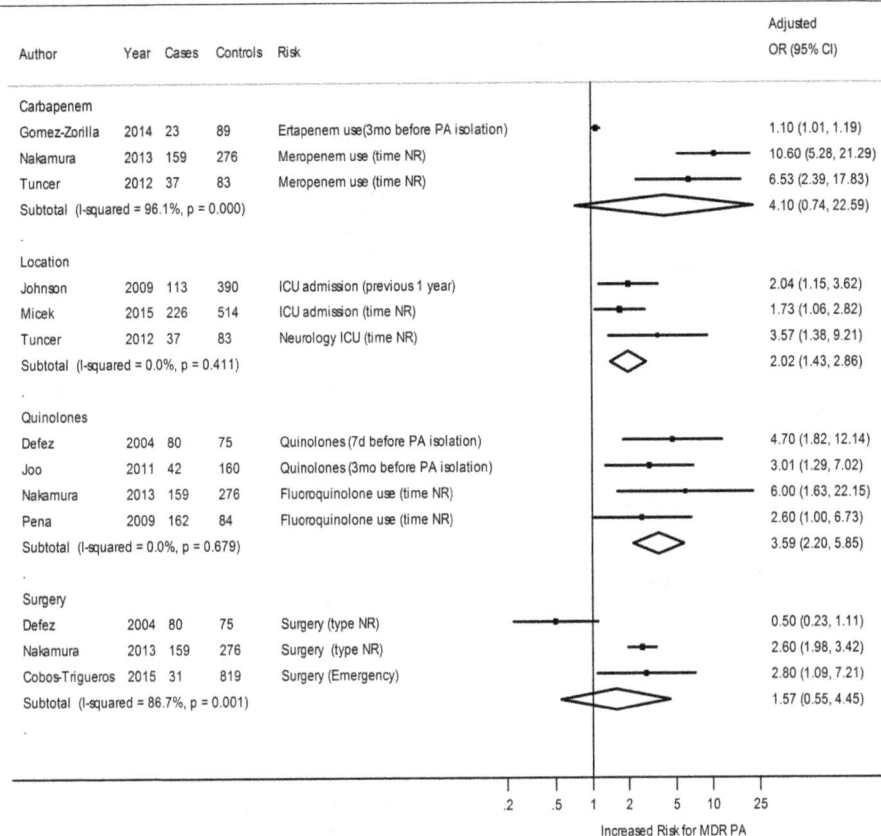

| Author | Year | Cases | Controls | Risk | Adjusted OR (95% CI) |
|--------|------|-------|----------|------|---------------------|
| **Carbapenem** | | | | | |
| Gomez-Zorilla | 2014 | 23 | 89 | Ertapenem use(3mo before PA isolation) | 1.10 (1.01, 1.19) |
| Nakamura | 2013 | 159 | 276 | Meropenem use (time NR) | 10.60 (5.28, 21.29) |
| Tuncer | 2012 | 37 | 83 | Meropenem use (time NR) | 6.53 (2.39, 17.83) |
| Subtotal (I-squared = 96.1%, p = 0.000) | | | | | 4.10 (0.74, 22.59) |
| **Location** | | | | | |
| Johnson | 2009 | 113 | 390 | ICU admission (previous 1 year) | 2.04 (1.15, 3.62) |
| Micek | 2015 | 226 | 514 | ICU admission (time NR) | 1.73 (1.06, 2.82) |
| Tuncer | 2012 | 37 | 83 | Neurology ICU (time NR) | 3.57 (1.38, 9.21) |
| Subtotal (I-squared = 0.0%, p = 0.411) | | | | | 2.02 (1.43, 2.86) |
| **Quinolones** | | | | | |
| Defez | 2004 | 80 | 75 | Quinolones (7d before PA isolation) | 4.70 (1.82, 12.14) |
| Joo | 2011 | 42 | 160 | Quinolones (3mo before PA isolation) | 3.01 (1.29, 7.02) |
| Nakamura | 2013 | 159 | 276 | Fluoroquinolone use (time NR) | 6.00 (1.63, 22.15) |
| Pena | 2009 | 162 | 84 | Fluoroquinolone use (time NR) | 2.60 (1.00, 6.73) |
| Subtotal (I-squared = 0.0%, p = 0.679) | | | | | 3.59 (2.20, 5.85) |
| **Surgery** | | | | | |
| Defez | 2004 | 80 | 75 | Surgery (type NR) | 0.50 (0.23, 1.11) |
| Nakamura | 2013 | 159 | 276 | Surgery (type NR) | 2.60 (1.98, 3.42) |
| Cobos-Trigueros | 2015 | 31 | 819 | Surgery (Emergency) | 2.80 (1.09, 7.21) |
| Subtotal (I-squared = 86.7%, p = 0.001) | | | | | 1.57 (0.55, 4.45) |

.2  .5  1  2  5  10  25

Increased Risk for MDR PA

**Fig. 2** Forest plot of risk factors for MDR versus non-MDR *P. aeruginosa* acquisition. CI = Confidence Interval; ICU = Intensive Care Unit; NR = Not Reported; OR = Odds Ratio; PA = *P. aeruginosa*

[13, 24, 32–34, 38]. XDR *P. aeruginosa* was compared with non-XDR *P. aeruginosa* (2 studies [32, 34]); non-XDR *P. aeruginosa* and non-*P. aeruginosa* (1 study [38]); non-*P. aeruginosa* (1 study [24]); susceptible *P. aeruginosa* (1 study [33]); and susceptible *P. aeruginosa* and non-*P. aeruginosa* (1 study [13]).The most frequently reported factors that significantly increased the risk of acquiring XDR *P. aeruginosa* included: prior fluoroquinolones use (2 studies), urinary catheter (2 studies). The following factors were not associated with an increased risk of XDR *P. aeruginosa*: ceftazidime use, days of ciprofloxacin use, number of different antibiotics used during time at risk (i.e. time between admission and isolation of bacteria in index cases).

### Studies of resistant *P. aeruginosa*
### Carbapenem-resistant *P. aeruginosa*
Twenty-three studies in 21 articles (*n* = 9877 subjects) that examined risk factors for acquisition of carbapenem-resistant *P. aeruginosa* [17, 19, 40, 42–47, 50, 51, 54–57, 59, 60, 61, 62, 64, 65]; two articles contributed to two studies each [44, 64]. Five were prospective studies and the remaining 16 had case-control or retrospective designs. The studies were conducted in

Brazil (8 studies), the USA (5 studies), Western Europe (4 studies), Asia (3 studies), and the USA and Western Europe (1 study). All studies were conducted in tertiary care or university hospitals. Three were multicenter studies. Table 2 summarizes baseline characteristics of included carbapenem resistant *P. aeruginosa* studies.

The descriptions of control groups varied across studies. For the purpose of analysis, we categorized the controls into two categories: susceptible *P. aeruginosa* and any control (non-*P. aeruginosa* with or without susceptible *P. aeruginosa*). The mean age ranged from 44 years to 67 years (cases) and from 41 years to 66 years (controls). Most studies included a mix of patients with respiratory, wound, genitourinary, and bloodstream as the source of infection.

### Carbapenem-resistant versus susceptible *P. aeruginosa*
In meta-analysis, prior use of piperacillin-tazobactam, vancomycin, and carbapenems were all significantly associated with acquisition of carbapenem-resistant *P. aeruginosa* (Additional file 1: Figures S1-S2). Other predictors including use of quinolones, hospital stay, and time at risk were not associated with a statistically

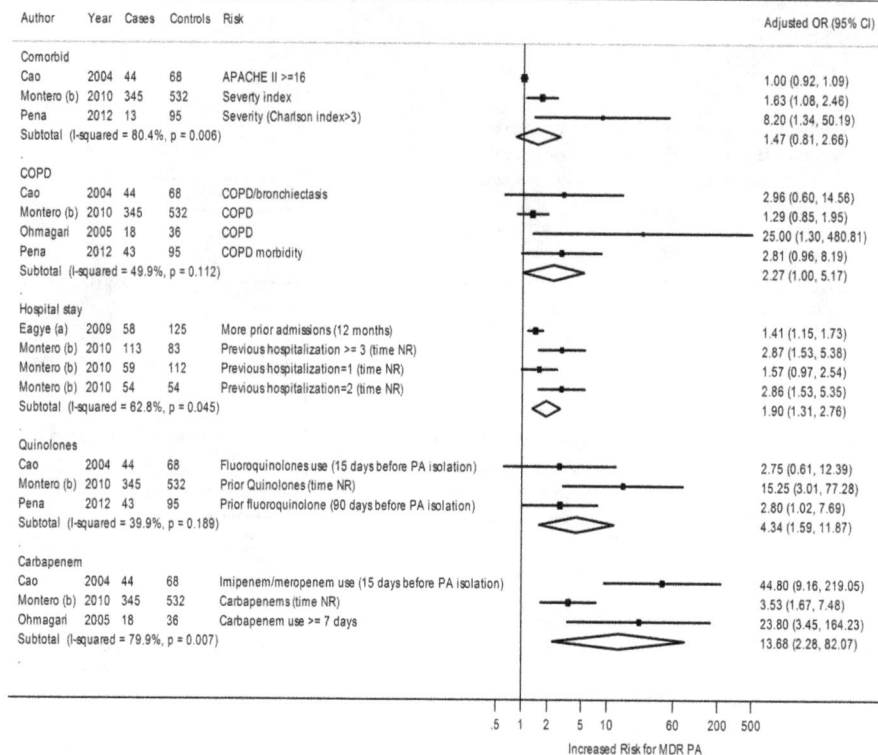

| Author | Year | Cases | Controls | Risk | | Adjusted OR (95% CI) |
|---|---|---|---|---|---|---|
| **Comorbid** | | | | | | |
| Cao | 2004 | 44 | 68 | APACHE II >=16 | | 1.00 (0.92, 1.09) |
| Montero (b) | 2010 | 345 | 532 | Severity index | | 1.63 (1.08, 2.46) |
| Pena | 2012 | 13 | 95 | Severity (Charlson index>3) | | 8.20 (1.34, 50.19) |
| Subtotal (I-squared = 80.4%, p = 0.006) | | | | | | 1.47 (0.81, 2.66) |
| **COPD** | | | | | | |
| Cao | 2004 | 44 | 68 | COPD/bronchiectasis | | 2.96 (0.60, 14.56) |
| Montero (b) | 2010 | 345 | 532 | COPD | | 1.29 (0.85, 1.95) |
| Ohmagari | 2005 | 18 | 36 | COPD | | 25.00 (1.30, 480.81) |
| Pena | 2012 | 43 | 95 | COPD morbidity | | 2.81 (0.96, 8.19) |
| Subtotal (I-squared = 49.9%, p = 0.112) | | | | | | 2.27 (1.00, 5.17) |
| **Hospital stay** | | | | | | |
| Eagye (a) | 2009 | 58 | 125 | More prior admissions (12 months) | | 1.41 (1.15, 1.73) |
| Montero (b) | 2010 | 113 | 83 | Previous hospitalization >= 3 (time NR) | | 2.87 (1.53, 5.38) |
| Montero (b) | 2010 | 59 | 112 | Previous hospitalization=1 (time NR) | | 1.57 (0.97, 2.54) |
| Montero (b) | 2010 | 54 | 54 | Previous hospitalization=2 (time NR) | | 2.86 (1.53, 5.35) |
| Subtotal (I-squared = 62.8%, p = 0.045) | | | | | | 1.90 (1.31, 2.76) |
| **Quinolones** | | | | | | |
| Cao | 2004 | 44 | 68 | Fluoroquinolones use (15 days before PA isolation) | | 2.75 (0.61, 12.39) |
| Montero (b) | 2010 | 345 | 532 | Prior Quinolones (time NR) | | 15.25 (3.01, 77.28) |
| Pena | 2012 | 43 | 95 | Prior fluoroquinolone (90 days before PA isolation) | | 2.80 (1.02, 7.69) |
| Subtotal (I-squared = 39.9%, p = 0.189) | | | | | | 4.34 (1.59, 11.87) |
| **Carbapenem** | | | | | | |
| Cao | 2004 | 44 | 68 | Imipenem/meropenem use (15 days before PA isolation) | | 44.80 (9.16, 219.05) |
| Montero (b) | 2010 | 345 | 532 | Carbapenems (time NR) | | 3.53 (1.67, 7.48) |
| Ohmagari | 2005 | 18 | 36 | Carbapenem use >= 7 days | | 23.80 (3.45, 164.23) |
| Subtotal (I-squared = 79.9%, p = 0.007) | | | | | | 13.68 (2.28, 82.07) |

.5  1  2  5  10    60  200  500

Increased Risk for MDR PA

**Fig. 3** Forest plot of risk factors for MDR versus susceptible *P. aeruginosa* acquisition. APACHE II = Acute Physiology And Chronic Health Evaluation II; CI = confidence interval; COPD = Chronic obstructive pulmonary disease; NR = Not Reported; OR = Odds Ratio; PA = *P. aeruginosa*

significant increased risk (Additional file 1: Figures S1-S2). Additional risk factors that significantly increased the risk of acquiring carbapenem-resistant *P. aeruginosa* are summarized in Additional file 1: Tables S6-S9.

### Carbapenem-resistant versus any control (unspecified or non- P. aeruginosa controls)

Four studies used other controls (3 studies that used Non-P.aeruginosa controls and one study did not specify the control) [17, 44, 45, 64]. No meta-analysis could be conducted as there were fewer than three studies for this comparison for the same type of predictor. All studies reported a statistically significant increased risk of carbapenem-resistant *P. aeruginosa*, compared with any control. The risk factors examined included prior use of antibiotics, comorbid score, length of hospital or ICU stay, hemodialysis, non-ambulatory status, transfer from another facility, indwelling urinary catheter, and mechanical ventilation.

### Other (non-carbapenem) resistant P. aeruginosa

Of the seven studies that reported data on acquisition of other (non-carbapenem) resistant *P. aeruginosa* in Table 3 [41, 45, 48, 49, 52, 53, 63], two reported data on piperacillin- or piperacillin-tazobactam-resistant *P. aeruginosa* [49, 63], three reported data on quinolone-resistant

*P. aeruginosa* [48, 52, 53], and two reported on *P. aeruginosa* resistant to the newer cephalosporins, namely, cefepime and ceftazidime [41, 45].

### Piperacillin- or piperacillin-tazobactam-resistant P. aeruginosa

No meta-analysis could be conducted as there were fewer than three studies for this comparison on any particular category of predictor [49, 63]. Two studies reported a statistically significant increased risk for piperacillin- or piperacillin-tazobactam-resistant *P. aeruginosa* for the following factors: admissions in prior year, ICU stay, time at risk, transfer, severe morbidity or higher comorbid score, and prior use of antibiotics (aminoglycosides, broad-spectrum cephalosporins, carbapenems, piperacillin-tazobactam, and quinolones).

### Quinolone-resistant P. aeruginosa

Three studies compared quinolone-resistant and susceptible *P. aeruginosa* [48, 53, 53]. In meta-analysis, prior use of quinolones predicted subsequent risk for acquisition of quinolone-resistant *P. aeruginosa* (Additional file 1: Figure S3). Other statistically significant risk factors for an increased acquisition of quinolone-resistant *P. aeruginosa* included indwelling airway, co-existing diabetes mellitus, and nosocomial residence (not defined) (Additional file 1: Table S10). The number of hospital days from admission to culture was not a significant predictor.

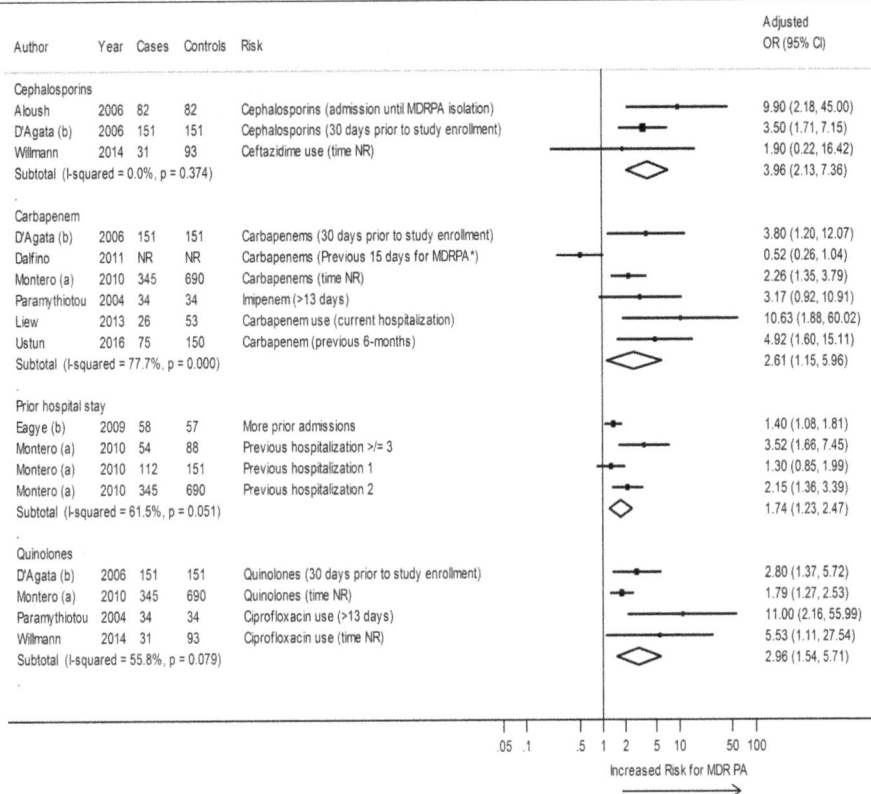

| Author | Year | Cases | Controls | Risk | Adjusted OR (95% CI) |
|--------|------|-------|----------|------|----------------------|
| **Cephalosporins** | | | | | |
| Aloush | 2006 | 82 | 82 | Cephalosporins (admission until MDRPA isolation) | 9.90 (2.18, 45.00) |
| D'Agata (b) | 2006 | 151 | 151 | Cephalosporins (30 days prior to study enrollment) | 3.50 (1.71, 7.15) |
| Willmann | 2014 | 31 | 93 | Ceftazidime use (time NR) | 1.90 (0.22, 16.42) |
| Subtotal (I-squared = 0.0%, p = 0.374) | | | | | 3.96 (2.13, 7.36) |
| **Carbapenem** | | | | | |
| D'Agata (b) | 2006 | 151 | 151 | Carbapenems (30 days prior to study enrollment) | 3.80 (1.20, 12.07) |
| Dalfino | 2011 | NR | NR | Carbapenems (Previous 15 days for MDRPA*) | 0.52 (0.26, 1.04) |
| Montero (a) | 2010 | 345 | 690 | Carbapenems (time NR) | 2.26 (1.35, 3.79) |
| Paramythiotou | 2004 | 34 | 34 | Imipenem (>13 days) | 3.17 (0.92, 10.91) |
| Liew | 2013 | 26 | 53 | Carbapenem use (current hospitalization) | 10.63 (1.88, 60.02) |
| Ustun | 2016 | 75 | 150 | Carbapenem (previous 6-months) | 4.92 (1.60, 15.11) |
| Subtotal (I-squared = 77.7%, p = 0.000) | | | | | 2.61 (1.15, 5.96) |
| **Prior hospital stay** | | | | | |
| Eagye (b) | 2009 | 58 | 57 | More prior admissions | 1.40 (1.08, 1.81) |
| Montero (a) | 2010 | 54 | 88 | Previous hospitalization >/= 3 | 3.52 (1.66, 7.45) |
| Montero (a) | 2010 | 112 | 151 | Previous hospitalization 1 | 1.30 (0.85, 1.99) |
| Montero (a) | 2010 | 345 | 690 | Previous hospitalization 2 | 2.15 (1.36, 3.39) |
| Subtotal (I-squared = 61.5%, p = 0.051) | | | | | 1.74 (1.23, 2.47) |
| **Quinolones** | | | | | |
| D'Agata (b) | 2006 | 151 | 151 | Quinolones (30 days prior to study enrollment) | 2.80 (1.37, 5.72) |
| Montero (a) | 2010 | 345 | 690 | Quinolones (time NR) | 1.79 (1.27, 2.53) |
| Paramythiotou | 2004 | 34 | 34 | Ciprofloxacin use (>13 days) | 11.00 (2.16, 55.99) |
| Willmann | 2014 | 31 | 93 | Ciprofloxacin use (time NR) | 5.53 (1.11, 27.54) |
| Subtotal (I-squared = 55.8%, p = 0.079) | | | | | 2.96 (1.54, 5.71) |

**Fig. 4** Forest plot of risk factors for MDR versus Non-*P. aeruginosa* acquisition. *Dalfino 2011, ICU stay was used for the control. CI = confidence interval; MDRPA = multi-drug resistant *P. aeruginosa*; NR = not reported; OR = Odds Ratio

### Third-generation cephalosporin-resistant P. aeruginosa

Two studies [41, 45] reported an increased risk for third-generation cephalosporin-resistant *P. aeruginosa* for the following factors: transfer from outside facility, prior use of antibiotics (e.g. extended-spectrum cephalosporins, extended-spectrum penicillin, or quinolones or amikacin). Both length of hospital stay before culture and prior use of carbapenem were not associated with an increased risk for resistance to higher generation cephalosporins in one study [41].

### Discussion

This systematic review of the literature summarizes risk factors that predict acquisition of MDR *P. aeruginosa*, XDR *P. aeruginosa*, and other resistant *P. aeruginosa*. Our meta-analysis identified that the risk factors for acquisition of MDR or XDR *P. aeruginosa* varied with regard to the type of control used for comparison. ICU stays (either as current or prior to current episode of infection) and use of quinolones was significantly associated with acquisition of MDR or XDR *P. aeruginosa*, compared with resistant or susceptible *P. aeruginosa*. Use of prior antibiotics including, cephalosporins, quinolones, or carbapenems, and prior hospital admissions predicted an increased risk of MDR or XDR *P. aeruginosa* versus non-*P. aeruginosa*.

The increasing rates of MDR or XDR, or resistant *P. aeruginosa* are a worldwide public health problem. Resistant strains of *P. aeruginosa* are associated with high mortality and increased resource utilization [66]. The emergence and spread of MDR *P. aeruginosa* may be associated with misuse or overuse of antimicrobials. Our meta-analysis found a consistent association between the use of quinolones and acquisition of MDR or XDR *P. aeruginosa P. aeruginosa*. However, association between carbapenem use and acquisition of MDR or XDR *P. aeruginosa* was not consistent across comparisons. While some primary studies did report a relationship between MDR or XDR *P. aeruginosa* and prior use of antibiotics [14, 30], our meta-analysis identified statistically significant associations between carbapenem use and acquisition of MDR or XDR *P. aeruginosa* and the significance of their association can vary by the type of comparator examined. Nonetheless, our results confirm that prior use of specific antimicrobials is an important risk factor for acquisition of MDR or XDR *P. aeruginosa*. Antimicrobial resistance occurs over time, often mediated by gene mutations and misuse or

**Table 2** Baseline characteristics of studies in carbapenem-resistant *P. aeruginosa*

| Author | Year | Design | Country | Case/Exposure | Control/Comparator | Total N | Age cases (Yr) | Age control (Yr) | Male cases (%) | Male control (%) |
|---|---|---|---|---|---|---|---|---|---|---|
| D'Agata (a) [17] | 2006 | CC, matched | USA, Italy | CRPA | Non-*P. aeruginosa* | 82 | 61 | 60 | 73 | 44 |
| DalBen [42] | 2013 | P, cohort | Brazil | MRAC and CRPA | Non-MRAC and non-CRPA | 325 | 44 | 41 | 59 | 41 |
| Djordjevic [43] | 2013 | P, cohort | Serbia | CRPA | CSPA | 261 | 59.2 | 61.4 | 80.8 | 64.9 |
| Eagye (a) [44] | 2009 | CC, control | USA | MRPA | MSPA | 183 | 66.4 | 66.1 | 58.6 | 59.2 |
| Eagye (b) [44] | 2009 | CC, control | USA | MRPA | Non-*P. aeruginosa* | 182 | 66.4 | 57.4 | 58.6 | 50.9 |
| Fortaleza (a) [45] | 2006 | CC, matched | Brazil | IRPA | Control (NR) | 324 | median 45 | median 44 | 68.5 | 60.2 |
| Furtado [46] | 2009 | CC, matched | Brazil | IRPA | Without IRPA | 245 | 50 | 54 | 68.3 | 59.3 |
| Furtado [47] | 2010 | CC, matched | Brazil | IRPA | Non-IRPA | 295 | 54 | 54 | 70.7 | 56.5 |
| Harris [50] | 2002 | CC, matched | USA | IRPA | Without IRPA | 866 | 55.7 | 49.4 | 39.1 | 39.1 |
| Harris [51] | 2011 | P, cohort | USA | IRPA | Non-IRPA | 3146 | 56.7 | 55.7 | 61.9 | 56.7 |
| Kohlenberg [54] | 2010 | CC, unmatched | Germany | CRPA | CSPA | 33 | median 60 | median 44.4 | 53.3 | 72.2 |
| Lautenbach [55] | 2010 | CC, unmatched | USA | IRPA | ISPA | 2542 | 61 (total) | 61 (total) | 63.3 | 56.1 |
| Lee [56] | 2015 | CC, matched | Taiwan | CRPA | All susceptible *P. aeruginosa* | 75 | 61.6 | 62 | 48 | 48 |
| Lin [57] | 2016 | CC, unmatched | Taiwan | CRPA | CSPA | 164 | 66.6 | 63.5 | 72 | 67.1 |
| Luyt [58] | 2014 | P, cohort | France | CRPA | CSPA | 169 | 57.6 | 57.9 | 65 | 66 |
| Onguru [59] | 2008 | P, cohort | Turkey | IRPA | ISPA | 170 | 45.9 | 49.7 | 72 | 66.3 |
| Pena [60] | 2007 | P, cohort | Spain | CRPA | CSPA | 254 | 59.8 | 57.1 | 60 | 65 |
| Pereira [61] | 2008 | CC, unmatched | Brazil | IRPA | ISPA | 59 | 51.8 | 50.7 | 70 | 55 |
| Tam [62] | 2007 | CC, unmatched | USA | CRPA | Pan-susceptible *P. aeruginosa* | 51 | 50 | 64 | 33 | 73 |
| Tuon [40] | 2012 | CC, unmatched | Brazil | CRPA | CSPA | 77 | 46.4 | 49 | 75.9 | 70.8 |
| Zavascki (a) [64] | 2005 | CC, unmatched | Brazil | IRPA | Non *P. aeruginosa* | 186 | 58 | 51 | 60 | 53 |
| Zavascki (b) [64] | 2005 | CC, unmatched | Brazil | IRPA | ISPA | 158 | 58 | 51 | 60 | 66 |
| Zhang [65] | 2009 | CC, unmatched | China | CRPA | CSPA | 34 | 61 | 50 | NR | NR |

*CC* case-control, *CRPA* carbapenem-resistant*P. aeruginosa*, *CSPA* carbapenem-susceptible *P.aeruginosa*, *ICU* Intensive Care Unit, *IRPA* imipenem-resistant *P. aeruginosa*, *ISPA* imipenem-susceptible *P.aeruginosa*, *MRAC* meropenem-resistant *Acinetobacter baumannii*, *MRPA* meropenem-resistant *P. aeruginosa*, *MSPA* meropenem-susceptible *P. aeruginosa*, *NR* not reported,k *P* parallel, *SICU* Surgical Intensive Care Unit, *YR* year

overuse of antimicrobials may accelerate this process. Understanding the epidemiology of MDR or XDR *P. aeruginosa* will be necessary to overcome infections with these resistant pathogens.

This review finding can be supported in the context of a recent review on MDR or XDR *P. aeruginosa*, which examined multivariate risk factors reported in eight included articles [67]. The authors of this review did not perform a meta-analysis but identified prior antimicrobial therapy, medical devices, patient-related characteristics, and environmental sources as risk factors for MDR or XDR *P. aeruginosa*. Our review, in which a meta-analysis was performed, demonstrated that admission location, prior admission, or use of quinolones was significantly associated with acquisition of MDR or XDR *P. aeruginosa*. In addition to reviewing MDR or XDR *P. aeruginosa*, we reviewed single drug-resistant *P. aeruginosa*. In meta-analysis, prior

use of piperacillin-tazobactam, vancomycin, or carbapenems were significantly associated with acquisition of carbapenem-resistant versus susceptible *P. aeruginosa*. In meta-analysis, prior fluoroquinolone use was a statistically significant predictor of subsequent quinolone-resistant versus susceptible *P. aeruginosa*.

There are limitations associated with this systematic literature review. To begin with, the study inclusion criteria were limited to published studies indexed in English. Secondly, studies eligible for inclusion were heterogeneous with respect to the definition of exposure, site of infection with *P. aeruginosa,* and risk factors included in the study. As a result, a combined meta-analysis may misrepresent the true picture. We mitigated these issues by using a random effects model in our analyses and by limiting analyses to similar comparators. However, in many instances there were risk factors that were statistically significant in two

**Table 3** Baseline characteristics of studies in resistant *P. aeruginosa*

| Author | Year | Design | Country | Case/Exposure | Control/Comparator | Total N | Age cases (Yr) | Age control (Yr) | Male cases (%) | Male controls (%) |
|---|---|---|---|---|---|---|---|---|---|---|
| Akhabue [41] | 2011 | CC, unmatched | USA | Cefepime-resistant P.aeruginosa | Cefepime-susceptible P.aeruginosa | 2529 | Median:61 (total) | Median:61 (total) | 62 | 56.4 |
| Fortaleza (b) [45] | 2006 | CC, matched | Brazil | Ceftazidime-resistant P.aeruginosa | Control | 165 | median 38 | median 44.5 | 72.7 | 62.7 |
| Gasink [48] | 2006 | CC, unmatched | USA | Fluoroquinolone-resistant P.aeruginosa | Fluoroquinolone-susceptible P.aeruginosa | 847 | 56 | 62 | NR | NR |
| Harris [49] | 2002 | CC, unmatched | USA | Piperacillin-tazobactam-resistant P. aeruginosa | Patients without Piperacillin-tazobactam-resistant P. aeruginosa | 1315 | 53.4 | 49.7 | 42.5 | 39.4 |
| Hsu [52] | 2005 | CC, unmatched | USA | Fluoroquinolone-resistant P.aeruginosa | Fluoroquinolone-susceptible P.aeruginosa | 177 | 73.8 | 68 | 43 | 49 |
| Khayr [53] | 2000 | CC, unmatched | USA | Ciprofloxacin-resistant P.aeruginosa | Ciprofloxacin-susceptible P.aeruginosa | 94 | Age > 65: 79% | Age > 65: 79% | 100 | 100 |
| Trouillet [63] | 2002 | CC, unmatched | France | Piperacillin-resistant P. aeruginosa | Piperacillin-susceptible P. aeruginosa | 135 | 64.6 | 65.5 | 67.6 | 64.4 |

*CC* case-control, *NR* not reported, *YR* year

studies, but unfortunately a third study was not available to permit the exploration of this factor through meta-analysis. Additionally, our study results may not be generalizable to all regions as studies from certain regions (for example, Western European nations for MDR or XDR *P. aeruginosa* and Brazil for carbapenem-resistant *P. aeruginosa*) were overrepresented in our sample published literature.

Confounding in observational studies reporting unadjusted data is a well-known source of bias. To mitigate this bias, we included risk factors that were analyzed in multivariate analyses. The choice of the control group (e.g. patients with infection with susceptible strains or patients without any infection at all) may also have influenced the results. We attempted to address this issue using similar comparison groups in the meta-analyses. As with any evidence synthesis, the limitations of the data available in primary studies will transfer into limitations of the systematic review. For example, the control group was not well defined in studies, specifically in studies that reported non- *P. aeruginosa* as controls. The description of these controls was unclear if the control group did or did not include MDR infection of a non-Pseudomonas bacteria. The results section describes variability across studies with regard to study characteristics, outcome assessment, and the relationship between risk factors and the outcome of acquisition of resistant *P. aeruginosa*. We could not conduct additional subgroup analyses by site of infection, or explain differences across studies using stratified analyses due to the small number of

available studies for any particular comparison. An insufficient number of studies (< 10 studies) precluded evaluatingthe potential for publication bias with funnel plots and Egger's tests for small study effects [68].

## Conclusions

Consistently, across comparisons, prior use of antibiotics and prior ICU stay was a significant risk predictor for acquisition of MDR or XDR *P. aeruginosa* infections. Depending on local epidemiology, this finding is useful in identifying patients at high risk for resistant *P. aeruginosa* that may benefit from alternate empiric treatment. Further, these findings emphasize the need for antimicrobial stewardship and infection control in hospitals and continued need for the development of new antimicrobial agents with activity against MDR *P. aeruginosa* [68]. The implementation of antimicrobial stewardship and infection control in hospitals can improve patient safety and care, reduce resource utilization, and reduce resistance. The increasing prevalence of antimicrobial resistance among hospitalized patients continues to pose a challenge for practitioners.

## Additional file

Additional file 1: **Table S1.** Search Strategy. **Table S2.** Patient–related Multivariate Risk Factors of Acquistion of MDR *P. aeruginosa*. **Table S3.** Antibiotic Treatment–related Multivariate Risk Factors of Acquistion of MDR *P. aeruginosa*. **Table S4.** Other Treatment–related Multivariate Risk Factors of Acquistion of MDR and XDR *P. aeruginosa*. **Table S5.**

Hospital–related Multivariate Risk Factors of Acquistion of MDR and XDR *P. aeruginosa*. **Table S6.** Patient–related Multivariate Risk Factors of Acquistion of Carbapenem-resistant *P. aeruginosa*. **Table S7.** Antibiotic Treatment–related Multivariate Risk Factors of Acquistion of Carbapenem-resistant *P. aeruginosa*. **Table S8.** Other Treatment–related Multivariate Risk Factors of Acquistion of Carbapenem-resistant *P. aeruginosa*. **Table S9.** Hospital–related Multivariate Risk Factors of Acquistion of Carbapenem-resistant *P. aeruginosa*. **Table S10.** Multivariate Risk Factors of Acquistion of Resistant *P. aeruginosa*. **Figure S1.** Meta-analysis of Risk Factors for Carbapenem versus Susceptible *P. aeruginosa* Acquisition. **Figure S2.** Meta-analysis of Prior Use of Carbapenem as a Risk Factor for Carbapenem versus Susceptible *P. aeruginosa* Acquisition. **Figure S3.** Meta-analysis of Prior Use of Fluoroquinolones as a Risk Factor for Quinolone-resistant versus Susceptible *P. aeruginosa* Acquisition.

## Abbreviations

AHRQ: Agency for Healthcare Research and Quality; APACHE II: Acute Physiology and Chronic Health Evaluation II; COPD: Chronic obstructive pulmonary disease; ESBL: Extended-spectrum beta-lactamase organisms; HAI: Hospital acquired infection; ICU: Intensive care unit; MDR: Multi-drug resistant; OR: Odds ratio; SAPS II: Simplified acute physiology score II; US: United States; XDR: Extensively drug resistant

## Funding

Funding for this review was provided to Tufts Medical Center by the Merck & Co., Inc., Kenilworth, NJ, USA. The funder played no role in the study search and selection, data synthesis and analysis.

## Authors' contributions

SM designed research; GR, EEA, and JC conducted research; GR and EEA analyzed data; and GR, EEA, and JC wrote the paper; SM and LP edited the paper; GR, EEA, and JC had primary responsibility for final content. All authors read and approved the final manuscript.

## Consent for publication

Not Applicable

## Competing interests

S. Merchant and L. Puzniak are employees of Merck & Co., Inc.

## Author details

[1]Center for Clinical Evidence Synthesis, Tufts Medical Center, 800 Washington Street, Box 63, Boston, MA 02111, USA. [2]Merck & Co., Inc., Kenilworth, NJ, USA.

## References

1.  Boucher HW, Talbot GH, Bradley JS, Edwards JE, Gilbert D, Rice LB, et al. Bad bugs, no drugs: no ESKAPE! An update from the Infectious Diseases Society of America. Clin Infect Dis. 2009;48(1):1):1–12.

2.  Peleg AY, Hooper DC. Hospital-acquired infections due to gram-negative bacteria. N Engl J Med. 2010;362(19):1804–13.

3.  Vincent JL, Rello J, Marshall J, Silva E, Anzueto A, Martin CD, et al. International study of the prevalence and outcomes of infection in intensive care units. JAMA. 2009;302(21):2323–9.

4.  Driscoll JA, Brody SL, Kollef MH. The epidemiology, pathogenesis and treatment of Pseudomonas aeruginosa infections. Drugs. 2007;67(3):351–68.

5.  Global Priority List of Antibiotic-Resistant Bacteria to Guide Research, Discovery, and Development of New Antibiotics. http://www.who.int/medicines/publications/global-priority-list-antibiotic-resistant-bacteria/en/ 2017 February 27 [cited 2017 Dec 5];

6.  Obritsch MD, Fish DN, MacLaren R, Jung R. National surveillance of antimicrobial resistance in Pseudomonas aeruginosa isolates obtained from intensive care unit patients from 1993 to 2002. Antimicrob Agents Chemother. 2004;48(12):4606–10.

7.  Nathwani D, Raman G, Sulham K, Gavaghan M, Menon V. Clinical and economic consequences of hospital-acquired resistant and multidrug-resistant Pseudomonas aeruginosa infections: a systematic review and meta-analysis. Antimicrob Resist Infect Control. 2014;3(1):32.

8.  Magiorakos AP, Srinivasan A, Carey RB, Carmeli Y, Falagas ME, Giske CG, et al. Multidrug-resistant, extensively drug-resistant and pandrug-resistant bacteria: an international expert proposal for interim standard definitions for acquired resistance. Clin Microbiol Infect. 2012;18(3):268–81.

9.  Raman G, Avendano E, Berger S, Menon V. Appropriate initial antibiotic therapy in hospitalized patients with gram-negative infections: systematic review and meta-analysis. BMC Infect Dis. 2015;15:395.

10. DerSimonian R, Laird N. Meta-analysis in clinical trials. Control Clin Trials. 1986;7(3):177–88.

11. Higgins JP, Thompson SG, Deeks JJ, Altman DG. Measuring inconsistency in meta-analyses. BMJ. 2003;327(7414):557–60.

12. Aloush V, Navon-Venezia S, Seigman-Igra Y, Cabili S, Carmeli Y. Multidrug-resistant Pseudomonas aeruginosa: risk factors and clinical impact. Antimicrob Agents Chemother. 2006;50(1):43–8.

13. Bodro M, Sabe N, Tubau F, Llado L, Baliellas C, Gonzalez-Costello J, et al. Extensively drug-resistant Pseudomonas aeruginosa bacteremia in solid organ transplant recipients. Transplantation. 2015;99(3):616–22.

14. Cao B, Wang H, Sun H, Zhu Y, Chen M. Risk factors and clinical outcomes of nosocomial multi-drug resistant Pseudomonas aeruginosa infections. J Hosp Infect. 2004;57(2):112–8.

15. Cilloniz C, Gabarrus A, Ferrer M, Puig dB, Rinaudo M, Mensa J, et al. Community-acquired pneumonia due to multidrug- and non-multidrug-resistant Pseudomonas aeruginosa. Chest. 2016;150(2):415–25.

16. Cobos-Trigueros N, Sole M, Castro P, Torres JL, Hernandez C, Rinaudo M, et al. Acquisition of Pseudomonas aeruginosa and its resistance phenotypes in critically ill medical patients: role of colonization pressure and antibiotic exposure. Crit Care. 2015;19:218.

17. D'Agata EM, Cataldo MA, Cauda R, Tacconelli E. The importance of addressing multidrug resistance and not assuming single-drug resistance in case-control studies. Infect Control Hosp Epidemiol. 2006;27(7):670–4.

18. Dalfino L, Mosca A, Brienza N, Spada M, Coppolecchia S, Miragliotta G, et al. Nosocomial infections in critically ill patients: When should multidrug-resistant Pseudomonas aeruginosa be suspected? Clin Microbiol Infect. 2011;17:S294–5. Conference: 21st ECCMID/27th ICC Milan Italy Conference Start: 20110507 Conference End: 20110510 Conference Publication: (var pagings)

19. Dantas RC, Ferreira ML, Gontijo-Filho PP, Ribas RM. Pseudomonas aeruginosa bacteraemia: independent risk factors for mortality and impact of resistance on outcome. J Med Microbiol. 2014;63(Pt:12):12–87.

20. Defez C, Fabbro-Peray P, Bouziges N, Gouby A, Mahamat A, Daures JP, et al. Risk factors for multidrug-resistant Pseudomonas aeruginosa nosocomial infection. J Hosp Infect. 2004;57(3):209–16.

21. Gomez-Zorrilla S, Camoez M, Tubau F, Periche E, Canizares R, Dominguez MA, et al. Antibiotic pressure is a major risk factor for rectal colonization by multidrug-resistant Pseudomonas aeruginosa in critically ill patients. Antimicrob Agents Chemother. 2014;58(10):5863–70.

22. Johnson LE, D'Agata EM, Paterson DL, Clarke L, Qureshi ZA, Potoski BA, et al. Pseudomonas aeruginosa bacteremia over a 10-year period: multidrug resistance and outcomes in transplant recipients. Transpl Infect Dis. 2009; 11(3):227–34.

23. Joo EJ, Kang CI, Ha YE, Kang SJ, Park SY, Chung DR, et al. Risk factors for mortality in patients with Pseudomonas aeruginosa bacteremia: clinical impact of antimicrobial resistance on outcome. Microb Drug Resist. 2011; 17(2):305–12.

24. Liew YX, Tan TT, Lee W, Ng JL, Chia DQ, Wong GC, et al. Risk factors for extreme-drug resistant Pseudomonas aeruginosa infections in patients with hematologic malignancies. Am J Infect Control. 2013;41(2):140–4.

25. Lodise TP, Miller CD, Graves J, Furuno JP, McGregor JC, Lomaestro B, et al. Clinical prediction tool to identify patients with Pseudomonas aeruginosa respiratory tract infections at greatest risk for multidrug resistance. Antimicrob Agents Chemother. 2007;51(2):417–22.

26. Micek ST, Wunderink RG, Kollef MH, Chen C, Rello J, Chastre J, et al. An international multicenter retrospective study of Pseudomonas aeruginosa nosocomial pneumonia: impact of multidrug resistance. Critical Care (London, England). 2015;19:219.

27. Montero M, Sala M, Riu M, Belvis F, Salvado M, Grau S, et al. Risk factors for multidrug-resistant Pseudomonas aeruginosa acquisition. Impact of antibiotic use in a double case-control study. Eur J Clin Microbiol Infect Dis. 2010;29(3):335–9.

28. Nakamura A, Miyake K, Misawa S, Kuno Y, Horii T, Kondo S, et al. Meropenem as predictive risk factor for isolation of multidrug-resistant Pseudomonas aeruginosa. J Hosp Infect. 2013;83(2):153–5.

29. Nseir S, Blazejewski C, Lubret R, Wallet F, Courcol R, Durocher A. Risk of acquiring multidrug-resistant gram-negative bacilli from prior room occupants in the intensive care unit. Clin Microbiol Infect. 2011;17(8):1201–8.

30. Ohmagari N, Hanna H, Graviss L, Hackett B, Perego C, Gonzalez V, et al. Risk factors for infections with multidrug-resistant Pseudomonas aeruginosa in patients with cancer. Cancer. 2005;104(1):205–12.

31. Paramythiotou E, Lucet JC, Timsit JF, Vanjak D, Paugam-Burtz C, Trouillet JL, et al. Acquisition of multidrug-resistant Pseudomonas aeruginosa in patients in intensive care units: role of antibiotics with antipseudomonal activity. Clin Infect Dis. 2004;38(5):670–7.

32. Park YS, Lee H, Chin BS, Han SH, Hong SG, Hong SK, et al. Acquisition of extensive drug-resistant Pseudomonas aeruginosa among hospitalized patients: risk factors and resistance mechanisms to carbapenems. J Hosp Infect. 2011;79(1):54–8.

33. Pena C, Gomez-Zorrilla S, Suarez C, Dominguez MA, Tubau F, Arch O, et al. Extensively drug-resistant Pseudomonas aeruginosa: risk of bloodstream infection in hospitalized patients. Eur J Clin Microbiol Infect Dis. 2012;31(10):2791–7.

34. Samonis G, Vardakas KZ, Kofteridis DP, Dimopoulou D, Andrianaki AM, Chatzinikolaou I, et al. Characteristics, risk factors and outcomes of adult cancer patients with extensively drug-resistant Pseudomonas aeruginosa infections. Infection. 2014;42(4):721–8.

35. Tumbarello M, Repetto E, Trecarichi EM, Bernardini C, De PG, Parisini A, et al. Multidrug-resistant Pseudomonas aeruginosa bloodstream infections: risk factors and mortality. Epidemiol Infect. 2011;139(11):1740–9.

36. Tuncer EG, Sonmezer MC, Tulek N, Erdinc SF, Bulut C, Berkem R, et al. Evaluation of risk factors for nosocomial multidrugresistant Pseudomonas aeruginosa infections. Clin Microbiol Infect. 2012;18:517. Conference: 22nd European Congress of Clinical Microbiology and Infectious Diseases London United Kingdom Conference Start: 20120331 Conference End: 20120403 Conference Publication: (var pagings).

37. Ustun C, Hosoglu S, Geyik MF. Risk factors for multi-drug-resistant Pseudomonas aeruginosa infections in a University Hospital - a case control study. Konuralp Tip Dergisi. 2016;8(2):2016.

38. Willmann M, Klimek AM, Vogel W, Liese J, Marschal M, Autenrieth IB, et al. Clinical and treatment-related risk factors for nosocomial colonisation with extensively drug-resistant Pseudomonas aeruginosa in a haematological patient population: a matched case control study. BMC Infect Dis. 2014;14:650.

39. Pena C, Suarez C, Tubau F, Dominguez A, Sora M, Pujol M, et al. Carbapenem-resistant Pseudomonas aeruginosa: factors influencing multidrug-resistant acquisition in non-critically ill patients. Eur J Clin Microbiol Infect Dis. 2009;28(5):519–22.

40. Tuon FF, Gortz LW, Rocha JL. Risk factors for pan-resistant Pseudomonas aeruginosa bacteremia and the adequacy of antibiotic therapy. Braz J Infect Dis. 2012;16(4):351–6.

41. Akhabue E, Synnestvedt M, Weiner MG, Bilker WB, Lautenbach E. Cefepime-Resistant Pseudomonas aeruginosa. Emerg Infect Dis. 2011;17(6):1037–43.

42. DalBen MF, Basso M, Garcia CP, Costa SF, Toscano CM, Jarvis WR, et al. Colonization pressure as a risk factor for colonization by multiresistant Acinetobacter spp and carbapenem-resistant Pseudomonas aeruginosa in an intensive care unit.[Erratum appears in Clinics (Sao Paulo). 2013 Dec; 68(12):1559]. Clinics (Sao Paulo, Brazil). 2013;68(8):1128–33.

43. Djordjevic Z, Folic M, Ruzic ZD, Ilic G, Jankovic S. Risk factors for carbapenem-resistant Pseudomonas aeruginosa infection in a tertiary care hospital in Serbia. J Infect Dev Ctries. 2013;7(9):686–90.

44. Eagye KJ, Kuti JL, Nicolau DP. Risk factors and outcomes associated with isolation of meropenem high-level-resistant Pseudomonas aeruginosa. Infect Control Hosp Epidemiol. 2009;30(8):746–52.

45. Fortaleza CM, Freire MP, Filho DC, de Carvalho RM. Risk factors for recovery of imipenem- or ceftazidime-resistant pseudomonas aeruginosa among patients admitted to a teaching hospital in Brazil. Infect Control Hosp Epidemiol. 2006;27(9):901–6.

46. Furtado GH, Bergamasco MD, Menezes FG, Marques D, Silva A, Perdiz LB, et al. Imipenem-resistant Pseudomonas aeruginosa infection at a medical-surgical intensive care unit: risk factors and mortality. J Crit Care. 2009;24(4):625–14.

47. Furtado GH, Gales AC, Perdiz LB, Santos AE, Wey SB, Medeiros EA. Risk factors for hospital-acquired pneumonia caused by imipenem-resistant Pseudomonas aeruginosa in an intensive care unit. Anaesth Intensive Care. 2010;38(6):994–1001.

48. Gasink LB, Fishman NO, Weiner MG, Nachamkin I, Bilker WB, Lautenbach E. Fluoroquinolone-resistant Pseudomonas aeruginosa: assessment of risk factors and clinical impact. Am J Med. 2006;119(6):526–5.

49. Harris AD, Perencevich E, Roghmann MC, Morris G, Kaye KS, Johnson JA. Risk factors for piperacillin-tazobactam-resistant Pseudomonas aeruginosa among hospitalized patients. Antimicrob Agents Chemother. 2002;46(3):854–8.

50. Harris AD, Smith D, Johnson JA, Bradham DD, Roghmann MC. Risk factors for imipenem-resistant Pseudomonas aeruginosa among hospitalized patients. Clin Infect Dis. 2002;34(3):340–5.

51. Harris AD, Johnson JK, Thom KA, Morgan DJ, McGregor JC, Ajao AO, et al. Risk factors for development of intestinal colonization with imipenem-resistant Pseudomonas aeruginosa in the intensive care unit setting. Infect Control Hosp Epidemiol. 2011;32(7):719–22.

52. Hsu DI, Okamoto MP, Murthy R, Wong-Beringer A. Fluoroquinolone-resistant Pseudomonas aeruginosa: risk factors for acquisition and impact on outcomes. J Antimicrob Chemother. 2005;55(4):535–41.

53. Khayr W, Rheault W, Waiters L, Walters A. Epidemiology of ciprofloxacin-resistant Pseudomonas aeruginosa in a veterans affairs hospital. Am J Ther. 2000;7(5):309–12.

54. Kohlenberg A, Weitzel-Kage D, van der Linden P, Sohr D, Vogeler S, Kola A, et al. Outbreak of carbapenem-resistant Pseudomonas aeruginosa infection in a surgical intensive care unit. J Hosp Infect. 2010;74(4):350–7.

55. Lautenbach E, Synnestvedt M, Weiner MG, Bilker WB, Vo L, Schein J, et al. Imipenem resistance in Pseudomonas aeruginosa: emergence, epidemiology, and impact on clinical and economic outcomes. Infect Control Hosp Epidemiol. 2010;31(1):47–53.

56. Lee CH, Su TY, Ye JJ, Hsu PC, Kuo AJ, Chia JH, et al. Risk factors and clinical significance of bacteremia caused by Pseudomonas aeruginosa resistant only to carbapenems. J Microbiol Immunol Infect. 2017;50(5):677–83.

57. Lin KY, Lauderdale TL, Wang JT, Chang SC. Carbapenem-resistant Pseudomonas aeruginosa in Taiwan: prevalence, risk factors, and impact on outcome of infections. J Microbiol Immunol Infect. 2016;49(1):52–9.

58. Luyt CE, Aubry A, Lu Q, Micaelo M, Brechot N, Brossier F, et al. Imipenem, meropenem, or doripenem to treat patients with Pseudomonas aeruginosa ventilator-associated pneumonia. Antimicrob Agents Chemother. 2014;58(3):1372–80.

59. Onguru P, Erbay A, Bodur H, Baran G, Akinci E, Balaban N, et al. Imipenem-resistant Pseudomonas aeruginosa: risk factors for nosocomial infections. J Korean Med Sci. 2008;23(6):982–7.

60. Pena C, Guzman A, Suarez C, Dominguez MA, Tubau F, Pujol M, et al. Effects of carbapenem exposure on the risk for digestive tract carriage of intensive care unit-endemic carbapenem-resistant Pseudomonas aeruginosa strains in critically ill patients. Antimicrob Agents Chemother. 2007;51(6):1967–71.

61. Pereira GH, Levin AS, Oliveira HB, Moretti ML. Controlling the clonal spread of Pseudomonas aeruginosa infection. Infect Control Hosp Epidemiol. 2008;29(6):549–52.

62. Tam VH, Chang KT, LaRocco MT, Schilling AN, McCauley SK, Poole K, et al. Prevalence, mechanisms, and risk factors of carbapenem resistance in bloodstream isolates of Pseudomonas aeruginosa. Diagn Microbiol Infect Dis. 2007;58(3):309–14.

63. Trouillet JL, Vuagnat A, Combes A, Kassis N, Chastre J, Gibert C. Pseudomonas aeruginosa ventilator-associated pneumonia: comparison of episodes due to piperacillin-resistant versus piperacillin-susceptible organisms. Clin Infect Dis. 2002;34(8):1047–54.

64. Zavascki AP, Cruz RP, Goldani LZ. Risk factors for imipenem-resistant Pseudomonas aeruginosa: a comparative analysis of two case-control studies in hospitalized patients. J Hosp Infect. 2005;59(2):96–101.

65. Zhang JF, Chen BL, Xin XY, Zhao HB, Wang HY, Song H, et al. Carbapenem resistance mechanism and risk factors of Pseudomonas aeruginosa clinical isolates from a University Hospital in Xi'an, China. Microb Drug Resist. 2009; 15(1):41–5.

66. Nicasio AM, Kuti JL, Nicolau DP. The current state of multidrug-resistant gram-negative bacilli in North America. Pharmacotherapy. 2008;28(2):235–49.

67. Buhl M, Peter S, Willmann M. Prevalence and risk factors associated with colonization and infection of extensively drug-resistant Pseudomonas aeruginosa: a systematic review. Expert Rev Anti-Infect Ther. 2015;13(9):1159–70.

68. Egger M, Davey SG, Schneider M, Minder C. Bias in meta-analysis detected by a simple, graphical test. BMJ. 1997;315(7109):629–34.

# 18

# Emergence of high drug resistant bacterial isolates from patients with health care associated infections at Jimma University medical center

Mulatu Gashaw[1,11*], Melkamu Berhane[2], Sisay Bekele[3], Gebre Kibru[1], Lule Teshager[1], Yonas Yilma[4], Yesuf Ahmed[5], Netsanet Fentahun[6], Henok Assefa[7], Andreas Wieser[8], Esayas Kebede Gudina[9] and Solomon Ali[1,10]

## Abstract

**Background:** The rates of resistant microorganisms which complicate the management of healthcare associated infections (HAIs) are increasing worldwide and getting more serious in developing countries. The objective of this study was to describe microbiological features and resistance profiles of bacterial pathogens of HAIs in Jimma University Medical Center (JUMC) in Ethiopia.

**Methods:** Institution based cross sectional study was carried out on hospitalized patients from May to September, 2016 in JUMC. Different clinical specimens were collected from patients who were suspected to hospital acquired infections. The specimens were processed to identify bacterial etiologies following standard microbiological methods. Antibacterial susceptibility was determined in vitro by Kirby-Bauer disk diffusion method following Clinical and Laboratory Standards Institute guidelines.

**Results:** Overall, 126 bacterial etiologies were isolated from 118 patients who had HAIs. Of these, 100 (79.4%) were gram negative and the remaining were gram positive. The most common isolates were *Escherichia coli* 31(24.6%), *Klebsiella* species 30(23.8%) and *Staphylococcus aureus* 26 (20.6%). Of 126 bacterial isolates, 38 (30. 2%), 52 (41.3%), and 24 (19%) were multidrug-resistant (MDR, resistant to at least one agent in three or more antimicrobial categories), extensively drug resistant (XDR, resistant to at least one agent in all but two or fewer antimicrobial categories (i.e. bacterial isolates remain susceptible to only one or two categories), pan-drug resistant (PDR, resistant to all antibiotic classes) respectively. More than half of isolated gram-negative rods (51%) were positive for extended spectrum beta-lactamase (ESBL) and/or AmpC; and 25% of gram negative isolates were also resistant to carbapenem antibiotics.

**Conclusions:** The pattern of drug resistant bacteria in patients with healthcare associated infection at JUMC is alarming. This calls for coordinated efforts from all stakeholders to prevent HAIs and drug resistance in the study setting.

**Keywords:** Antimicrobial agents, Drug resistant isolates, Multidrug resistance, Extensively resistance, Pandrug resistance, Carbapenem resistance, Extended spectrum beta-lactamase

* Correspondence: mulatugashaw@gmail.com; mulatu.gashaw@ju.edu.et
[1]School of Medical Laboratory Science, Jimma University, Jimma, Ethiopia
[11]Institute of Health, Jimma University, P.O. Box 1368, Jimma, Ethiopia
Full list of author information is available at the end of the article

## Introduction

The emergence and rapid spread of multidrug resistant pathogenic bacteria is becoming a global health challenge [1]. Recent studies showed an increasing rate of bacterial resistance against available antibiotics. The problem is more pronounced in developing countries attributed to limited antibiotic option, irrational drug use, poor drug quality, poor sanitation, malnutrition, poor and inadequate health care systems, and lack of control for antibiotic use and stewardship program [2, 3].

In the past few decades, antimicrobial drugs have saved many lives and reduced the grief of many million people globally [3]. However, the extraordinary benefits of antimicrobials in reducing morbidity and mortality have been challenged by the emergence of drug resistant bacteria. The recent emergence and spread of these resistant bacteria have become a serious public health concern [4]. Especially, the spread of such bacteria in resource limited countries would have devastating consequences considering the health infrastructure, antibiotic options available and over all resource constraints observed in such countries [5].

In recent years, high dissemination of ESBL producing, carbapenem, and methicillin resistant bacteria are observed worldwide [6, 7]. It is described that the problem of ESBL-producing organisms is more intense in developing countries [8]. However, the magnitude of the problem is still probably underestimated due to inadequate or ineffective detection in some clinical settings [3, 7, 9]. ESBLs are a group of plasmid-mediated, diverse, complex and rapidly evolving enzymes which are capable of hydrolyzing penicillin's, broad-spectrum cephalosporin's and monobactam's [10]. Accordingly, ESBL enzyme producing bacteria have a capacity to resist the action of penicillin's, broad-spectrum cephalosporin's and monobactam's [11]. Furthermore, there is an evidence indicating that most of ESBL producing bacteria are also resistant for carbapenem antibiotics [12, 13]. ESBLs production is most commonly seen among Gram negative bacteria including *Escherichia coli, Klebsiella pneumoniae, Proteus mirabilis and Pseudomonas aeruginosa* [14].

Infections resulting from antibiotic resistant bacteria are more difficult and, in some instances, impossible to treat with current available antibiotics. Such infections lead to higher morbidity and mortality, imposing huge healthcare cost [15, 16]. In recent years, varieties of bacteria are becoming resistant against two or more classes of antibiotics as a result of selective pressure or horizontal gene transfer. For instance, the magnitude of resistance seen among *E. coli, S. aureus, Klebsiella* species, *P. aeruginosa, A. baumannii,* and *Enterobacter* species is more threatening as these bacteria are the commonest etiologies for commonly observed hospital and community acquired infections [17, 18].

In Ethiopia, the patterns of antibiotic resistance among commonly seen bacterial etiologies have been described previously in different settings [19–21]. However, most of these studies did not address the magnitude of ESBL producing and carbapenem resistance patterns comprehensively. It is also known that bacterial antibiotic resistance is a dynamic process. Resistance patterns seen in the past might not be representing the current situation due to the strong correlation between efficiency of antibiotic use and antibiotic resistance. As a result, information about the current antibiotic resistance pattern of bacteria is very vital to understand the dynamic and trend of resistance.

Clinical characteristics of patients with HAIs at Jimma University Medical Center have recently been published. The incidence and overall prevalence of HAIs at the hospital were 28.15 per 1000 patient days and 19.41% respectively [22]. In the current study, we aimed to determine the MDR, XDR, PDR, ESBL mediated and carbapenem resistance patterns of bacteria isolated from patients with HAIs at the hospital.

## Methods and materials

Institution based cross-sectional study was carried out in all wards of JUMC from May, 2016 to September, 2016. Totally, 1015 patients were admitted, of these 197 patients had sign of healthcare associated infection during the study time and all were taken as study participants. Microbiological investigation was done for 192 participants suspected to have healthcare associated infection; no microbiological test was done for the other five cases due to inability to obtain proper specimen. Different clinical specimens (blood, urine, wound swab, pus, and sputum) were collected aseptically from the patients with signs of healthcare associated infection. Bacterial identification was performed by standard microbiological methods which are adopted from CLSI guideline.

### Phenotypic determination of antibiotic susceptibility patterns

Antibacterial susceptibility of Penicillin (10 µg), Oxacillin (1 µg), Gentamycin (10 µg), Chloramphenicol (30 µg), Tetracycline (30 µg) Erythromycin (15 µg), Trimethoprim-sulfamethoxazole (1.25 g), Clindamycin (2 µg), Cefoxitin (30 µg), Ciprofloxacin (5 µg), Nitrofurantoin (300 µg), Norfloxacin (10 µg), Ampicillin (10 µg), Amoxicillin-clavulanic acid (10 µg), Ceftriaxone (30 µg), Ceftazidime (30 µg), Cefepime (30 µg), and Meropenem (10 µg), (Oxoid, UK) were determined in vitro by Kirby-Bauer disk diffusion method following Clinical and Laboratory Standards Institute guidelines [23].

## ESBL and/or AmpC detection

The presence of an ESBL and/or AmpC was determined with Cefpodoxime (10 µg), Cefotaxime (30 µg), Cefepime (30 µg) and Ceftazidime (30 µg) containing antibiotic discs (Mast Group, UK) by disc diffusion confirmation test. After the discs were inserted on inoculated plates, then they were incubated at 35–37 °C for 18–24 h aerobically. Finally, zones of inhibition were read and recorded on excel sheet. The data from the excel sheet was transported to Mast group ESBL/AmpC and CARBA plus calculator spreadsheet (Mast group, UK) and reported as negative or positive for ESBL or/and AmpC and finally the results were recorded.

The results were registered as resistant, intermediate and susceptible; but for the sake of analysis intermediate and resistant isolates were grouped together as resistant. Classification of MDR, XDR and PDR were carried out according to Magiorakos et al, definitions [4]. All the antibiotic disks were from Oxoid (Oxoid, UK) and Mast discs (Mast group, UK). The inhibition zone diameter was measured using caliper and recorded on excel sheet.

## Data quality control

Standard operating procedures (SOPs) were strictly followed while we did all bacteriological procedures starting from sample collection, isolation, identification and antibiotic susceptibility testing. Susceptible American Type Culture Collection (ATCC) 25,922 *E. coli* and ATCC 25923 *Staphylococcus aureus* were used as control strains and the test results were only accepted when the inhibition zone diameters of the above mentioned control strains were within performance ranges as described by CLSI [23]. ESBL positive ATCC 700603 *Klebsiella pneumoniae* and both ESBL and carbapenemase negative *E. coli* ATCC 25922 control strains were used in this study as positive and negative control respectively. To standardize the inoculum density of bacterial suspension for a susceptibility test, 0.5 McFarland standards, which is comparable with the approximate number of bacterial suspension ($1.0 \times 10^8$ to $2.0 \times 10^8$ bacteria/mL), was used [23].

## Data analysis and statistical tests

Data were double entered to Epi Data version 3.1 and transferred to SPSS version 20 and Microsoft Excel software for analysis and the results were presented as tables, pie-charts and graphs. *P*-values < 0.05 were considered as statistically significant.

## Ethical consideration

The study was approved by the Institutional Review Board of Institute of Health, Jimma University. Informed written consent was also obtained from participants and/or guardians after explaining the objective of the study. All the laboratory results were communicated as early as possible with the treating physicians for better management of the patients.

## Result

### Socio-demography and background information of the participants

From 1015 patients who were enrolled in the study; only 197 admitted patients had developed sign of healthcare associated infection with in the study time. Of these, 118 (59.9%) patients had culture confirmed healthcare associated infections. Sociodemographic and clinical characteristics of study participants have recently been published. The incidence and overall prevalence of HAIs at the hospital were 28.15 per 1000 patient days and 19.41% respectively [22].

### Isolation rate

Totally 240 clinical samples were obtained from 192 patients who were clinically diagnosed with healthcare associated infection. The most common sources of specimen were urine (55%) followed by wound swab/pus (24.2%), blood (15%), and sputum (5.8%). A total of 126 bacterial pathogens were isolated from 118 patient samples. A single organism was isolated from 110 (93.2%) patient samples, and two organisms were isolated from 8 (6.8%) patient samples who had been admitted to ICU. The overall culture positivity rate of participants was 118/192(61.5%). Most commonly isolated bacteria were *E. coli* 31(24.6%), *Klebsiella* species 30(23.8%) and *S. aureus* 26 (20.6%) (Fig. 1).

### Drug resistance patterns of isolates to different classes of antibiotics

Antibiotic resistance patterns of the isolated pathogen of nosocomial origin are shown in Table 1. Half of *S. aureus* isolates were resistant to gentamicin 50.0% (13/26); and 53.84% (14/26) and 57.7% (15/26) of the isolates were resistant to methicillin /cefoxitin/oxacillin and ceftriaxone/chloramphenicol in vitro respectively; and all of *S. aureus* isolates were resistant against penicillin (Table 1). From a total of 26 *S. aureus* isolates, 3(11.5%), 10(38.5%) 10 (38.5%) and 3(11.6%) were MoDR, MDR, XDR and PDR respectively (Table 2).

From Gram negative bacteria, *E. coli* and *Klebsiella* species were the most frequent isolates. More than 90% of *E. coli* isolates were resistant against ampicillin, tetracycline and trimethoprim-sulfamethoxazole (Table 1). Conversely, only 16.1% of *E.coli* isolates were resistant against meropenem. Likewise, the resistance rate of *Klebsiella* species were 100% for ampicillin, 90% for tetracycline, 80% for trimethoprim

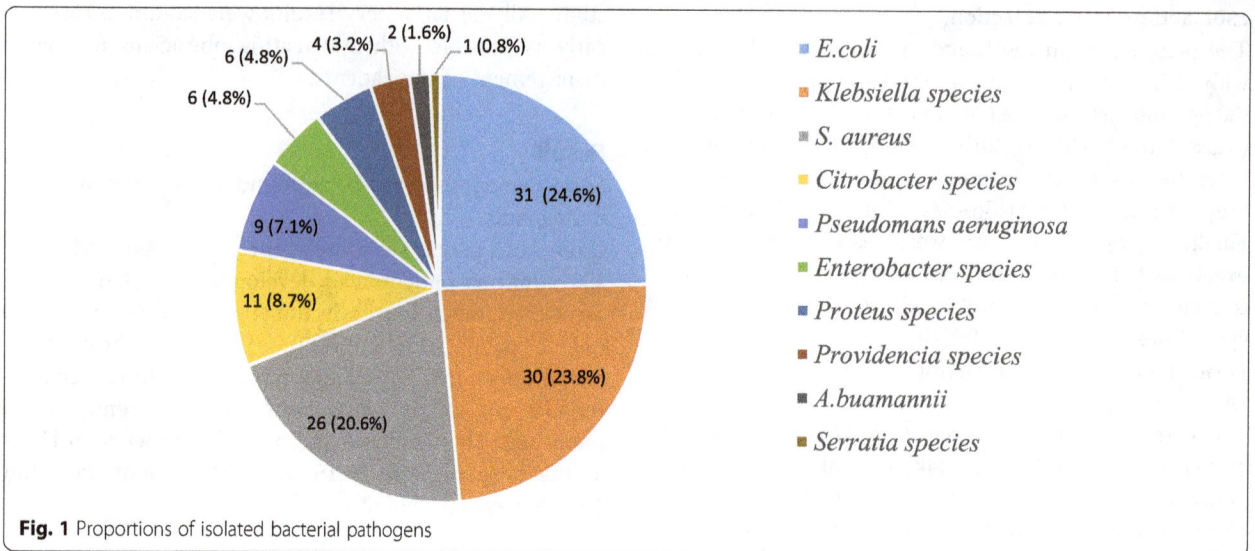

**Fig. 1** Proportions of isolated bacterial pathogens

-sulfamethoxazole, 40% for ciprofloxacin and 30% for meropenem (Table 1).

### Classification of isolates based on their drug resistance pattern

As shown in Table 2, among 126 bacterial isolates, 38 (30.2%), 52 (41.3%), and 24 (19%) were MDR, XDR, and PDR respectively. Eight of the isolates were resistant to a single antimicrobial class and only four *Klebsiella* isolates were susceptible to all classes of the antimicrobials. The predominant isolates (*E. coli*, *Klebsiella* species and *S. aureus*) showed very high antimicrobial resistance patterns. The overall MDR rate of the isolated bacteria was 30.16%. All bacteria isolated from ICU and pediatrics wards, 87.5% of bacteria isolated from Gynecology and obstetrics wards, 88% of bacteria isolated from Medical wards and 85.7% of bacteria isolated from surgical wards were MDR. The overall prevalence of PDR among all isolates was 19.0%. *Citrobacter species* (45.4%) and *Pseudomonas aeruginosa* (33.3%) have shown high pandrug resistance rate. On the

**Table 1** Frequency of antimicrobial resistant bacterial isolates for selected antimicrobial classes

| Antibiotic classes | Antibiotics | S. aureus (n = 26) | E. coli (n = 31) | Klebsiella species (n = 30) | Citrobacter species (n = 11) | P. aeruginosa (n = 9) | Enterobacter species (n = 6) | Proteus species (n = 6) | Providencia species (n = 4) | A. buamannii (n = 2) | Serratia species (n = 1) |
|---|---|---|---|---|---|---|---|---|---|---|---|
| Penecillins 3rd and 4th generation cephalosporins | Penicillin | 26 | – | – | – | – | – | – | – | – | – |
| | Ampicillin | – | 29 | 30 | 11 | 9 | 6 | 5 | 4 | 2 | 1 |
| | Ceftriaxone | 15 | 15 | 16 | 7 | 9 | 4 | 4 | 2 | 2 | 1 |
| | Ceftazidime | – | 16 | 17 | 8 | 8 | 5 | 4 | 2 | 2 | 1 |
| | Cefepime | – | 14 | 15 | 6 | 5 | 2 | 4 | 2 | 2 | 1 |
| Anti-staphylococcal β-lactams | Oxacillin | 14 | – | – | – | – | – | – | – | – | – |
| Cephamycins | Cefoxitin | 14 | 19 | 23 | 6 | 8 | 6 | 4 | 1 | 2 | 1 |
| Aminoglycosides | Gentamycin | 13 | 22 | 21 | 7 | 8 | 3 | 3 | 1 | 2 | 1 |
| Phenicols | Chloramphenicol | 15 | 19 | 20 | 8 | 9 | 1 | 3 | 3 | 2 | 1 |
| Macrolides | Erythromycin | 19 | – | – | – | – | – | – | – | – | – |
| Lincosamides | Clindamycin | 17 | – | – | – | – | – | – | – | – | – |
| Tetracycline | Tetracycline | 17 | 29 | 27 | 7 | 9 | 4 | 6 | 4 | 2 | 1 |
| Folate pathway inhibitors | Trimethoprim-sulfamethoxazole | 19 | 28 | 24 | 9 | 4 | 2 | 6 | 3 | 2 | 1 |
| Fluoroquinolones | Ciprofloxacin | 16 | 14 | 12 | 6 | 6 | 3 | 3 | 2 | 1 | 1 |
| Carbapenems | Meropenem | – | 5 | 9 | 2 | 4 | 1 | 0 | 1 | 2 | 1 |
| Penecillins + β-lactamase inhibitors | Amoxicillin-clavulanic acid | – | 28 | 29 | 9 | 9 | 6 | 6 | 4 | 2 | 1 |

**Table 2** Frequency distribution of MultiS, MoDR, MDR, XDR, and PDR pattern of isolated bacteria

| Isolated organisms | Total | MultiS | MoDR | MDR | XDR | PDR |
|---|---|---|---|---|---|---|
| S. aureus | 26 | 0 | 3 | 10 | 10 | 3 |
| E. coli | 31 | 0 | 3 | 11 | 10 | 7 |
| Klebsiella species | 30 | 4 | 2 | 9 | 13 | 2 |
| Citrobacter species | 11 | 0 | 0 | 2 | 4 | 5 |
| Enterobacter species | 6 | 0 | 0 | 2 | 3 | 1 |
| Proteus species | 6 | 0 | 0 | 2 | 4 | 0 |
| Providencia species | 4 | 0 | 0 | 0 | 3 | 1 |
| Pseudomonas aeruginosa | 9 | 0 | 0 | 2 | 4 | 3 |
| Acinetobacter baumannii | 2 | 0 | 0 | 0 | 1 | 1 |
| Serratia species | 1 | 0 | 0 | 0 | 0 | 1 |
| Total | 126 | 4 | 8 | 38 | 52 | 24 |

MultiS, susceptible to all antibiotic classes; MoDR, resistant to single antibiotic class; MDR, resistant to at least one agent in three or more antimicrobial categories; XDR, resistant to at least one agent in all but two or fewer antimicrobial categories (i.e. bacterial isolates remain susceptible to only one or two categories); PDR, resistant to all antibiotic classes. Source: Based on definitions by Magiorakos et al. [4]

other hand, *Klebsiella* species (6.6%) and *S.aureus* (11.5%) have shown the least PDR rate. *E.coli* (22.6%) and *Enterobacter species* (16.7%) have also shown a moderate PDR rate.

## Prevalence of ESBL, AmpC, and Carbapenemase producing isolates

Of the 1 hundred isolated gram-negative rods, 36 and 7% were positive for extended spectrum beta-lactamase (ESBL) and AmpC respectively. Eight percent of the isolates were positive for both extended spectrum beta-lactamase (ESBL) and AmpC. With regard to the proportion of carbapenemase producing isolates, 25% of gram negative isolates have shown carbapenem resistance (Table 3). To be precise, 16.1% of *E.coli* and 30.0% of *Klebsiella* species were carbapenem resistant isolates (Table 3).

## Antimicrobial resistance pattern and impact on clinical outcome

Of 118 patients with culture confirmed healthcare associated infection, 13 patients (11.02%) died and all of the isolated microorganisms from these 13 patients were multidrug resistant (MDR) as shown in Table 4. The mean hospital stays of the patients infected with MDR bacteria were $15.4 \pm 9.6$ days (range 3–49 days). There is statistically significant association between mean duration of stay and infection with MDR bacteria (Table 4).

## Discussion

The overall rate of MDR, XDR and PDR bacterial isolates from JUMC were found to be 30.16, 41.27 and 19.0% respectively. Furthermore, the observed MDR rate is significantly associated with prolonged hospital stay and all patients, who died, were infected with MDR bacterial species (even if, it is not statistically significant). On the other hand, the observed XDR and PDR rate at the hospital indicates that the problem of AMR is increasing at an alarming rate and pathogenic bacteria that circulate in JUMC are becoming more resistant to all available antibiotics. The occurrence of PDR pathogenic bacteria would also have huge potential threat and implications for patient care in the hospital and the community at large. As we are living in the era of very connected world, it is highly likely for these PDR bacteria to be disseminated to other parts of Ethiopia and other parts of the world as well.

To the best of our knowledge, there is no previous report from Ethiopia on the rate of XDR and PDR pathogenic bacteria to compare with this result. It is possible to list some reasons which might have contributed for this observed high XDR and PDR rate. The first reason might be associated with lack of AMR surveillance and stewardship program at JUMC and in Ethiopia in general. There is enough evidence that indicates AMR surveillance and stewardship program helps to understand

**Table 3** Prevalence of ESBL, AmpC, and Carbapenem resistant isolates of gram negative rods

| Isolated organisms | Total | ESBL & AmpC producing isolates | | | | Carbapenemase resistance | |
|---|---|---|---|---|---|---|---|
| | | Not ESBL & AmpC, N (%) | ESBL, N (%) | AmpC, N (%) | ESBL & AmpC, N (%) | Yes, N (%) | No, N (%) |
| E. coli | 31 | 12(38.7) | 14(45.2) | 3 (9.7) | 2 (6.5) | 5 (16.1) | 26 (83.9) |
| Klebsiella species | 30 | 14 (46.7) | 13 (43.3) | 2 (6.7) | 1 (3.3) | 9 (30.0) | 21 (70.0) |
| Citrobacter species | 11 | 5 | 4 | 0 | 2 | 2 | 9 |
| Enterobacter species | 6 | 2 | 3 | 0 | 1 | 1 | 5 |
| Proteus species | 6 | 5 | 1 | 0 | 0 | 0 | 6 |
| Providencia species | 4 | 1 | 2 | 1 | 0 | 1 | 3 |
| Pseudomonas aeruginosa | 9 | 5 | 1 | 1 | 2 | 4 | 5 |
| Acinetobacter baumannii | 2 | 2 | 0 | 0 | 0 | 2 | 0 |
| Serratia species | 1 | 1 | 0 | 0 | 0 | 1 | 0 |
| Total | 100 | 49 | 36 | 7 | 8 | 25 | 75 |

**Table 4** Antimicrobial resistance and associated factors

| Variable | Non MDR (N = 12) (%) | MDR (N = 106) (%) | P |
|---|---|---|---|
| History of treatment[a] | | | |
| No | 9 (75.0) | 85 (80.19) | |
| Yes | 3 (25.0) | 21 (19.81) | 0.672 |
| Patient outcome | | | |
| Progress | 12 (100) | 93 (87.74) | |
| Died | 0 | 13 (12.26) | 0.198 |
| Duration of stay in Hospital | | | |
| <=15 days | 8 (66.6) | 25 (23.58) | |
| > 15 days | 4 (33.4) | 81 (76.42) | 0.002 |

Non-MDR: susceptible to all antibiotic classes/resistant to one/two antibiotic classes; MDR: resistant to at least one agent in three or more antimicrobial categories Magiorakos et al. [4]

[a] taking antibiotics in the last 3 months of the study period

the pattern of resistance and improve the utilization of antibiotics to prevent occurrence of antibiotic resistance.

The second reason might be associated with lack of comprehensive national antibiotic policies and problems in implementations of policies. In Ethiopia, there is no clear antibiotic policy and controlling mechanism about antibiotic usage. It is a common practice in Ethiopia to buy any antibiotic from private drug vendors and pharmacies without any prescription. This might have contributed for emergence and dissemination of antibiotic resistant bacteria at different settings. The third reason might be associated with lack of system to assess the quality and reliability of imported antibiotics in Ethiopia. For instance, one previous study which assessed the quality of anti-tuberculosis drugs in Ethiopia in 2013 has indicated that around 17% of anti TB drugs were fake drugs [24]. It is easy to imagine the role of these fake drugs on anti TB drug resistance. Likewise, though there is no previous research done in Ethiopia to assess the quality of antibiotics dispensed in private and government pharmacies, it is highly likely that some of them might be sub-standard, given that substantial proportion of the antibiotics in private pharmacies are supplied through unknown routes [25, 26].

The emergence of ESBL producing gram negative rods have become a rising concern in the developing world [27]. In this study, phenotypically, the most common ESBL producing microorganisms were E. coli and Klebsiella species which are 51.6% (16/31) and 46.7% (14/30) respectively; which is comparable with the studies done in Nigeria, Nepal and Burma in which ESBL producing Enterobacteriaceae were 44.3, 43.7 and 38.0% respectively [14, 28, 29]. However, the other studies done in India and Nepal

showed that 30.18 and 18.4% of *Klebsiella pneumoniae* produce ESBL respectively which is lower than our report [30, 31]. Even though the prevalence of ESBLs is not well documented, in many parts of the world 10–40% of strains of *Escherichia coli* and *Klebsiella pneumoniae* are estimated to produce ESBLs [27]. High proportion of ESBL producing isolates was documented in the current study which might be due to the fact that our study participants were all hospitalized; since hospitalization was identified as the strongest independent risk factor to express ESBL [32].

Regarding to carbapenem resistance, 19 (21.4%), 4 (44.4%) and 2 (100%) of the *Enterobacteriaceae*, *P. aeruginosa* and *A. buamannii* were carbapenem resistant respectively which are found in the priority one list according to WHO classification [33]. In addition to that, 53.8% of the other commonly isolated *S. aureus* were methicillin resistant which also needs high attention. Therefore, high attention should be given to these pathogens which are considered as priority one and two according to WHO [33]. To compare with other similar studies, the rate of carbapenem resistance among *E.coli* (16.1%) and *Klebsiella* species (30%) is consistent with multinational study done in Europe [34]. In contrary, 25% carbapenem resistance rate observed in this study is lower than a report from Brazil which was 100% [35]. This could be explained by the difference in utilization of carbapenem antibiotics to treat different infections in the respective setups [36, 37]. The observed high carbapenem resistance rate can also be due to prescription of antibiotics without the knowledge of their susceptibility pattern, or introduction and dissemination of carbapenem resistant bacteria strains from other areas with high resistance rate might also be possible as JUMC is frequently visited by different European, Chinese and Korean nationalities due to different collaborative researches, training and service activities.

As reported by other studies, meropenem was the most effective antibiotic against most gram-negative rods [38]. To control high rate of antibiotic resistant isolates coordinated and urgent action is needed to prevent the development of drug resistance in the setting. Surveillance on antibiotic resistance will also be most useful to decide the correct empirical treatment and will help to control and prevent infections caused by resistant pathogens. Furthermore, our data suggest that the most effective antibiotics for gram-negative bacilli in vitro are meropenem followed by cefepime and for gram-positive organisms less resistance was observed against gentamycin.

## Conclusion

In this study, high antimicrobial resistance rate was demonstrated. The observed high PDR, ESBL and carbapenem resistance rate is worrisome. Coordinated effort is needed from all stakeholders working in health system in Ethiopia to tackle this important public health problem. An immediate action should be taken at the hospital to start antibiotic stewardship program to reduce the observed antibiotic resistance and prevent further complications.

## Abbreviations
HAI: Health care associated infection; MDR: Resistant to at least one agent in three or more antimicrobial categories; MoDR: Resistant to single antibiotic class; MultiS: Susceptible to all antibiotic classes; PDR: Resistant to all antibiotic classes; XDR: Resistant to at least one agent in all but two or fewer antimicrobial categories (i.e. bacterial isolates remain susceptible to only one or two categories)

## Acknowledgements
We would like to thank Jimma University for funding this research and we would also like to thank all laboratory personnels working at Jimma University Medical Center, bacteriology laboratory for their unreserved support during data collection.

## Funding
This project was funded by Jimma University through the Institute of Health, Research and Postgraduate Office.

## Authors' contributions
MG, SA, EKG & MB conceived, designed, instrument development, supervision of data collection, analysis and manuscript writing. SB, GK, LT, YY, YA, NF, HA, and AW, participated in study design, development of instruments, supervision of data collection and editing and revision of the manuscript. All authors read and approved the final manuscript.

## Consent for publication
Not applicable – This manuscript does not contain any individual person's data.

## Competing interests
The authors declare that they have no competing interests.

## Author details
[1]School of Medical Laboratory Science, Jimma University, Jimma, Ethiopia. [2]Department of Pediatrics and Child Health, Jimma University, Jimma, Ethiopia. [3]Department of Ophthalmology, Jimma University, Jimma, Ethiopia. [4]Department of Surgery, Jimma University, Jimma, Ethiopia. [5]Department of Obstetrics and Gynecology, Jimma University, Jimma, Ethiopia. [6]Department of Health Education and Behavioral Health, Jimma University, Jimma, Ethiopia. [7]Department of Epidemiology and Statistics, Jimma University, Jimma, Ethiopia. [8]Head of the parasitology laboratory and deputy head of the molecular diagnostics laboratory at the Max von Pettenkofer-Institute, Ludwigs-Maximilians-University (LMU), München, Germany. [9]Department of Internal Medicine, Jimma University, Jimma, Ethiopia. [10]WHO-TDR clinical research former fellow at AERAS Africa and Rockville, Rockville, MD, USA. [11]Institute of Health, Jimma University, P.O. Box 1368, Jimma, Ethiopia.

## References
1. Chakraborty A, Pal NK, Sarkar S, Gupta MS. Antibiotic resistance pattern of Enterococci isolates from nosocomial infections in a tertiary care hospital in Eastern India. J Natl Sci Biol Med. 2015;6(2):394.
2. Colodner R, Rock W, Chazan B, Keller N, Guy N, Sakran W, et al. Risk factors for the development of extended-spectrum beta-lactamase-producing bacteria in nonhospitalized patients. Eur J Clin Microbiol Infect Dis. 2004; 23(3):163–7.
3. Ayukekbong JA, Ntemgwa M, Atabe AN. The threat of antimicrobial resistance in developing countries: causes and control strategies. Antimicrob Resist Infect Control. 2017;6(1):47.
4. Magiorakos AP, Srinivasan A, Carey R, Carmeli Y, Falagas M, Giske C, et al. Multidrug-resistant, extensively drug-resistant and pandrug-resistant bacteria: an international expert proposal for interim standard definitions for acquired resistance. Clin Microbiol Infect. 2012;18(3):268–81.
5. Lashinsky JN, Henig O, Pogue JM, Kaye KS. Minocycline for the Treatment of Multidrug and Extensively Drug-Resistant A. baumannii: A Review. Infect Dis Ther. 2017;6:1–13.
6. Bouchillon S, Johnson B, Hoban D, Johnson J, Dowzicky M, Wu D, et al. Determining incidence of extended spectrum β-lactamase producing Enterobacteriaceae, vancomycin-resistant enterococcus faecium and methicillin-resistant Staphylococcus aureus in 38 centres from 17 countries: the PEARLS study 2001–2002. Int J Antimicrob Agents. 2004;24(2):119–24.
7. Organization WH. Antimicrobial resistance: global report on surveillance: World Health Organization; 2014.
8. Pitout JD, Laupland KB. Extended-spectrum β-lactamase-producing Enterobacteriaceae: an emerging public-health concern. Lancet Infect Dis. 2008;8(3):159–66.
9. Fridkin S, Baggs J, Fagan R, Magill S, Pollack LA, Malpiedi P, et al. Vital signs: improving antibiotic use among hospitalized patients. MMWR Morb Mortal Wkly Rep. 2014;63(9):194–200.
10. Fernando M, Luke W, Miththinda J, Wickramasinghe R, Sebastiampillai B, Gunathilake M, et al. Extended spectrum beta lactamase producing organisms causing urinary tract infections in Sri Lanka and their antibiotic susceptibility pattern–a hospital based cross sectional study. BMC Infect Dis. 2017;17(1):138.
11. Tang SS, Apisarnthanarak A, Hsu LY. Mechanisms of β-lactam antimicrobial resistance and epidemiology of major community-and healthcare-associated multidrug-resistant bacteria. Adv Drug Deliv Rev. 2014;78:3–13.
12. Miriagou V, Cornaglia G, Edelstein M, Galani I, Giske C, Gniadkowski M, et al. Acquired carbapenemases in gram-negative bacterial pathogens: detection and surveillance issues. Clin Microbiol Infect. 2010;16(2):112–22.
13. Kumarasamy KK, Toleman MA, Walsh TR, Bagaria J, Butt F, Balakrishnan R, et al. Emergence of a new antibiotic resistance mechanism in India, Pakistan, and the UK: a molecular, biological, and epidemiological study. Lancet Infect Dis. 2010;10(9):597–602.
14. Ogefere HO, Aigbiremwen PA, Omoregie R. Extended-Spectrum Beta-lactamase (ESBL)–producing gram-negative isolates from urine and wound specimens in a tertiary health Facility in Southern Nigeria. Trop J Pharm Res. 2015;14(6):1089–94.
15. Kollef KE, Schramm GE, Wills AR, Reichley RM, Micek ST, Kollef MH. Predictors of 30-day mortality and hospital costs in patients with ventilator-associated pneumonia attributed to potentially antibiotic-resistant gram-negative bacteria. CHEST Journal. 2008;134(2):281–7.
16. Mauldin PD, Salgado CD, Hansen IS, Durup DT, Bosso JA. Attributable hospital cost and length of stay associated with health care-associated infections caused by antibiotic-resistant gram-negative bacteria. Antimicrob Agents Chemother. 2010;54(1):109–15.
17. Silvestri L, van Saene H. Hospital-acquired infections due to gram-negative bacteria. N Engl J Med. 2010;363(15):1482–6.
18. Finley RL, Collignon P, Larsson DJ, McEwen SA, Li X-Z, Gaze WH, et al. The scourge of antibiotic resistance: the important role of the environment. Clin Infect Dis. 2013;57(5):704–10.
19. Abera B, Kibret M, Mulu W. Extended-Spectrum beta (β)-lactamases and Antibiogram in Enterobacteriaceae from clinical and drinking water Sources from Bahir Dar City, Ethiopia. PloS one. 2016;11(11):e0166519.
20. Desta K, Woldeamanuel Y, Azazh A, Mohammod H, Desalegn D, Shimelis D, et al. High Gastrointestinal Colonization Rate with Extended-Spectrum β-Lactamase-Producing Enterobacteriaceae in Hospitalized Patients: Emergence of Carbapenemase-Producing K. pneumoniae in Ethiopia. PloS one. 2016;11(8):e0161685.
21. Mulualem Y, Kasa T, Mekonnen Z, Suleman S. Occurrence of extended spectrum beta (b)-lactamases in multidrug resistant Escherichia coli isolated from a clinical setting in Jimma university specialized hospital, Jimma, Southwest Ethiopia. East Afr J Public Health. 2012;9(2):58–61.
22. Ali S, Birhane M, Bekele S, Kibru G, Teshager L, Yilma Y, et al. Healthcare associated infection and its risk factors among patients admitted to a tertiary hospital in Ethiopia: longitudinal study. Antimicrob Resist Infect Control. 2018;7(1):2.

23. Wayne P. Clinical and laboratory standards institute. Perform Stand Antimicrob Susceptibility Testing. 2007;17.

24. Bate R, Jensen P, Hess K, Mooney L, Milligan J. Substandard and falsified anti-tuberculosis drugs: a preliminary field analysis. Int J Tuberc Lung Dis. 2013;17(3):308–11.

25. WHO. 1 in 10 medical products in developing countries is substandard or falsified. Geneva: World Health Organization; 2017.

26. WHO. Global Surveillance and Monitoring System for substandard and falsifed medical products. Geneva: World Health Organization; 2017. Licence: CC BY-NC-SA 3.0 IGO

27. Rupp ME, Fey PD. Extended spectrum β-lactamase (ESBL)-producing Enterobacteriaceae. Drugs. 2003;63(4):353–65.

28. Parajuli NP, Acharya SP, Mishra SK, Parajuli K, Rijal BP, Pokhrel BM. High burden of antimicrobial resistance among gram negative bacteria causing healthcare associated infections in a critical care unit of Nepal. Antimicrob Resist Infect Control. 2017;6(1):67.

29. Myat TO, Hannaway RF, Zin KN, Htike WW, Win KK, Crump JA, et al. ESBL-and carbapenemase-producing enterobacteriaceae in patients with bacteremia, Yangon, Myanmar, 2014. Emerg Infect Dis. 2017;23(5):857.

30. Shukla I, Tiwari R, Agrawal M. Prevalence of extended spectrum-lactamase producing Klebsiella pneumoniae in a tertiary care hospital. Indian J Med Microbiol. 2004;22(2):87.

31. Chaudhary P, Bhandari D, Thapa K, Thapa P, Shrestha D, Chaudhary H, et al. Prevalence of extended Spectrum Beta-lactamase producing Klebsiella Pneumoniae isolated from urinary tract infected patients. J Nepal Health Res Counc. 2016;14(33):111–5.

32. Bisson G, Fishman NO, Patel JB, Edelstein PH, Lautenbach E. Extended-spectrum β-lactamase–producing Escherichia coli and Klebsiella species: risk factors for colonization and impact of antimicrobial formulary interventions on colonization prevalence. Infect Control Hospital Epidemiol. 2002;23(5):254–60.

33. Organization WH. Global priority list of antibiotic-resistant bacteria to guide research, discovery, and development of new antibiotics. Geneva: World Health Organization; 2017.

34. Grundmann H, Glasner C, Albiger B, Aanensen DM, Tomlinson CT, Andrasević AT, et al. Occurrence of carbapenemase-producing Klebsiella pneumoniae and Escherichia coli in the European survey of carbapenemase-producing Enterobacteriaceae (EuSCAPE): a prospective, multinational study. Lancet Infect Dis. 2017;17(2):153–63.

35. Gonçalves IR, Ferreira M, Araujo B, Campos P, Royer S, Batistão D, et al. Outbreaks of colistin-resistant and colistin-susceptible KPC-producing Klebsiella pneumoniae in a Brazilian intensive care unit. J Hosp Infect. 2016;94(4):322–9.

36. Kebede HK, Gesesew HA, Woldehaimanot TE, Goro KK. Antimicrobial use in paediatric patients in a teaching hospital in Ethiopia. PLoS One. 2017;12(3):e0173290.

37. Yadesa TM, Gudina EK, Angamo MT. Antimicrobial use-related problems and predictors among hospitalized medical in-patients in Southwest Ethiopia: prospective observational study. PLoS One. 2015;10(12):e0138385.

38. Alexopoulou A, Vasilieva L, Agiasotelli D, Siranidi K, Pouriki S, Tsiriga A, et al. Extensively drug-resistant bacteria are an independent predictive factor of mortality in 130 patients with spontaneous bacterial peritonitis or spontaneous bacteremia. World J Gastroenterol. 2016;22(15):4049.

# 19

# Predictive factors for multidrug-resistant gram-negative bacteria among hospitalised patients with complicated urinary tract infections

Aina Gomila[1,2,3*] [iD], Evelyn Shaw[1,2,3], Jordi Carratalà[1,2,3,4], Leonard Leibovici[5], Cristian Tebé[3], Irith Wiegand[6], Laura Vallejo-Torres[7], Joan M. Vigo[8], Stephen Morris[7], Margaret Stoddart[9], Sally Grier[9], Christiane Vank[6], Nienke Cuperus[10], Leonard Van den Heuvel[10], Noa Eliakim-Raz[5], Cuong Vuong[6], Alasdair MacGowan[9], Ibironke Addy[6] and Miquel Pujol[1,2,3] on behalf of COMBACTE-MAGNET WP5- RESCUING Study

## Abstract

**Background:** Patients with complicated urinary tract infections (cUTIs) frequently receive broad-spectrum antibiotics. We aimed to determine the prevalence and predictive factors of multidrug-resistant gram-negative bacteria in patients with cUTI.

**Methods:** This is a multicenter, retrospective cohort study in south and eastern Europe, Turkey and Israel including consecutive patients with cUTIs hospitalised between January 2013 and December 2014. Multidrug-resistance was defined as non-susceptibility to at least one agent in three or more antimicrobial categories. A mixed-effects logistic regression model was used to determine predictive factors of multidrug-resistant gram-negative bacteria cUTI.

**Results:** From 948 patients and 1074 microbiological isolates, *Escherichia coli* was the most frequent microorganism (559/1074), showing a 14.5% multidrug-resistance rate. *Klebsiella pneumoniae* was second (168/1074) and exhibited the highest multidrug-resistance rate (54.2%), followed by *Pseudomonas aeruginosa* (97/1074) with a 38.1% multidrug-resistance rate. Predictors of multidrug-resistant gram-negative bacteria were male gender (odds ratio [OR], 1.66; 95% confidence interval [CI], 1.20–2.29), acquisition of cUTI in a medical care facility (OR, 2.59; 95%CI, 1.80–3.71), presence of indwelling urinary catheter (OR, 1.44; 95%CI, 0.99–2.10), having had urinary tract infection within the previous year (OR, 1.89; 95%CI, 1.28–2.79) and antibiotic treatment within the previous 30 days (OR, 1.68; 95%CI, 1.13–2.50).

**Conclusions:** The current high rate of multidrug-resistant gram-negative bacteria infections among hospitalised patients with cUTIs in the studied area is alarming. Our predictive model could be useful to avoid inappropriate antibiotic treatment and implement antibiotic stewardship policies that enhance the use of carbapenem-sparing regimens in patients at low risk of multidrug-resistance.

**Keywords:** Multidrug-resistance, Complicated urinary tract infection, Gram-negative bacteria, Predictive model of multidrug-resistance gram-negative bacteria

* Correspondence: agomilagrange@gmail.com
[1]Department of Infectious Diseases, Hospital Universitari de Bellvitge, Institut Català de la Salut (ICS-HUB), Feixa Llarga s/n, L'Hospitalet de Llobregat, 08907 Barcelona, Spain
[2]Spanish Network for Research in Infectious Diseases (REIPI RD12/0015), Instituto de Salud Carlos III, Madrid, Spain
Full list of author information is available at the end of the article

## Background

Urinary tract infections (UTIs) are one of the most common bacterial infections [1]. Complicated urinary tract infections (cUTIs), occurring in individuals with functional or structural urinary tract abnormalities, are a leading cause of hospital admissions, hospital-acquired infections, and antibiotic use [2].

The prevalence of cUTIs is difficult to assess accurately. Data from the most recent point prevalence survey of healthcare-associated infections (HAIs) in European acute care hospitals showed that UTI was the third most common cause, accounting for 19% of estimated 3.2 million overall cases of HAIs [3]. This figure, although huge, clearly underestimates the overall cUTI incidence in Europe because it did not include patients developing cUTIs in the community and in long-term care facilities (LTCFs). In LTCFs, cUTIs occur in more than one million patients annually [4]. Aging, comorbidities, and an increasing number of invasive urologic procedures for both diagnosis and treatment have been related to this high prevalence of cUTIs in the European population.

Antibiotic resistance has become a major healthcare problem in Europe and worldwide [5, 6]. Currently, multidrug-resistant (MDR) gram-negative bacteria (GNB) pose a threat in hospitals and nursing homes [7]. According to the recent Annual Report of the European Antimicrobial Resistance Surveillance Network (EARS-Net) [8], MDR rates showed large variations across Europe, being higher in southern and south-eastern Europe than in northern Europe. Patients with suspected cUTIs are frequently treated empirically with broad-spectrum antibiotics. Developing a model that helps select patients at high risk for MDR could be useful when choosing empirical antibiotic regimens and in antibiotic stewardship policies.

Considering the lack of contemporary data on hospitalised patients with cUTIs, we aimed to determine the prevalence of MDR among hospitalised patients with cUTIs in countries with high MDR-GNB prevalence and develop a predictive model to determine the risk of MDR-GNB infections, which would be useful to select more targeted antibiotic regimens avoiding the frequent treatment with broad-spectrum antibiotics.

## Methods

### Study design

The COMBACTE-MAGNET, WP5 RESCUING Study was a multicenter, retrospective, observational cohort study including hospitalised patients with cUTI from January 2013 to December 2014. Data was collected from patients who were diagnosed with cUTI as the primary cause of hospitalisation and from patients who were hospitalised for other reasons but who developed cUTIs during their hospitalization [9]. This study conformed to the STROBE guidelines for reporting observational studies [10].

### Setting and patients

The study was conducted in Bulgaria (2 hospitals), Greece (2 hospitals), Hungary (3 hospitals), Israel (3 hospitals), Italy (3 hospitals), Romania (2 hospitals), Spain (3 hospitals) and Turkey (2 hospitals). Patients were identified by searching for the appropriate International Classification of Diseases (ICD)-9 Clinical Modification (CM) or ICD-10 CM Codes [11, 12] at discharge from hospital (diagnoses are detailed in Additional file 1). All patients who met the criteria for cUTI were selected for data collection. In order to avoid selection bias, each hospital included 50 to 60 consecutive patients with cUTI until achieving the total estimated sample size of 1000 patients.

Complicated urinary tract infection inclusion criteria followed the Food and Drug Administration (FDA) guidance on cUTI [13], and consisted on:

- Patients with UTI and at least one of the following underlying conditions: a) indwelling urinary catheter; b) urinary retention (at least 100 mL of residual urine after voiding); c) neurogenic bladder; d) obstructive uropathy (e.g., nephrolithiasis, fibrosis); e) renal impairment caused by intrinsic renal disease (estimated glomerular filtration rate < 60 mL/min); f) renal transplantation; g) urinary tract modifications, such as an ileal loop or pouch; or h) pyelonephritis.
- And at least one of the following signs or symptoms: a) chills or rigors associated with fever or hypothermia (temperature > 38 °C or < 36 °C); b) flank pain (pyelonephritis) or pelvic pain (cUTI); c) dysuria, urinary frequency, or urinary urgency; or d) costovertebral angle tenderness on physical examination.
- And urine culture with $\geq 10^5$ colony-forming units/mL of uropathogen (no more than two species) or;
- At least one blood culture growing possible uropathogens (no more than two species) with no other evident site of infection.

The exclusion criteria were as follows: a) patients aged < 18 years, b) diagnosis of prostatitis according to FDA guidance, c) polymicrobial infections including Candida spp., d) polymicrobial infections including more than two bacterial species, or e) cUTI with Candida spp. as sole uropathogen, d) patients with uncomplicated cystitis.

If a patient had more than one episode of cUTI during the same hospitalisation, only the first episode was included.

### Data collection and validation

Data on demographic characteristics, comorbidities, place of acquisition of infection, signs and symptoms of infection, laboratory and microbiology, imaging tests, management of infection including antibiotic therapy and interventional procedures, details of discharge and outcome of infection, including death if applicable, were reviewed by professionals who received web-database training sessions. For data collection, an access-controlled web-based electronic case report form was used. At each site, a screening log was kept of the patients with infections detected according to the ICD codes, detailing the excluded patients and the reasons for exclusion. To confirm data quality, study sites were monitored and audited by a contract research organization (CRO) from Utrecht, Netherlands.

### Definitions

Acquisition of cUTI in a medical care facility was considered if it was:

- Hospital-acquired: if it started ≥48 h after hospital admission.
- Healthcare-associated: if it was detected at hospital admission or within the first 48 h of hospitalization, with the patient fulfilling any of the following criteria: 1) receiving intravenous therapy, wound care, or specialized nursing care at home in the previous 30 days; 2) admission in the hospital or haemodialysis ward or receiving intravenous chemotherapy in the previous 30 days; 3) hospitalization for ≥2 days in the previous 90 days; 4) residence in a long-term care facility; 5) underwent invasive urinary procedure within the previous 30 days; or 6) having a long-term indwelling urinary catheter.

We used the following categories for cUTIs:

- UTI related to indwelling urinary catheterization, including long-term, short-term, or intermittent catheterization
- Pyelonephritis with no other urinary tract modification, defined as sepsis, flank pain or costovertebral angle tenderness
- UTI related to anatomical urinary tract modification, including any urinary diversion procedure, nephrostomy or stents, or renal transplants
- UTI related to obstructive uropathy, including any obstruction intrinsic or extrinsic to the urinary tract, such as lithiasis, tumor, ureteral herniation, or prostate hyperplasia
- UTI related to other events that do not fall under any other category

Multidrug resistance was defined according to an international expert proposal by Magiorakos et al. [14], as non-susceptibility to at least one agent in three or more antimicrobial categories (extended-spectrum penicillins, carbapenems, cephalosporins, aminoglycosides, and fluoroquinolones). Extensively drug-resistance (XDR) was defined as non-susceptibility to at least one agent in all but two or fewer antimicrobial categories (i.e., bacterial isolates remaining susceptible to only one or two categories) tested for a determined microorganism.

### Outcomes

The primary outcome was the presence of MDR, as previously defined.

Secondary outcomes included the following:

- Estimation of the MDR prevalence in each country and participating hospital
- Definition of the most prevalent microbiology according to source of infection
- Assessment of the resistance rate of the main GNB to the different antimicrobial classes

### Statistical methods

The chi-square or Fisher's exact test was used to compare categorical data, and Student's t-test or the Mann-Whitney U test to compare continuous data, as appropriate. The quantile-quantile normality plot and Kolmogorov-Smirnov test were used to assess whether a continuous variable was normally distributed.

#### Predictive model of MDR in patients with cUTI

Countries and hospitals presented a non-homogeneous MDR baseline risk. To account for such variations, a mixed-effects logistic regression model to predict the risk of MDR in patients with cUTIs, including all different epidemiological and clinical variables, was built using hospitals as clusters. First, a stepwise selection method based on the Akaike Information Criterion was performed to identify variables that explained the bulk of MDR infections. Adequacy of the final model was assessed by collinearity, influential observations, and residuals. To evaluate discrimination properties, the Hosmer-Lemeshow goodness-of-fit test was used. Moreover, the bootstrapping resampling method was used to improve the robustness of estimated standard errors. Results were given as odds ratios (OR) and 95% confidence intervals (95% CI). All tests were two-tailed, and a $p$-value of < 0.05 was considered statistically significant.

All data were analyzed using R software (2017). R Foundation for Statistical Computing, Vienna, Austria.

### Results

#### Patients' epidemiological characteristics and univariate analysis of MDR-GNB

Fifty-two cases were excluded due to lack of information on the presence of MDR, leaving a final sample of 948 patients. Among them, 1074 bacterial isolates were obtained.

The patients' clinical characteristics are shown in Table 1. Females comprised 56%, the mean age was 65.8 ± 18.2 years, 34.4% were admitted due to conditions other than cUTIs, 17.4% came from LTCFs, and 46% were functionally dependent. Factors associated with MDR by univariate

**Table 1** Patients' epidemiological characteristics and univariate analysis of multidrug-resistance in gram-negative bacteria

|  | Entire Cohort (n = 948) | Susceptible (n = 691) | MDR (n = 257) | p-Value |
|---|---|---|---|---|
| Male gender, n (%) | 420 (44.3) | 270 (39.1) | 150 (58.4) | < 0.001 |
| Mean age (SD), years | 65.8 (18.2) | 65.6 (18.6) | 66.5 (16.8) | 0.526 |
| Elective admission, n (%) | 141 (14.9) | 97 (14) | 44 (17.1) | 0.236 |
| Admission reason: conditions other than cUTI, n (%) | 326 (34.4) | 214 (31) | 112 (43.6) | < 0.001 |
| Place of residency: long-term care facility, n (%) | 165 (17.4) | 98 (14.2) | 67 (26.1) | < 0.001 |
| Underlying disease, n (%) |  |  |  |  |
| Acute myocardial infarction | 79 (8.3) | 56 (8.1) | 23 (8.9) | 0.676 |
| Congestive heart failure | 182 (19.2) | 134 (19.4) | 48 (18.7%) | 0.804 |
| Peripheral vascular disease | 70 (7.4) | 55 (8) | 15 (5.8) | 0.267 |
| Cerebrovascular disease | 182 (19.2) | 122 (17.7) | 60 (23.3) | 0.048 |
| Dementia | 130 (13.7) | 93 (13.5) | 37 (14.4) | 0.709 |
| Chronic pulmonary disease | 135 (14.2) | 91 (13.2) | 44 (17.1) | 0.122 |
| Connective tissue disease | 21 (2.2) | 15 (2.2) | 6 (2.3) | 0.879 |
| Peptic ulcer | 46 (4.9) | 34 (4.9) | 12 (4.7) | 0.873 |
| Diabetes mellitus | 250 (26.4) | 186 (26.9) | 64 (24.9) | 0.531 |
| Chronic kidney disease | 263 (27.7) | 191 (27.6) | 72 (28) | 0.909 |
| Hemiplegia | 86 (9.1) | 58 (8.4) | 28 (10.9) | 0.233 |
| Leukaemia | 9 (0.9) | 6 (0.9) | 3 (1.2) | 0.673 |
| Lymphoma | 13 (1.4) | 11 (1.6) | 2 (0.8) | 0.338 |
| Chronic liver disease | 50 (5.3) | 35 (5.1) | 15 (5.8) | 0.637 |
| Solid tumour | 114 (12.3) | 75 (11.1) | 39 (15.4) | 0.075 |
| Metastatic tumour | 47 (5) | 35 (5.1) | 12 (4.7) | 0.803 |
| Valvulopathy | 88 (9.3) | 69 (10) | 19 (7.4) | 0.221 |
| HIV infection | 10 (1.1) | 8 (1.2) | 2 (0.8) | 0.611 |
| Charlson index ≥ 3, n (%) | 418 (44.1) | 299 (43.3) | 119 (46.3) | 0.403 |
| Organ transplant, n (%) | 65 (6.9) | 45 (6.5) | 20 (7.8) | 0.492 |
| Immunosuppression, n (%) | 94 (9.9) | 64 (9.3) | 30 (11.7) | 0.270 |
| Steroids, n (%) | 68 (7.2) | 46 (6.7) | 22 (8.6) | 0.313 |
| Functional capacity: dependent, n (%) | 436 (46.1) | 298 (43.3%) | 138 (53.9) | 0.003 |
| Prior UTI (within the previous year), n (%) | 247 (26.1) | 167 (24.2) | 80 (31.2) | 0.027 |
| Prior antibiotics (within the previous 30 days), n (%) | 190 (20.1) | 120 (17.4) | 70 (27.6) | 0.001 |
| Prior quinolone | 64 (6.8) | 38 (5.5) | 26 (10.2) | 0.010 |
| Prior Penicillin | 55 (5.8) | 35 (5.1) | 20 (7.9) | 0.103 |
| Prior cephalosporin | 42 (4.4) | 27 (3.9) | 15 (5.9) | 0.188 |
| Prior Carbapenem | 22 (2.3) | 10 (1.4) | 12 (4.7) | 0.003 |
| Prior other antibiotics | 51 (5.4) | 31 (4.5) | 20 (7.9) | 0.042 |
| Acquisition in a medical care facility, n (%) | 410 (43.2) | 244 (35.3) | 166 (64.6) | < 0.001 |
| Source of cUTI, n (%) |  |  |  |  |
| Indwelling urinary catheterisation | 308 (32.5) | 189 (27.4) | 119 (46.3) | < 0.001 |
| Pyelonephritis with normal tract anatomy | 196 (20.7) | 164 (23.7) | 32 (12.5) | < 0.001 |
| Obstructive uropathy | 152 (16) | 114 (16.5) | 38 (14.8) | 0.523 |
| Urinary tract diversion | 84 (8.9) | 64 (9.3) | 20 (7.8) | 0.476 |

**Table 1** Patients' epidemiological characteristics and univariate analysis of multidrug-resistance in gram-negative bacteria *(Continued)*

| | Entire Cohort (*n* = 948) | Susceptible (*n* = 691) | MDR (*n* = 257) | *p*-Value |
|---|---|---|---|---|
| Other | 208 (21.9) | 160 (23.2) | 48 (18.7) | 0.139 |
| Shock/severe sepsis, n (%) | 140 (15.9) | 104 (16.2) | 36 (14.9) | 0.635 |

*MDR* multidrug resistance, *SD* standard deviation, *cUTI* complicated urinary tract infection, *HIV* human immunodeficiency virus, *UTI* urinary tract infection

analysis were male gender, admission due to reasons other than cUTIs, residing in LTCF, dependent functional capacity, UTI within the previous year, antibiotic treatment within the previous 30 days, acquisition of cUTI in a medical care facility, and presence of an indwelling urinary catheter.

## Most frequent bacterial aetiology and patterns of antimicrobial resistance

Of all bacterial isolates (*n* = 1074), the most frequent was *Escherichia coli*, isolated in 52% of samples, followed by *Klebsiella pneumoniae* in 15.6%, *Pseudomonas aeruginosa* in 9%, *Proteus mirabilis* in 7.3%, and *Enterococcus* spp. in 3.2%. Only these 5 bacteria were evaluated due to their clinical significance. *Escherichia coli* was mainly related to pyelonephritis with normal urinary tract (76.5%), while *K. pneumoniae* was more frequently associated with urinary tract diversion (22.6%). *Pseudomonas aeruginosa*, *P. mirabilis* and *Enterococcus* spp. were significantly related to the presence of an indwelling urinary catheter (18.8%, 25.6% and 5.8% respectively) (Table 2).

Significant differences in MDR rate occurred between the different participating hospitals, ranging from < 20% in some countries such as Hungary and Spain to almost 60% in other countries such as Bulgaria and Greece (Fig. 1a). The MDR rates by hospital varied in accordance with the country's trend (Fig. 1b).

The antimicrobial resistance patterns according to the most frequent GNB are shown in Table 3. *Escherichia coli* had a fluoroquinolone resistance rate of 39.5%, a third-generation cephalosporin (3GC) resistance rate of 24.2% and a MDR rate of 14.5%. *Klebsiella pneumoniae* exhibited the highest MDR rate (54.2%), followed by *P. aeruginosa* (38.5%) and *P. mirabilis* (24.1%). By antibiotic class, fluoroquinolones had the highest resistance rates (39.5% in *E. coli*, 56.5% in *K. pneumoniae*, 42.1% in *P. aeruginosa*, and 55.7% in *P. mirabilis*), followed by 3GC and aminoglycosides (Table 3). Resistance to carbapenems was 32.6% in *P. aeruginosa*, 19.6% in *K. pneumoniae* and 2.3% in *E. coli*.

## Predictive model of MDR-GNB in patients with cUTIs

Identified predictive factors for MDR risk are reported in Table 4. The resulting equation and an illustrative example for calculating MDR-GNB risk are described in Additional file 1. The proposed model had good discrimination for MDR prediction, with a 0.80 statistic (area under the receiver operating characteristic curve) (Fig. 2). Calibration was also excellent, with a good observed/expected ratio of MDR risk by deciles of predicted risk (Fig. 3a) and by hospital (Fig. 3b).

The factors that best predicted the bulk of MDR presence were male gender (odds ratio [OR], 1.66; 95% confidence interval [CI], 1.20–2.29), acquisition of cUTI in a medical care facility (OR, 2.59; 95% CI, 1.80–3.71), presence of an indwelling urinary catheter (OR, 1.44; 95% CI, 0.99–2.10), having a UTI within the previous year (OR, 1.89; 95% CI, 1.28–2.79), and antibiotic treatment within the previous 30 days (OR, 1.68; 95% CI, 1.13–2.50) (Table 4).

**Table 2** Most frequent bacterial aetiology of complicated urinary tract infections according to source of infection (sources = 948, isolations = 1074)

| Source (*n* = 948) | *E. coli* *n* = 559 (52%) | *K. pneumoniae* *n* = 168 (15.6%) | *P. aeruginosa* *n* = 97 (9%) | *P. mirabilis* *n* = 79 (7.3%) | *Enterococcus* spp. *n* = 34 (3.2%) |
|---|---|---|---|---|---|
| Indwelling urinary catheterisation (*n* = 308), n (%) | 124 (40.3%) | 63 (20.4%) | 58 (18.8%) | 40 (25.6%) | 18 (5.8%) |
| Pyelonephritis with normal tract anatomy (*n* = 196), n (%) | 150 (76.5%) | 25 (12.7%) | 4 (2.0%) | 13 (6.6%) | 0 (0.0) |
| Obstructive uropathy (*n* = 152), n (%) | 98 (64.4%) | 26 (17.1%) | 12 (7.9%) | 11 (7.2%) | 5 (3.3%) |
| Urinary tract diversion (*n* = 84), n (%) | 48 (57.1%) | 19 (22.6%) | 10 (11.9%) | 2 (2.4%) | 4 (4.8%) |
| Others (*n* = 208), n (%) | 139 (66.8%) | 35 (16.8%) | 13 (6.2%) | 13 (6.2%) | 7 (3.4%) |

*E. coli*, Escherichia coli; *K. pneumoniae*, Klebsiella pneumoniae; *P. aeruginosa*, Pseudomonas aeruginosa; *P. mirabilis*, Proteus mirabilis; *Enterococcus* spp., Enterococcus species. First column include all sources of infection (*n* = 948), and first raw include the five more frequent bacteria taking as denominator the total number of isolations (*n* = 1074). All other isolates up to the total number are not included in the table. Denominators in central boxes are the total number of each row (sources)

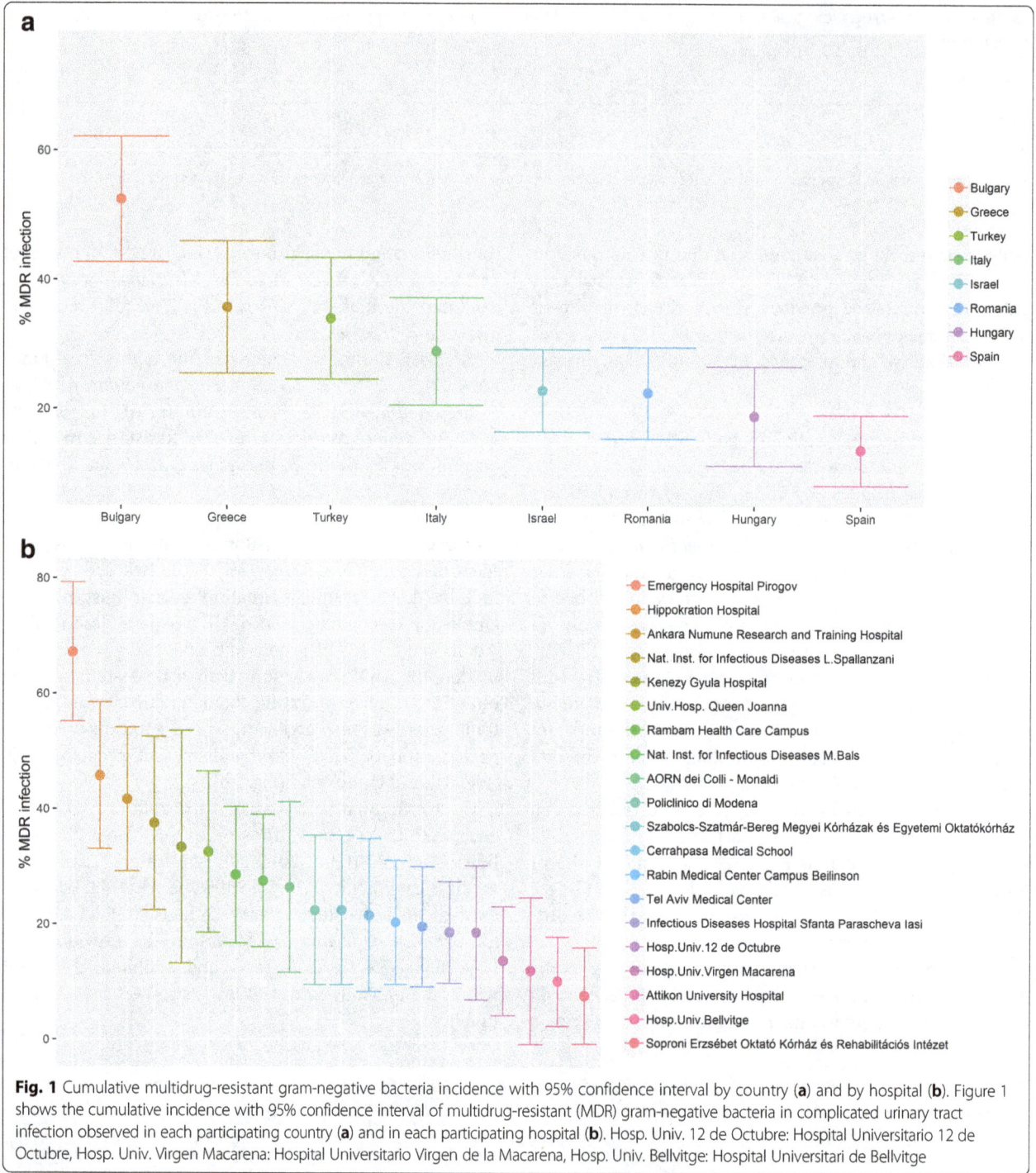

**Fig. 1** Cumulative multidrug-resistant gram-negative bacteria incidence with 95% confidence interval by country (**a**) and by hospital (**b**). Figure 1 shows the cumulative incidence with 95% confidence interval of multidrug-resistant (MDR) gram-negative bacteria in complicated urinary tract infection observed in each participating country (**a**) and in each participating hospital (**b**). Hosp. Univ. 12 de Octubre: Hospital Universitario 12 de Octubre, Hosp. Univ. Virgen Macarena: Hospital Universitario Virgen de la Macarena, Hosp. Univ. Bellvitge: Hospital Universitari de Bellvitge

## Discussion

This large, multicenter, retrospective cohort study of hospitalised patients with cUTIs provides a comprehensive update about antibiotic resistance in countries with high MDR incidence. In this cohort, *K. pneumoniae* had the highest MDR rate among all the GNB analysed, and fluoroquinolones had the highest resistance rates. We developed a model to predict the risk of cUTIs caused by

MDR organisms, in order to avoid inappropriate treatment and help establish antibiotic stewardship policies.

In our cohort, *E. coli* continues to be the most frequent cause of cUTI, as previously observed [15, 16]. Although it was associated with low MDR levels, it showed a fluoroquinolone resistance rate of almost 40% and a 3GC resistance rate of 24%. Previous studies already described an increased resistance rate of *E. coli* to fluoroquinolones and

**Table 3** Patterns of antimicrobial resistance to main antibiotic groups by the four most frequent gram-negative bacteria

| | AMG-R n (%) | FQ-R n (%) | 3GC-R n (%) | P/T-R n (%) | CARB-R n (%) | MDR n (%) | XDR n (%) |
|---|---|---|---|---|---|---|---|
| E. coli (n = 559) | 108 (19.3) | 221 (39.5) | 135 (24.2) | 57 (10.2) | 13 (2.3) | 81 (14.5) | 2 (0.4) |
| K. pneumoniae (n = 168) | 77 (45.8) | 95 (56.5) | 98 (58.3) | 64 (38.1) | 33 (19.6) | 91 (54.2) | 23 (13.7) |
| P. aeruginosa (n = 97) | 36 (37.9) | 40 (42.1) | 47 (49.5) | 30 (31.6) | 31 (32.6) | 36 (38.5) | 16 (16.8) |
| P. mirabilis (n = 79) | 29 (36.7) | 44 (55.7) | 20 (25.4) | 9 (11.4) | 4 (5.0) | 19 (24.1) | 1 (1.3) |

AMG-R aminoglycoside-resistant, FQ-R fluoroquinolone-resistant, 3GC-R third-generation cephalosporin-resistant, P/T-R piperacillin/tazobactam-resistant, CARB-R carbapenem-resistant, MDR multidrug-resistant, XDR extensively drug-resistant, E. coli, Escherichia coli; K. pneumoniae, Klebsiella pneumoniae; P. aeruginosa, Pseudomonas aeruginosa; P. mirabilis, Proteus mirabilis

trimethoprim-sulfamethoxazole, precluding their use as empiric treatment in mild and severe infections [16, 17]. Similar to our results, the Study for Monitoring Antimicrobial Resistance Trends (SMART) in the United States showed a 35% resistance rate of E. coli to ciprofloxacin [18]. This high fluoroquinolone resistance rate contrasts with the 20% reported by the EARS-Net in 2016 [8]. However, the rate was obtained by including northern European countries that had low antimicrobial resistance rates. On the contrary, the south-eastern countries showed rates similar to those observed in our study. Besides, the EARS-Net included only invasive isolates, a sample profile quite different to ours. MDR rates similar to our results were also observed in the Asia-Pacific region [19].

In our cohort, K. pneumoniae was the second most frequent microorganism, showing a remarkably carbapenem-resistance rate of almost 20% and having ileal loop or urinary diversion as the most frequent source of infection.

**Table 4** Predictive model of multidrug-resistant gram-negative bacteria in patients with complicated urinary tract infection: a mixed-effects logistic regression model

| Factors | OR | 95% CI | p-Value |
|---|---|---|---|
| (Intercept) | 0.1 | 0.06–0.16 | < 0.001 |
| Gender (male) | 1.66 | 1.20–2.29 | 0.002 |
| Acquisition in a medical facility | 2.59 | 1.80–3.71 | < 0.001 |
| Indwelling urinary catheter | 1.44 | 0.99–2.10 | 0.06 |
| UTI within the previous year | 1.89 | 1.28–2.79 | 0.001 |
| Antibiotics within the previous 30 days | 1.68 | 1.13–2.50 | 0.011 |

OR odds ratio, CI confidence interval, UTI urinary tract infection
Potential predictors included in the predictive model were age, sex, source of infection, place of residency, functional capacity score, personal history of myocardial infarction, congestive heart failure, peripheral vascular disease, cerebrovascular disease, dementia, chronic pulmonary disease, ulcer disease, diabetes mellitus, chronic kidney disease, hemiplaegia, solid tumor, liver disease, metastatic tumor, Charlson score, infection acquisition site, presence of indwelling urinary catheter, urinary retention, organ transplant, kidney organ transplant, immunosuppressive therapy, active chemotherapy, corticosteroid therapy, UTI within the previous year, previous 30-day antibiotic treatment (including previous treatment with quinolones, penicillins, cephalosporins, carbapenems, and other antibiotics), infection severity, neurogenic bladder, obstructive uropathy, other urinary tract modification, and chronic renal impairment

The countries with the highest rate of carbapenem-resistant K. pneumoniae were Greece and Turkey, while those with the lowest were Spain and Hungary. This study did not analyse the type of resistance mechanisms present in Enterobacteriaceae; nevertheless, phenotypic resistance to carbapenems commonly results from acquiring carbapenemases that affect even the latest generations of penicillins and cephalosporins, in addition to other antibiotic families such as aminoglycosides and fluoroquinolones. The European survey of carbapenemase-producing Enterobacteriaceae (EuSCAPE), performed in 2013–2014 in Europe, Turkey, and Israel, showed that K. pneumoniae and

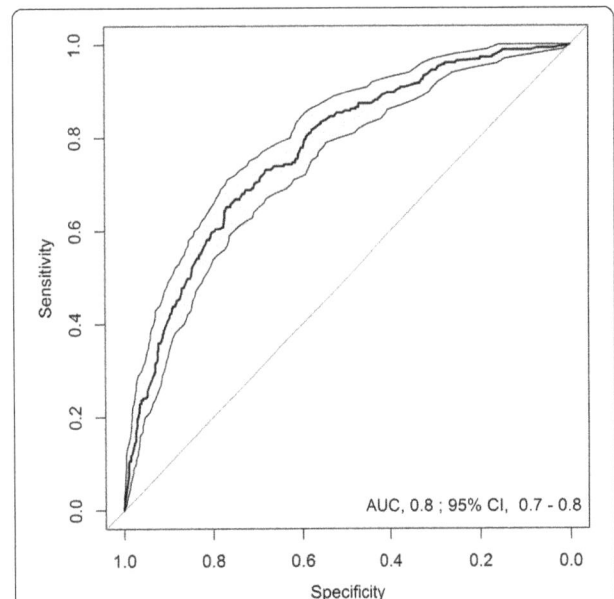

**Fig. 2** Receiver operating characteristic curve of the predictive model of multidrug-resistance in gram-negative bacteria. Figure 2 shows the evaluation of the discriminative power of the mixed-effects logistic regression predictive model for multidrug-resistant gram-negative bacteria among patients with complicated urinary tract infection by the receiver operating characteristic curve using observed multidrug-resistance incidence as the gold standard. AUC, area under the curve; CI, confidence interval

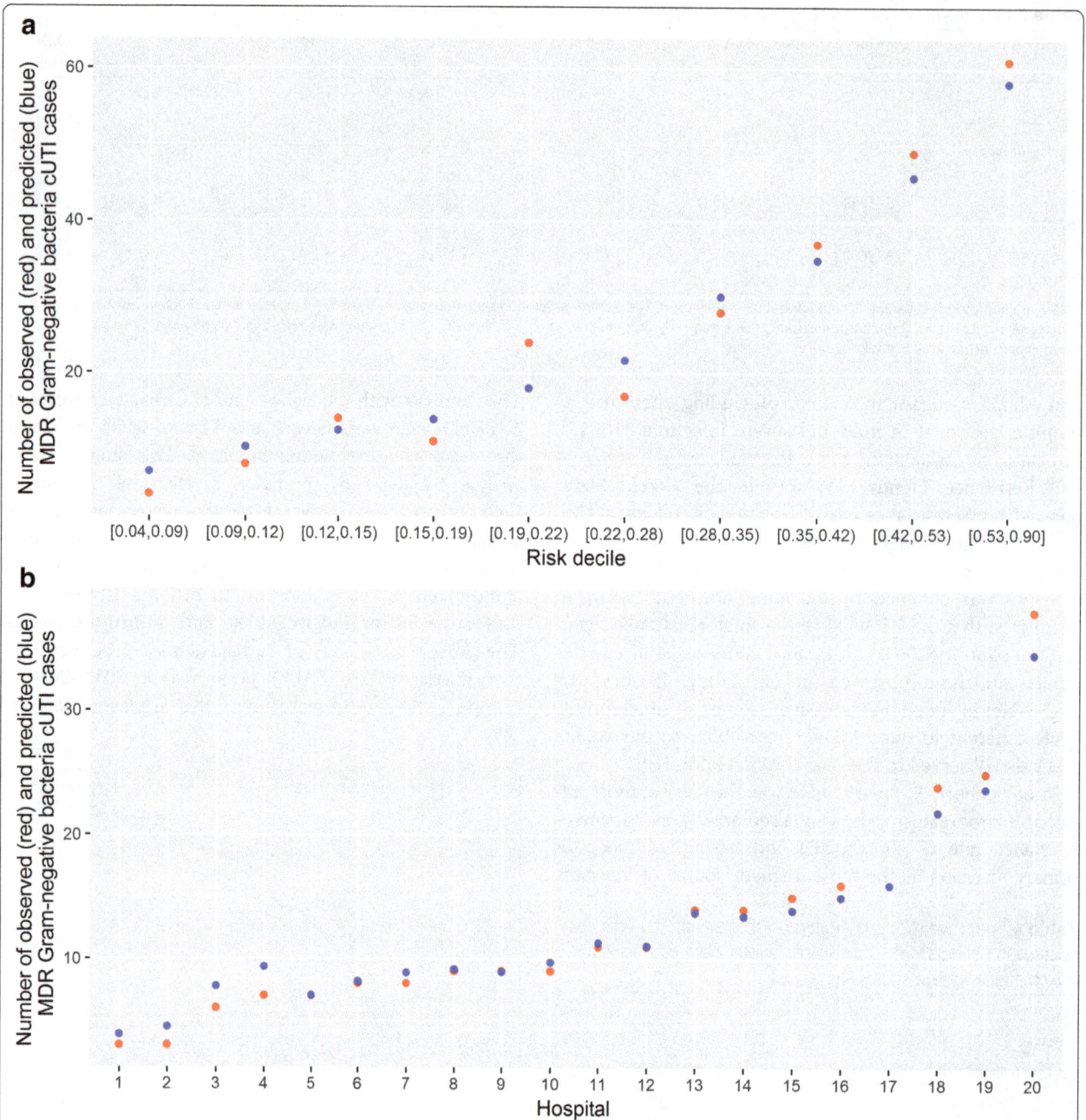

**Fig. 3** Observed versus predicted multidrug-resistant gram-negative bacteria risk, stratified by deciles of predicted risk (**a**) and by hospital (**b**). **a** shows the observed to expected events by probability deciles and (**b**) shows the observed to expected events by hospital. Events are defined as multidrug-resistant (MDR) gram-negative bacteria complicated urinary tract infections. Hospitals included in (**b**) are: 1. Soproni Erzsébet Oktató Kórház és Rehabilitációs Intézet, 2. Hospital Universitari de Bellvitge, 3. Attikon University Hospital, 4. Hospital Universitario Virgen de la Macarena, 5. Hospital Universitario 12 de Octubre, 6. Infectious Diseases Hospital Sfanta Parascheva Iasi, 7. Tel Aviv Medical Center, 8. Rabin Medical Center Campus Beilinson, 9. Cerrahpasa Medical School, 10. Szabolcs-Szatmár-Bereg Megyei Kórházak és Egyetemi Oktatókórház, 11. Policlinico di Modena, 12. AORN dei Colli – Monaldi, 13. National Institute for Infectious Diseases Matei Bals, 14. Rambam Health Care Campus, 15. University Hospital Queen Joanna, 16. Kenezy Gyula Hospital, 17. National Institute for Infectious Diseases Lazzaro Spallanzani, 18. Ankara Numune Research and Training Hospital, 19. Hippokration Hospital, 20. Emergency Hospital Pirogov

*E. coli* produced carbapenemases, mainly KPC-type and OXA-48-like, in the countries represented in our study [20]. However, 29% of *K. pneumoniae* isolates had unidentified mechanisms of carbapenem resistance, and

almost 10% of *K. pneumoniae* isolates were resistant to all antibiotics tested, consistent with our findings.

*P. aeruginosa* isolates showed a carbapenem-resistance rate that reached 32%. In this case, the presence of a urinary catheter was the most frequently associated factor. Countries with the greatest rates of carbapenem-resistant *P. aeruginosa* included Italy and Turkey, while those with the lowest rates were Israel and Hungary. The mechanisms of MDR in *P. aeruginosa* have been related to the production of cephalosporinases, combined with mutations that decrease carbapenem permeability of the bacterial cell wall [21–23]. The selective antibiotic pressure caused by broad-spectrum antibiotics favours the emergence of MDR strains, and once it is produced, its reversion is very slow [24].

We have developed and internally validated a clinical predictive model for hospitalised patients with suspected cUTIs that helps determine the risk of MDR-GNB infections, considering the country's baseline risk. This model may be useful in reducing inappropriate empirical antibiotic treatment that leads to poor clinical outcomes in these patients [25]. It may also help implement antibiotic stewardship programs that enhance the use of carbapenem-sparing antibiotic regimens in patients at low risk for MDR [24, 26]. The severity of infection based on physician's clinical judgement and severity scores needs to be assessed, since non-severe cUTI will probably benefit more from receiving treatment based on susceptibility testing [27]. Importantly, however, more severe cases with potentially serious consequences of treatment failure could benefit from applying our model.

The most reliable factor that predicted MDR was the acquisition of cUTIs in medical care facilities, mostly LTCFs. Most patients admitted to LTCFs are old, have comorbidities, and are functionally dependent. These patients frequently receive repeated courses of antibiotics for various reasons, including cUTIs. Thus, LTCFs have been identified as important reservoirs of MDR-GNB [28]. Besides patients having had a UTI within the previous year and having received antibiotics within the previous month, other predictive factors for MDR identified by our model have been also described by other authors [29, 30]. All of them reflect high cumulative exposure to antibiotics and, consequently, selection of MDR endogenous flora.

Male UTI is usually considered complicated due to the more complex urinary tract anatomy. This implies longer antibiotic treatments and frequent relapse of infection, resulting in repeated antibiotic exposure and higher risk of MDR [31].

The presence of a urinary catheter has been associated with a higher risk of UTI [32, 33] and infections caused by microorganisms with higher intrinsic resistance, such as *P. aeruginosa* and *Enterococcus* spp. [1]. Our study reaffirmed this observation since *P. aeruginosa* was significantly associated with urinary catheter use. The catheter inhibits the defence mechanisms of the urinary tract epithelium against bacteria and facilitates the rapid invasion of the bladder by microorganisms colonizing the device. The urinary catheter also promotes the development of bacterial biofilm, where antibiotics do not achieve significant concentrations [34].

The main limitation of this study is that the model has been validated in a group of hospitals from south and eastern Europe, Turkey and Israel and the results may not be generalizable to other populations. Therefore, further external validation is necessary to confirm our results. Also, the retrospective design and approach for identifying cases could have led to underestimate non-severe cases occurring in patients admitted due to other reason than cUTI and who developed cUTI during the hospitalisation. On the other hand, difficult to treat MDR-GNB cUTIs could have been more easily identified. The main strength of the study is its large-scale, multicenter, and multinational design including 948 patients and the case-validation system. Furthermore, the effect of possible differences in MDR baseline risk by each hospital on the main outcome was considered to create the predictive model.

## Conclusions

The current high rate of MDR-GNB infections among hospitalised patients with cUTIs is alarming in south and eastern Europe, Turkey and Israel. A high MDR rate has been observed among *K. pneumoniae* and *P. aeruginosa* isolates. Our study developed a predictive model that could be useful in determining the risk for MDR-GNB cUTI, with the purpose of targeting patients at high risk with broad-spectrum antibiotics and guiding the implementation of antibiotic stewardship policies that enhance the use of carbapenem-sparing antibiotic regimens in patients at low risk for MDR-GNB.

**Abbreviations**

95%CI: 95% confidence interval; CRO: Contract research organization; cUTIs: Complicated urinary tract infections; EARS-Net: European Antimicrobial Resistance Surveillance Network; EuSCAPE: European survey of carbapenemase-producing Enterobacteriaceae; FDA: Food and Drug Administration; GNB: Gram-negative bacteria; HAIs: Healthcare-associated infections; ICD-9 (– 10) CM: International Classification of Diseases-9 (– 10) Clinical Modification; KPC: *Klebsiella pneumoniae* carbapenemase; LTCFs: Long-term care facilities; MDR: Multidrug-resistance; OR: Odds ratio; OXA: Oxacillinase; SMART: Study for Monitoring Antimicrobial Resistance Trends; STROBE: Strengthening the Reporting of Observational studies in Epidemiology; UTIs: Urinary tract infections; XDR: Extensively drug-resistance

**Acknowledgements**

COMBACTE-MAGNET, RESCUING Study Group members: Tanya Babitch, Dora Tancheva, Rossitza Vatcheva-Dobrevska, Sotirios Tsiodras, Emmanuel Roilides, Istvan Várkonyi, Judit Bodnár, Aniko Farkas, Yael Zak-Doron, Yehuda Carmeli, Emanuele Durante Mangoni, Cristina Mussini, Nicola Petrosillo, Andrei Vata, Adriana Hristea, Julia Origüen, Jesus Rodriguez-Baño, Arzu Yetkin, and Nese Saltoglu.

**Funding**

This research project received support from the Innovative Medicines Initiative Joint Undertaking under grant agreement n° 115523 | 115620 | 115737 resources of which are composed of financial contribution from the European Union

Seventh Framework Programme (FP7/2007–2013) and EFPIA companies in kind contribution. The research leading to these results was conducted as part of the COMBACTE-MAGNET consortium. For further information please refer to www.COMBACTE.com.

**Authors' contributions**

AG, LL and MP conceived and designed the study. AG, JC and MP were major contributors in writing the manuscript. ES, LL, IW, CV, CV, IA participated in the design of the study and coordination and helped to draft the manuscript. CT performed the statistical analysis of data. All authors read and approved the final manuscript.

**Consent for publication**

No applicable.

**Competing interests**

Authors IA, CV, IW, and CV belong to EFPIA (European Federation of Pharmaceutical Industries and Association) member companies in the IMI JU and costs related to their part in the research were carried by the respective company as in kind contribution under the IMI JU scheme. Other authors declare no potential conflicts.

**Author details**

[1]Department of Infectious Diseases, Hospital Universitari de Bellvitge, Institut Català de la Salut (ICS-HUB), Feixa Llarga s/n, L'Hospitalet de Llobregat, 08907 Barcelona, Spain. [2]Spanish Network for Research in Infectious Diseases (REIPI RD12/0015), Instituto de Salud Carlos III, Madrid, Spain. [3]Institut d'Investigació Biomèdica de Bellvitge (IDIBELL), Feixa Llarga s/n, L'Hospitalet de Llobregat, 08907 Barcelona, Spain. [4]University of Barcelona, Barcelona, Spain. [5]Department of Medicine E, Beilinson Hospital, Rabin Medical Center, Petah Tikva; Sackler Faculty of Medicine, Tel Aviv University, Tel Aviv, Israel. [6]AiCuris Anti-infective Cures GmbH, Wuppertal, Germany. [7]UCL Department of Applied Health Research, University College London, London, UK. [8]Informatics Unit, Fundació Institut Català de Farmacologia, Barcelona, Spain. [9]Department of Medical Microbiology, Southmead Hospital, North Bristol NHS Trust, Bristol, UK. [10]Julius Center for Health Sciences and Primary Care, University Medical Center Utrecht, Utrecht, Netherlands.

**References**

1. Flores-Mireles AL, Walker JN, Caparon M, Hultgren SJ. Urinary tract infections: epidemiology, mechanisms of infection and treatment options. Nat Rev Microbiol. 2015;13(5):269–84.

2. Tandogdu Z, Wagenlehner FME. Global epidemiology of urinary tract infections. Curr Opin Infect Dis. 2016;29(1):73–9.

3. European Centre for Disease Prevention and Control. Point prevalence survey of healthcare-associated infections and antimicrobial use in European acute care hospitals 2011–2012. Available at: https://ecdc.europa. eu/sites/portal/files/media/en/publications/Publications/healthcare-associated-infections-antimicrobial-use-PPS.pdf. Accessed 8 May, 2018.

4. European Centre for Disease Prevention and Control (ECDC). Point prevalence survey of healthcare-associated infections and antimicrobial use in European long-term care facilities. April–May 2013. Stockholm; 2014. Available at: https://ecdc.europa.eu/sites/portal/files/media/en/publications/Publications/healthcare-associated-infections-point-prevalence-survey-long-term-care-facilities-2013.pdf. Accessed 8 May, 2018.

5. Levy SB, Marshall B. Antibacterial resistance worldwide: causes, challenges and responses. Nat Med. 2004;10(12s):S122–9.

6. Centers for Disease Control and Prevention (CDC). Antibiotic resistance threats in the United States, 2013. Available at: http://www.cdc.gov/drugresistance/threat-report-2013/index.html. Accessed 8 May, 2018.

7. Mody L, Krein SL, Saint S, Min LC, Montoya A, Lansing B, et al. A targeted infection prevention intervention in nursing home residents with indwelling devices: a randomized clinical trial. JAMA Intern Med. 2015;175(5):714–23.

8. Surveillance Report. Surveillance of antimicrobial resistance in Europe 2016. Available at: https://ecdc.europa.eu/sites/portal/files/documents/AMR-surveillance-Europe-2016.pdf. Accessed 8, May, 2018.

9. Shaw E, Addy I, Stoddart M, Vank C, Grier S, Wiegand I, et al. Retrospective observational study to assess the clinical management and outcomes of hospitalised patients with complicated urinary tract infection in countries with high prevalence of multidrug resistant gram-negative bacteria (RESCUING). BMJ Open. 2016;6(7):e011500.

10. von Elm E, Altman DG, Egger M, Pocock SJ, Gøtzsche PC, Vandenbroucke JP, et al. Strengthening the reporting of observational studies in epidemiology (STROBE) statement: guidelines for reporting observational studies. BMJ. 2007;335(7624):806–8.

11. International Classification of Diseases, Ninth Revision, Clinical Modification, ICD-9-CM. Available at: https://www.cdc.gov/nchs/icd/icd9cm.htm. Accessed 14 Mar 2018.

12. International Classification of Diseases, Tenth Revision, Clinical Modification, ICD-10-CM. Available at: https://www.cdc.gov/nchs/icd/icd10cm.htm. Accessed 14 Mar 2018.

13. Complicated Urinary Tract Infections: Developing Drugs for Treatment. Guidance for Industry. U.S. Department of Health and Human Services, Food and Drug Administration Center for Drug Evaluation and Research (CDER), 2015. http://www.fda.gov/downloads/Drugs/Guidances/ucm070981.pdf. Accessed 8 May 2018.

14. Magiorakos AP, Srinivasan A, Carey RB, Carmeli Y, Falagas ME, Giske CG, et al. Multidrug-resistant, extensively drug-resistant and pandrug-resistant bacteria: an international expert proposal for interim standard definitions for acquired resistance. Clin Microbiol Infect. 2012;18(3):268–81.

15. Nicolle LE, AMMI Canada Guidelines Committee* ACG. Complicated urinary tract infection in adults. Can J Infect Dis Med Microbiol. 2005;16:349–60.

16. Bader MS, Loeb M, Brooks AA. An update on the management of urinary tract infections in the era of antimicrobial resistance. Postgrad Med. 2017;129(2):242–58.

17. Bader MS, Hawboldt J, Brooks A. Management of complicated urinary tract infections in the era of antimicrobial resistance. Postgrad Med. 2010;122(6):7–15.

18. Bouchillon SK, Badal RE, Hoban DJ, Hawser SP. Antimicrobial susceptibility of inpatient urinary tract isolates of gram-negative bacilli in the United States: results from the study for monitoring antimicrobial resistance trends (SMART) program: 2009–2011. Clin Ther. 2013;35(6):872–7.

19. Hsueh P, Hoban DJ, Carmeli Y, Chen S, Desikan S, Alejandria M, et al. Consensus review of the epidemiology and appropriate antimicrobial therapy of complicated urinary tract infections in Asia-Pacific region. J Inf Secur. 2011;63(2):114–23.

20. Grundmann H, Glasner C, Albiger B, Aanensen DM, Tomlinson CT, Andrasević AT, et al. Occurrence of carbapenemase-producing Klebsiella pneumoniae and Escherichia coli in the European survey of carbapenemase-producing Enterobacteriaceae (EuSCAPE): a prospective, multinational study. Lancet Infect Dis. 2017;17(2):153–63.

21. Bonomo RA, Burd EM, Conly J, Limbago BM, Poirel L, Segre JA, et al. Carbapenemase-Producing Organisms: A Global Scourge. Clin Infect Dis. 2018;66(8):1290–7.

22. Vasoo S, Barreto JN, Tosh PK. Emerging Issues in Gram-Negative Bacterial Resistance: An Update for the Practicing Clinician. Mayo Clin Proc. 2015; 90(3):395–403.

23. Exner M, Bhattacharya S, Christiansen B, Gebel J, Goroncy-Bermes P, Hartemann P, et al. Antibiotic resistance: What is so special about multidrug-resistant Gram-negative bacteria? GMS Hyg Infect Control. 2017;12:Doc05.

24. Palacios-Baena ZR, Gutiérrez-Gutiérrez B, Calbo E, Almirante B, Viale P, Oliver A, et al. Empiric therapy with Carbapenem-sparing regimens for bloodstream infections due to extended-Spectrum β-lactamase-producing Enterobacteriaceae: results from the INCREMENT cohort. Clin Infect Dis. 2017;65(10):1615–23.

25. Zilberberg MD, Nathanson BH, Sulham K, Fan W, Shorr AF. Carbapenem resistance, inappropriate empiric treatment and outcomes among patients hospitalized with Enterobacteriaceae urinary tract infection, pneumonia and sepsis. BMC Infect Dis. 2017;17(1):279.

26. Ostrowsky B, Banerjee R, Bonomo RA, Cosgrove SE, Davidson L, Doron S, et al. Infectious Diseases Physicians: Leading the Way in Antimicrobial Stewardship. Clin Infect Dis. 2018;66(7):995–1003.

27. Eliakim-Raz N, Babitch T, Shaw E, Addy I, Wiegand I, Vank C, et al. Risk factors for treatment failure and mortality among hospitalised patients with complicated urinary tract infection: a multicentre retrospective cohort study, RESCUING Study Group. Clin Infect Dis. 2018; https://doi.org/10.1093/cid/ciy418.

28. Magiorakos AP, Burns K, Rodríguez-Baño J, Borg M, Daikos G, Dumpis U, et al. Infection prevention and control measures and tools for the prevention of entry of carbapenem-resistant Enterobacteriaceae into healthcare settings: guidance from the European Centre for Disease Prevention and Control. Antimicrob Resist Infect Control. 2017;6:113.

29. Vazquez-Guillamet MC, Vazquez R, Micek ST, Kollef-Marin H. Predicting resistance to piperacillin-Tazobactam, Cefepime and Meropenem in septic patients with bloodstream infection due to gram-negative Bacteria. Clin Infect Dis. 2017;65(10):1607–14.

30. Bischoff S, Walter T, Gerigk M, Ebert M, Vogelmann R. Empiric antibiotic therapy in urinary tract infection in patients with risk factors for antibiotic resistance in a German emergency department. BMC Infect Dis. 2018;18(1):56.

31. Karlowsky JA, Lagacé-Wiens PRS, Simner PJ, DeCorby MR, Adam HJ, Walkty A, et al. Antimicrobial resistance in urinary tract pathogens in Canada from 2007 to 2009: CANWARD surveillance study. Antimicrob Agents Chemother. 2011;55(7):3169–75.

32. Hooton TM, Bradley SF, Cardenas DD, Colgan R, Geerlings SE, Rice JC, et al. Diagnosis, prevention, and treatment of catheter-associated urinary tract infection in adults: 2009 international clinical practice guidelines from the Infectious Diseases Society of America. Clin Infect Dis. 2010;50(5):625–63.

33. Pallett A, Hand K. Complicated urinary tract infections: Practical solutions for the treatment of multiresistant gram-negative bacteria. J Antimicrob Chemother. 2010;65 Suppl 3:iii25–33.

34. Tenke P, Kovacs B, Bjerklund Johansen TE, Matsumoto T, Tambyah PA, Naber KG. European and Asian guidelines on management and prevention of catheter-associated urinary tract infections. Int J Antimicrob Agents. 2008;31:68–78.

# 20

# Incidence and outcomes of multidrug-resistant gram-negative bacteria infections in intensive care unit from Nepal

Shraddha Siwakoti[1]*⊙, Asish Subedi[2], Abhilasha Sharma[1], Ratna Baral[1], Narayan Raj Bhattarai[1] and Basudha Khanal[1]

## Abstract

**Background:** Infections caused by multi-drug resistant gram-negative bacterial infections are the principle threats to the critically ill patients of intensive care units. Increasing reports of these infections from the Nepalese intensive care unit underline the clinical importance of these pathogens. However, the impact of these infections on the patient's clinical outcome has not yet been clearly evaluated. The objective of our study was to determine the incidence and associated clinical outcome of multi-drug resistant gram-negative bacterial infections in intensive care unit from a tertiary care center of Nepal.

**Methods:** A prospective cohort study was conducted among adult patients admitted in intensive care unit of B. P Koirala Institute of Health Sciences from July to December 2017. Patients infected with multi-drug resistant gram-negative bacteria, non-multi-drug resistant gram-negative bacteria and those without infection were included. Identification of gram-negative bacteria and their antibiotic susceptibility pattern was performed with standard microbiological methods. Demographic, clinical profiles and outcomes (in-hospital-mortality, intensive care unit and hospital length of stay) were documented.

**Results:** The incidence rate of multi-drug resistant gram-negative bacteria infections was 47 per 100 admitted patients (64/137) with 128 episodes. *Acinetobacter species* (41%, 52/128) was the commonest followed by *Klebsiella pneumoniae* (28%, 36/128) and *Pseudomonas spp* (21%, 27/128). Patients with multi-drug resistant gram-negative bacteria in comparison to non-multi-drug resistant gram-negative bacteria had high healthcare-associated infections (95%, 61/64 versus 20%, 2/10; $p = < 0.001$). In-hospital-mortality was 38% (24/64), 20% (2/10) and 10% (4/41) in multi-drug resistant, non-multi-drug resistant and uninfected group respectively ($p = 0.007$). After adjustment for independent risk factors, compared to uninfected patients, the odds ratio (CI) for in-hospital-mortality in multi-drug resistant and non-multi-drug resistant group was (4.7[1.4–15.5], $p = 0.01$) and 2.60 [0.38–17.8], $p = 0.32$) respectively. Multi-drug resistant patients also had longer intensive care unit and hospital stay, however, it was statistically insignificant.

**Conclusion:** The incidence of multi-drug resistant gram-negative bacterial infections was remarkably high in our intensive care unit and showed a significant association with healthcare-associated infections and in-hospital-mortality.

**Keywords:** ICU, Multidrug-resistant gram-negative bacteria, Healthcare-associated infection, Incidence, Outcome

* Correspondence: shraddha.siwakoti@bpkihs.edu
[1]Department of Microbiology, B. P. Koirala Institute of Health Sciences, Dharan 56700, Nepal
Full list of author information is available at the end of the article

## Background

The prevalence of infection is high among patients admitted to intensive care units (ICUs) and it is a major cause of mortality [1, 2]. The extended prevalence of infection in intensive care study reported infection in 51% of patients with gram-negative bacteria (GNB) isolation from 62% of infectious episodes [2]. As a disastrous effect of infection, antimicrobial resistance is an increasing concern in ICUs worldwide [3]. The global scenario shows that gram-positive infections are common in the developed countries ICUs [4]. However, multidrug-resistant gram-negative bacteria (MDR-GNB) infections dominate in the Asia-Pacific region [4, 5] including Nepal [6, 7]. Among MDR-GNB, extended-spectrum beta-lactamases (ESBL) organisms, carbapenemase producing enterobacteriaceae, carbapenem-resistant *Acinetobacter species*, multidrug-resistant *Pseudomonas aeruginosa* are the major culprits. Unfortunately, new antibacterial agents have not been developed in pace with the growth of multidrug-resistant (MDR) organisms [8]. There are now a rising number of reports globally [9] and also from Nepal [6, 7] of MDR-GNB infections in ICUs for which the treatment options are limited. The impact of the MDR-GNB infections can be determined from analyzing clinical outcomes, in-hospital-mortality and the length of ICU or hospital stay [10]. The association of MDR-GNB with a prolonged hospital length of stay (LOS) and mortality remains controversial. Several studies [10, 11] have reported the direct association whereas, others [12, 13] have shown that MDR-GNB infections are not associated with increased hospital LOS and mortality. Previous studies from Nepal have reported a high incidence of MDR-GNB infections from ICU [6, 7], but the impact of these infections on clinical outcome has not been evaluated. Therefore, the objective of our study was to determine the incidence of MDR-GNB infections in the critically ill patients from adult ICU, as well as the clinical outcomes with regard to in-hospital-mortality, ICU and hospital LOS.

## Methods

### Study design

This prospective cohort study was conducted in seven bedded general adult ICU under the care of the department of Anesthesiology and Critical care unit, B.P Koirala Institute of Health Sciences (BPKIHS), Nepal.

### Study population

All consecutive adult patients admitted to the medical ICU from July to December 2017 were eligible for the study. Patients infected with MDR-GNB, non-MDR-GNB and those without infection were included.

### Microbiological procedures

Pathogenic bacteria isolated from the clinical specimens from the ICU were further characterized by conventional biochemical tests to identify the specific GNB by using standard microbiologic methods [14]. Antibiotic susceptibility test of GNB strains was done by the Kirby Bauer disc diffusion method on Mueller Hinton agar (MHA) as per the Clinical Laboratory Standard Institute (CLSI) guidelines [15]. Antibiotics of following concentrations were used: ampicillin (10 μg), amikacin (30 μg), gentamycin (10 μg), tobramycin(10 μg), ciprofloxacin (5 μg), levofloxacin (5 μg), chloramphenicol (30 μg), co-trimoxazole (25 μg), ceftazidime (30 μg), cefotaxime (30 μg), cefepime (30 μg), piperacillin (100 μg), carbenicillin (100 μg.), piperacillin-tazobactam (100/10 μg), imipenem (10 μg), tigecycline (30 μg), polymyxin B (300unit), and colistin sulphate (10 μg) from HiMedia Laboratories, India. Disk zone diameters were interpreted according to the CLSI 2017 recommendations. Quality control for culture plates and antibiotic susceptibility was performed using *Escherichia coli* ATCC 25922 and *Pseudomonas aeruginosa* ATCC 27853. All the strains were subjected to various phenotypic methods for the screening and confirmation of the beta lactamases. Strains showing decreased sensitivity to ceftazidime/ cefotaxime were considered as screen positive for ESBL production and were subjected to the following confirmatory phenotypic tests as per the CLSI guidelines [15].

• ESBL- A difference in the zone size of 5 mm between ceftazidime and ceftazidime+ clavulanic acid and cefotaxime and cefotaxime+clavulanic acid discs was considered as confirmed ESBL producer [15].

• Carbapenemase- The screen positive for carbapenemase production was considered for strains showing resistance to carbapenems. A positive modified hodge test (MHT) with appearance of clover leaf at the streaking line was considered as carbapenemase producer as per the CLSI guidelines [15]. A difference in the zone size of 7 mm between Imipenem and Imienem+ EDTA disc in the EDTA disk synergy test was considered as MBL producer [16].

### Definitions

Infection-An episode of infection was defined as the isolation of GNB in the presence of compatible signs or symptoms. Healthcare-associated infections (HCAI) and those infections present on admission were included.

Infection occurring > 48 h after admission to the hospital was defined as HCAI.

MDR was defined as non-susceptibility to at least one agent in three or more antimicrobial categories [17].

Diagnostic criteria recommended by CDC was implemented to classify different infections. Pneumonia was considered if purulent tracheobronchial secretion or new pathogenic bacteria isolated from sputum or tracheal aspirate culture with ≥10 [4] colony forming unit/ml and at least two of the following criteria were met: fever (> 38°C); leukocytes > 12,000 or < 4000 cells/ml; new or progressive pulmonary infiltrates on chest X-rays; new onset or worsening cough or dyspnea or tachypnea; or worsening gas exchange.

An episode of blood stream infection (BSI) was defined as one positive blood culture with a recognized pathogen or two positive cultures with same organism drawn on separate occasions with one of the following signs and symptoms: (fever(> 38°C), chills and rigor and hypotension.

An episode of urinary tract infection (UTI) was defined as a positive urine culture of ≥10 [5] colony forming units/ml and with no more than two species of microorganisms, and at least one of following signs or symptoms: fever (> 38°C); dysuria; suprapubic tenderness; costovertebral angle pain or tenderness with no other recognized cause.

An episode of surgical site infection (SSI) was defined as infection which occurred within 30 days after the operation involving skin, subcutaneous tissue or deep soft tissue of the incision and at least one of the following: purulent drainage with or without laboratory confirmation; organisms isolated from an aseptically obtained culture of fluid or tissue; or one of the signs or symptoms of infection: pain or tenderness, localised swelling, redness, or heat.

Based on the presence or absence of infection, patients were categorized into three groups: Uninfected patients- Patients without infection; Non-MDR-GNB patients-Infections attributed to susceptible GNB and MDR-GNB patients- Infections attributed to MDR-GNB.

Patients were included more than once in the analysis for separate episodes of infection.

In cases of polymicrobial infections, the episode was defined as an MDR-GNB case if 1 of the isolates was an MDR-GNB strain.

Previous antibiotic therapy was defined as antibiotic used within 30 days prior to positive culture for GNB.

Empiric antibiotic therapy was considered inappropriate if it did not include at least one antibiotic active against the GNB in vitro. Empirical antibiotic treatment protocols were same for all the groups and the antibiotic was changed after the culture and sensitivity report.

## Data collection
Patient demographic characteristics, underlying conditions and reason for hospital admission were recorded in the participant record form at the time of admission. Patient were routinely followed up again each morning and data on clinical or laboratory parameters were collected, including previous antibiotic therapy, clinical manifestations, HCAI,

pathogens and antibiotic resistance. The baseline severity of illness were assessed with acute physiology chronic health evaluation II (APACHE II) score [18] and Charlson comorbidity index (CCI) score [19]. Further, the data were collected regarding clinical outcomes that included the ICU stay, hospital stay, discharge and in-hospital-mortality.

## Statistical analysis
Data were entered in the MS Excel 2007 and analyzed with STATA version 14 (stata corporation, college station, Tx, USA). Normal distribution of data was tested using histogram, skewness-kurtosis, and shapiro–wilk test. We used kruskal–wallis test for non-parametric data to compare between three groups. Categorical data were analyzed using the chi-square test or fisher's exact test as appropriate. Univariate and multivariate logistic regression analysis was used to compare in-hospital-mortality between the groups. Data are reported as median (IQR), number (percentage), odds ratio (95% confidence interval). Values of $p$ < 0.05 was considered statistically significant.

## Results
A total of 137 patients were admitted to the ICU during the 6 months study period. There were128 episodes of MDR-GNB infections in 64 patients with an incidence rate of 47 per 100 ICU admissions. There were 41 uninfected and 10 infected cases with 19 episodes of non-MDR-GNB infections (Fig. 1).

Among the GNB infection episodes, incidences of MDR for each of the bacterial strains were reported as 100% (4/4) for *Enterobacter spp*, 100% (2/2) for *Citrobacter spp*, 93% (52/56) for *Acinetobacter spp*, 86% (36/42) for *Klebsiella pneumoniae*, 84% (27/32) for *Pseudomonas spp* and 64%(7/11) for *Escherichia coli*. Polymicrobial infection was present in 28% (18/64) MDR-GNB patients and 10% (1/10) in non-MDR-GNB patients. The detailed results of GNB pattern in the non-MDR-GNB and MDR-GNB group are presented in Table 1.

In the MDR group, bacteria were most frequently isolated from the lower respiratory tract infection (LRTI) (72%, 92/128) followed by BSI (14%, 18/128), UTI and SSI each with (3%, 4/128). Whereas, in the non-MDR group, BSI (53%, 10/19) was the commonest followed by LRTI (42%, 8/19) and UTI (5%, 1/19). MDR-GNB showed variable degree of resistance to different classes of antibiotics as shown in Table 2.

Demographic and clinical characteristics are provided in Table 3.

Patients with MDR-GNB in comparison to non-MDR-GNB were found to have high incidence of previous antibiotic therapy (95%, 61/64 versus 60%, 6/10; p = < 0.001) and HCAI (95%, 61/64 versus 20%, 2/10; $p$ = < 0.001).

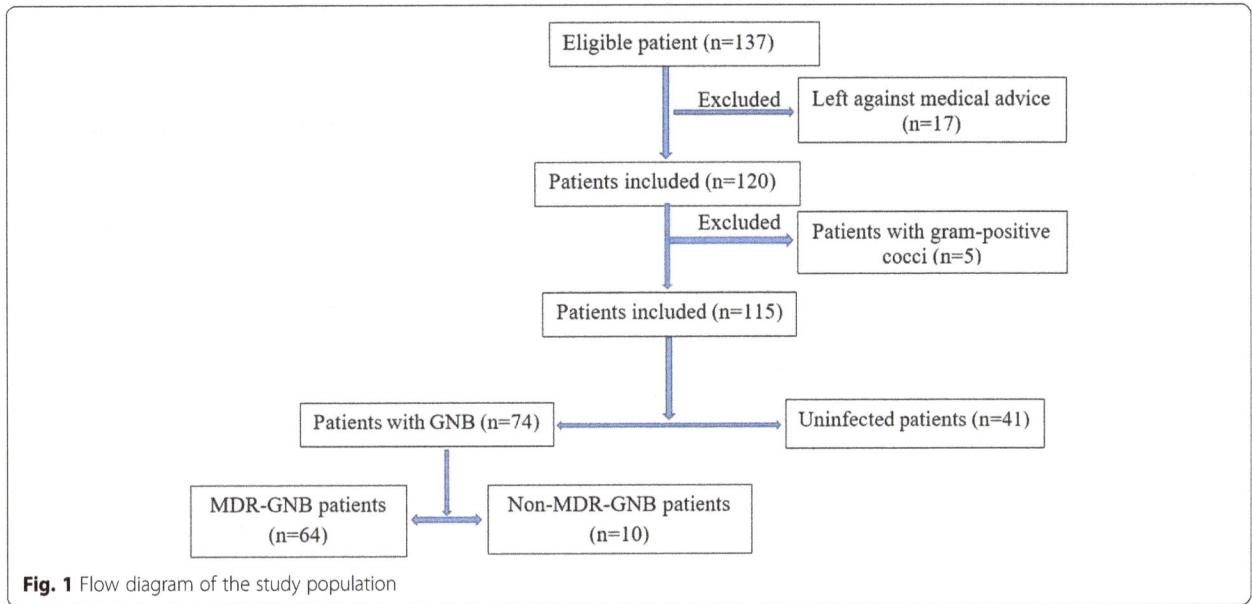

**Fig. 1** Flow diagram of the study population

With respect to the clinical outcome, in-hospital-mortality among patients in the MDR group (38%, 24/64) was significantly higher than those in the non-MDR group (20%, 2/10) and uninfected group (10%, 4/41) ($p = 0.007$) as depicted in Table 4. However, no difference was detected when MDR-GNB group was compared to non-MDR-GNB group ($p = 0.47$).

The findings of univariate and multivariate logistic regression for variables associated with in-hospital- mortality are described in Table 5.

After adjustment for independent risk factors, compared to uninfected patients, the odds ratio (CI) for in-hospital-mortality in MDR-GNB group was (4.7[1.4–15.5], $p = 0.01$), while in patients with non-MDR-GNB it was (2.60 [0.38–17.8], $p = 0.32$).

## Discussion

The increasing incidence of MDR-GNB infections reported from the different ICU's in Nepal is of great concern [6, 7]. However, most prior work from Nepal has

been focused on their incidence and the common mechanism of drug resistance [6, 7]. To our knowledge, this is the first study from Nepal that highlights the association between MDR-GNB infections and various clinical outcomes in ICU admitted patients.

The present study found that MDR-GNB infections was not uncommon in ICU and it accounted for 47 MDR-GNB cases per 100 ICU admission. Despite significant advances in ICU in current years, the incidence of MDR-GNB HCAI remains higher in the ICU compared with other hospital units [20]. In our study, 95% cases of MDR-GNB were associated with HCAI. Similar findings were reported by other recent studies from Nepal which were done by Parajuli et al., Bhandari et al. and khanal et al. which reported 96% [6], 79% [21] and 69% [7] of GNB causing HCAI from ICU were MDR. Rampant antibiotic use, increased prevalence of drug resistance and nonadherence to infection control strategies are the emerging problems in Nepalese ICU's predisposing for the emergence and spread of HCAI [6]. Likewise,

**Table 1** Gram-negative bacilli (GNB) infections from ICU ($n = 147$)

| Gram negative bacilli isolates | Total GNB | Non-MDR-GNB | MDR-GNB | | | Total MDR |
| --- | --- | --- | --- | --- | --- | --- |
| | | | Resistance mechanisms | | | |
| | | | ESBL | CP(MBL) | Other | |
| Acinetobacter spp | 56 | 4(21%) | 6 | 34 | 12 | 52(41%) |
| Pseudomonas spp | 32 | 5(26%) | 3 | 19 | 5 | 27(21%) |
| Klebsiella pneumoniae | 42 | 6(32%) | 12 | 19 | 5 | 36(28%) |
| Escherichia coli | 11 | 4(21%) | 6 | 1 | – | 7(5.5%) |
| Enterobacter spp | 4 | – | 2 | 2 | – | 4(3%) |
| Citrobacter spp | 2 | – | 2 | | – | 2(1.5%) |
| Total | 147 | 19(100%) | 31(24%) | 75(59%) | 22(17%) | 128(100%) |

**Table 2** Antibiotic sensitivity of multidrug-resistant gram negative bacilli ($n = 128$)

| Antimicrobial agents | Resistance (%) among bacterial isolates | | | | | |
|---|---|---|---|---|---|---|
| | Acinetobacter spp ($n = 52$) | Pseudomonas spp ($n = 27$) | Klebsiella pneumoniae ($n = 36$) | Escherichia coli ($n = 7$) | Enterobacter spp ($n = 4$) | Citrobacter spp ($n = 2$) |
| Levofloxacin | 85 | 88 | 73 | 57 | 100 | 50 |
| Ciprofloxacin | 92 | 90 | 82 | 86 | 100 | 100 |
| Amikacin | 93 | 89 | 76 | 71 | 100 | 50 |
| Gentamycin | 93 | 89 | 79 | 71 | 100 | 50 |
| Tobramycin | – | 87 | – | – | – | – |
| Chloramphenicol | – | – | 73 | 57 | 100 | 0 |
| Cotrimoxazole | 90 | – | 73 | 71 | 100 | 50 |
| Ampicillin | – | – | – | 100 | 100 | 100 |
| Piperacillin | 93 | 90 | 79 | | 100 | 100 |
| Piperacillin- Tazobactam | 86 | 82 | 73 | 100 | 100 | 100 |
| Amoxicillin-clavulanate | – | – | 76 | 100 | 100 | 100 |
| Ceftazidime | 93 | 92 | 92 | 100 | 100 | 100 |
| Cefotaxime | 93 | 92 | 92 | 100 | 100 | 100 |
| Cefepime | 87 | 90 | 86 | 100 | 100 | 100 |
| Imipenem | 81 | 82 | 69 | 14 | 100 | 0 |
| Tigecycline | 58 | 63 | 57 | 14 | 67 | 0 |
| Polymixin B | 0 | 0 | 0 | 0 | 0 | 0 |
| Colistin Sulphate | 0 | 0 | 0 | 0 | 0 | 0 |

in a study from India, 58% MDR-GNB were isolated from the ICUs specimens from the total received specimens [22]. Another study from India on epidemiology of MDR-GNB isolated from ventilator-associated pneumonia in ICU patients found 88% of total isolates to be GNB, among which 72% were MDR [23]. A systematic review of the burden of MDR HCAI among ICU patients in Southeast Asia showed substantially higher incidence of MDR *Acinetobacter baumannii* (58%) than reported from other parts of globe [24]. These scenario shows high prevalence of MDR-GNB infections in ICUs of Asia including Nepal. The present study showed high frequency of bacterial isolates producing beta-lactamases (MBL 59%, ESBL 24%). Current studies from Nepal also have reported high incidence of ESBL (43% [6], 40% [21], 25% [7]) and MBL (65% [21], 50% [6], 37% [7]) from ICU. Prevalence of ESBL and carbapenemases producing GNB from ICU was 22.7% and 9.6% respectively in a recent study from India [25]. Studies from the west also have shown an increasing trend of ESBL with ICU GNB isolates [20]. Sader and colleagues reported on the prevalence and trends of MDR-GNB occurring in the ICU of the hospitals in the United States and Europe from January 2009 to December 2011 [20]. Over the 3-year study period, rates of ESBL-producing strains of *Escherichia coli* and *Klebsiella spp* from the ICU increased from 11.9 to 17.4% and 27.5–41.8% respectively from 2009 to 2011 [20]. Alike, a SENTRY study also

reported that GNB resistance to imipenem increased from 34.5% in 2006 to 59.8% in 2009 across the world [26]. This globally increasing trend of carbapenemase resistance in the ICUs poses a significant concern since it limits the range of therapeutic alternative forcing the clinicians to use agents like colistin which is expensive and associated with significant toxicity [8]. The reports of infections caused by MDR non-fermentative gram-negative bacteria and enterobacteriaceae are increasingly documented from the Nepalese ICU. In this study, 93% of *Acinetobacter spp*, 86% of *Klebsiella pneumoniae*, 84% of *Pseudomonas spp* and 64% of *Escherichia coli* were MDR and a similar result was also reported from Nepal [7]. Excessive use of broad spectrum antibiotics as observed in this study along with inadherence to infection control measures are the main causes for this terrifying rates of MDR infections in our ICU.

In the present study, multivariate analysis showed strong association between MDR-GNB patients and in-hospital-mortality even after adjusting all the confounding factors (Odds ratio: 4.7, $p$-0.01). Ben-David D et al. [11], in a retrospective study on the outcome of carbapenem-resistant *Klebsiella pneumoniae*, (CRKP) BSI, also found mortality to be significantly higher among patients with CRKP compared with those with susceptible *K. pneumoniae* BSI (48% vs.17%). A study by Cosgrove et al. [10] on the impact of the emergence of resistance to third-generation cephalosporins in

**Table 3** Baseline and Clinical characteristics of patients

| Variables | Uninfected patients; $n = 41$ | Patients with MDR-GNB; $n = 64$ | Patients with non-MDR-GNB; $n = 10$ | $p$-value |
|---|---|---|---|---|
| Age (years) | 43.5(28–56) | 53(27–65) | 55(40–60) | 0.27 |
| Age categories | | | | |
| < 65 | 25(61%) | 49(76%) | 8(80%) | 0.18 |
| > 65 | 16(39%) | 15(23%) | 2(20%) | |
| Sex(M/F) | 19/23 | 28/35 | 4/6 | 0.95 |
| Reason for admission | | | | |
| Cardiovascular | 9(22%) | 16(25%) | 6 (60%) | 0.89 |
| Respiratory | 27(66%) | 44 (69%) | 3(30%) | |
| Digestive/Liver | 1(2%) | 2(3%) | 0 (0%) | |
| Renal | 1(2%) | 2(3%) | 1 (10%) | |
| Neurological | 3(7%) | 0 (0%) | 0(0%) | |
| Medical/Surgical admission | 35/6 | 50/14 | 7/3 | 0.47 |
| CCI Score | 0(0–2) | 1(0–3) | 1(0–1) | 0.77 |
| APACHE Score | | | | |
| At 24 h | 13.5(11–16) | 16(12–21) | 13(12–15) | 0.15 |
| At 48 h | 13(11–15) | 17(12–20) | 13(12–14) | 0.08 |
| Duration of ventilation | 0(0–7) | 10(6–16) | 7.5(6–11) | 0.22 |
| Previous antibiotic therapy | 17(41%) | 61(95%) | 6(60%) | < 0.001 |
| Aminoglycoside | 5(12%) | 18(28%) | 2(20%) | 0.13 |
| Fluoroquinolone | 3(7%) | 20(31%) | 2(20%) | 0.009 |
| Macrolide | 3(7%) | 13(20%) | 2(20%) | 0.15 |
| Beta-lactam/Beta-lactamase inhibitor | 4(10%) | 27(42%) | 4(40%) | 0.001 |
| Cephalosporin | 5(12%) | 10(16%) | 0(0%) | 0.49 |
| Carbapenem | 1(2%) | 22((34%) | 0(0%) | < 0.001 |
| Tigecycline | 0(0%) | 4(6%) | 0(0%) | 0.29 |
| Clindamycin | 0(0%) | 6(9%) | 0(0%) | 0.12 |
| Vancomycin or teicoplanin | 0(0%) | 23(36%) | 1(10%) | < 0.001 |
| Metronidazole | 0(0%) | 7(11%) | 0(0%) | 0.06 |
| Duration of prior antibiotics used (days) | 0(0–6) | 7(6–8) | 4(0–5) | < 0.001 |
| Health-care-associated infection | | 61(95%) | 2(20%) | < 0.001 |

Note: Values are in median (IQR), number, number (%)

*Enterobacter spp* on patient outcomes also found a significant increase in mortality (Relative risk, 5.02). This may possibly due to that appropriate antibiotic therapy will be started later for MDR-GNB infections in compared to infections caused by antibiotic-sensitive bacteria. In contrary to our findings some of the earlier studies did not find significant associations between MDR-GNB and mortality [12, 13]. However, variation in the clinical virulence of the varieties of GNB prevalent in different geographical areas may be the reasons for these conflicting results. Further, the patients infected by MDR-GNB, compared with those with non-MDR-GNB

**Table 4** Clinical outcome of patients

| Outcome | Uninfected patients $n = 41$ | Patients with MDR-GNB $n = 64$ | Patients with non-MDR-GNB $n = 10$ | $p$-value |
|---|---|---|---|---|
| In-hospital-mortality | 4(10%) | 24 (38%) | 2 (20%) | 0.007 |
| Discharged | 37 (90%) | 40 (62%) | 8 (80%) | 0.007 |
| ICU stay | 9(5–12) | 13(8–18) | 9(7–12) | 0.43 |
| Hospital stay | 11(8–17) | 14(10–21) | 9(7–15) | 0.93 |

Note: Values are in median (IQR), number, number (%)

**Table 5** Univariate and Multivariate logistic regression for variables associated with hospital mortality

| Variables | Univariate analysis | | Multivariate analysis | |
| --- | --- | --- | --- | --- |
| | Odds ratio (95% CI) | p value | Odds ratio (95% CI) | p value |
| MDR GNB[a] | 5.46(1.72–17.26) | 0.004 | 4.71(1.42–15.54) | 0.01 |
| Non- MDR GNB[a] | 2.37(0.36–15.26) | 0.36 | 2.60(0.38–17.83) | 0.32 |
| Age | 1.00(0.98–1.03) | 0.50 | 1.001(0.96–1.03) | 0.95 |
| Male | 0.70(0.29–1.66) | 0.42 | 0.59(0.23–1.53) | 0.28 |
| CCI Score | 1.15(0.84–1.56) | 0.36 | 1.05(0.63–1.72) | 0.84 |
| APACHE 24 h | 1.07(1.00–1.16) | 0.04 | 1.04(0.91–1.20) | 0.48 |
| APACHE 48 h | 1.09(1.00–1.17) | 0.02 | 0.38(0.89–1.17) | 0.72 |

Note: [a]In reference to patients without infection

isolates, had a longer average stay in ICU and hospital, however, it did not reached the statistically significant level. As a consequence of prolonged hospitalization, MDR-GNB patients may have the economic impact due to increase in financial burden.

This study had certain limitations, including small sample size and lack of data on inappropriate empiric antibiotic therapy that could possibly influence in-hospital-mortality. Also, genotypic screening for resistance genes could not be performed due to the limited resources.

## Conclusion

The present study revealed a high incidence of MDR-GNB infections in ICU. HCAI and in-hospital-mortality were significantly associated with MDR-GNB infection. Likewise, MDR-GNB patients needed prolong ICU and hospital stay, however, it was statistically insignificant. Our study highlights the alarming need of multidisciplinary efforts to address the situation and recommends the implementation of antimicrobial stewardship, continuous surveillance, strict adherence to hand hygiene and contact precautions and regular environmental cleaning to contain the development and spread of antimicrobial resistance among the local isolates.

## Abbreviations

APACHE II: Acute physiology and chronic health evaluation II; BPKIHS: B.P Koirala Institute of Health Sciences; BSI: Blood stream infection; CCI: Charlson comorbidity index; CDC: Centers for Disease Control and Prevention (CDC); CLSI: Clinical Laboratory Standard Institute; ECDC: European Centre for Disease Prevention and Control; ESBL: Extended-spectrum beta-lactamases; HCAI: Healthcare-associated infections; ICU: Intensive care unit; IRC: Institutional review committee; LOS: Length of stay; LRTI: Lower respiratory tract infection; MDRGNB: Multi-drug resistant gram-negative bacilli; MHA: Mueller Hinton agar (MHA); MHT: Modified hodge test; SSI: Surgical site infection; UTI: Urinary tract infection; XDR: Extensively drug resistant

## Acknowledgements
All staffs of the Department of Microbiology.

## Authors' contributions
Conceptualization: SS, AS[1], AS[2], RB, NRB, BK. Investigation and Methodology: SS, RB, AS[2]. Resources: SS, NRB, BK. Supervision: BK, NRB, AS[2]. Statistical analysis: AS[2]. Writing original draft: SS. Writing-review and editing: NRB, AS[1], AS[2], BK. All authors read and approved the final manuscript.

## Consent for publication
Informed consent for publication of the findings were taken from patient or from their closest relative.

## Competing interests
The authors declare that they have no competing interests.

## Author details
[1]Department of Microbiology, B. P. Koirala Institute of Health Sciences, Dharan 56700, Nepal. [2]Department of Anaesthesiology and Critical care, B. P. Koirala Institute of Health Sciences, Dharan, Nepal.

## References
1. Vincent JL, Sakr Y, Sprung CL, et al. Sepsis in European intensive care units: results of the SOAP study. Crit Care Med. 2006;34:344–53 PMID: 16424713.
2. Vincent JL, Rello J, Marshall J, et al. International study of the prevalence and outcomes of infection in intensive care units. JAMA. 2009;302:2323–9. https://doi.org/10.1001/jama.2009.1754.
3. Cohen J. Confronting the threat of multidrug-resistant gram-negative bacteria in critically ill patients. J Antimicrob Chemother. 2013;68:490–1. https://doi.org/10.1093/jac/dks460.
4. Chaudhry D, Prajapat B. Intensive care unit bugs in India: How do they differ from the Western world? J Assoc Chest Physicians. 2017;5:10–7. https://doi.org/10.4103/2320-8775.196645.
5. Mendes RE, Mendoza M, Banga Singh KK, et al. Regional resistance surveillance program results for 12 Asia Pacific nations (2011). Antimicrob Agents Chemother. 2013; 5 7(11):5721–5726. doi: https://doi.org/10.1128/AAC.01121-13.
6. Parajuli NP, Acharya SP, Mishra SK, et al. High burden of antimicrobial resistance among gram-negative bacteria causing healthcare associated infections in a critical care unit of Nepal. Antimicrob Resist Infect Control. 2017;6:67. https://doi.org/10.1186/s13756-017-0222-z.
7. Khanal S, Joshi DR, Bhatta DR, et al. -lactamase-producing multidrug-resistant bacterial pathogens from tracheal aspirates of intensive care unit patients at National Institute of neurological and allied sciences. Nepal ISRN Microbiology. 2013; https://doi.org/10.1155/2013/847569.
8. Boucher HW, Talbot GH, Bradley JS, et al. Bad bugs, no drugs: no ESKAPE! An update from the Infectious Diseases Society of America. Clin Infect Dis. 2009;48:1–12.
9. Falagas ME, Bliziotis IA, Kasiakou SK, et al. Outcome of infections due to pan-drug resistant (PDR) gram-negative bacteria. BMC Infect Dis. 2005;5:24. https://doi.org/10.1186/1471-2334-5-24.
10. Cosgrove SE. The relationship between antimicrobial resistance and patient outcomes: mortality, length of hospital stay, and health care costs. Clin Infect Dis. 2006;42:82–9. https://doi.org/10.1086/499406.
11. Ben-David D, Kordevani R, Keller N, et al. Outcome of carbapenem resistant

Klebsiella pneumoniae bloodstream infections. Clin Microbiol Infect. 2012; 18(1):54–60. https://doi.org/10.1111/j.1469-0691.2011.03478.x.

12. Blot S, Vandewoude K, De Bacquer D, et al. Nosocomial bacteremia caused by antibiotic-resistant gram-negative bacteria in critically ill patients: clinical outcome and length of hospitalization. Clin Infect Dis. 2002;34(12):1600–6. https://doi.org/10.1086/340616.

13. Menashe G, Borer A, Yagupsky P, et al. Clinical significance and impact on mortality of ESBL-producing gram-negative isolates in nosocomial bacteremia. Scand J Infect Dis. 2001;33(3):188–93 PMID: 11303808.

14. Washington CW Jr, Stephen DA, William MJ, et al. Koneman's color atlas and text book of diagnostic microbiology. 6th ed. Philadelphia: Lippincott Williams and Wilkins; 2006.

15. Clinical and Laboratory Standards Institute. Performance standards for antimicrobial susceptibility testing; 27th ed. CLSI supplement. *CLSI Document M100-S27*. Wayne, PA: Clinical and Laboratory Standards Institute; 2017.

16. Yong D, Lee K, Yum JH, et al. Imipenem-EDTA disk method for differentiation of metallo-beta-lactamase-producing clinical isolates of pseudomonas spp. and Acinetobacter spp. J Clin Microbiol. 2002;40(10): 3798–801 PMID: 12354884.

17. Magiorakos AP, Srinivasan A, Carey RB, et al. Multidrug-resistant, extensively drugresistant and pandrug-resistant bacteria: an international expert proposal for interim standard definitions for acquired resistance. Clin Microbiol Infect. 2012;18(3):268–81. https://doi.org/10.1111/j.1469-0691.2011.03570.x.

18. Knaus WA, Draper EA, Wagner DP, et al. APACHE II: a severity of disease classification system. Crit Care Med. 1985;13:818–29 https://doi.org/10.1097/00003246-198510000-00009.

19. Charlson ME, Pompei P, Ales KL, et al. A new method of classifying prognostic comorbidity in longitudinal studies: development and validation. J Chronic Dis. 1987;40:373–83 PMID: 3558716.

20. Sader HS, Farrell DJ, Flamm RK, Jones RN. Antimicrobial susceptibility of gram-negative organisms isolated from patients hospitalized in intensive care units in United States and European hospitals (2009-2011). Diagn Microbiol Infect Dis. 2014;78(4):443–8.

21. Bhandari P, Thapa G, Pokhrel BM, et al. Nosocomial Isolates and Their Drug Resistant Pattern in ICU Patients at National Institute of Neurological and Allied Sciences, Nepal. Int J Microbiol. 2015;2015:572163 https://doi.org/10.1155/2015/572163.

22. Subhedar V, Jain SK. Gram negative super bugs: a new generation of ICU infections, an emerging challenge for health care settings. Am J Microbiol Res. 2016;4:47–50.

23. Gupta R, Malik A, Rizvi M, et al. Epidemiology of multidrug-resistant gram-negative pathogens isolated from ventilator-associated pneumonia in ICU patients. J Glob Antimicrob Resist. 2017;9:47–50. https://doi.org/10.1016/j.jgar.2016.12.016.

24. Teerawattanapong N, Panich P, Kulpokin D, et al. A systematic review of the burden of multidrug-resistant healthcare-associated infections among intensive care unit patients in Southeast Asia: the rise of multidrug-resistant Acinetobacter baumannii. Infect Control Hosp Epidemiol. 2018;39(5):525–33. https://doi.org/10.1017/ice.2018.58.

25. Arora A, Jain C, Saxena S, Kaur R. Profile of drug resistant gram negative bacteria from ICU at a tertiary Care Center of India. Asian J Med Health. 2011;3(3):1–7. https://doi.org/10.9734/AJMAH/2017/31434.

26. Gales AC, Jones RN, Sader HS. Contemporary activity of colistin and polymyxin B against a worldwide collection of gram-negative pathogens: results from the SENTRY antimicrobial surveillance program (2006-09). J Antimicrob Chemother. 2011;66(9):2070–4.

# 21

# Factors associated with bacteraemia due to multidrug-resistant organisms among bacteraemic patients with multidrug-resistant organism carriage

Hélène Mascitti[1], Clara Duran[1], Elisabeth-Marie Nemo[1], Frédérique Bouchand[2], Ruxandra Câlin[1], Alexis Descatha[1], Jean-Louis Gaillard[3], Christine Lawrence[3], Benjamin Davido[1], François Barbier[4] and Aurélien Dinh[1*] (ID)

## Abstract

**Background:** Infections caused by multidrug-resistant organisms (MDRO) are emerging worldwide. Physicians are increasingly faced with the question of whether patients need empiric antibiotic treatment covering these pathogens. This question is especially essential among MDRO carriers. We aim to determine the occurrence of MDRO bacteraemia among bacteraemic patients colonized with MDRO, and the associated factors with MDRO bacteraemia among this population.

**Methods:** We performed a retrospective monocentric study among MDRO carriers hospitalized with bacteraemia between January 2013 and August 2016 in a French hospital. We compared characteristics of patients with MDRO and non-MDRO bacteraemia.

**Results:** Overall, 368 episodes of bacteraemia were reviewed; 98/368 (26.6%) occurred among MDRO carriers. Main colonizing bacteria were extended-spectrum beta-lactamase (ESBL)-producing *Escherichia coli* (40/98; 40.8%), ESBL-producing *Klebsiella pneumoniae* (35/98; 35.7%); methicillin-resistant *Staphylococcus aureus* (26/98; 26.5%) and multidrug-resistant *Pseudomonas aeruginosa* (PA) (12/98; 12.2%).

There was no significant difference considering population with MDRO bacteraemia vs. non-MDRO bacteraemia, except for immunosuppression [OR 2.86; $p = 0.0207$], severity of the episode [OR 3.13; $p = 0.0232$], carriage of PA [OR 5.24; $p = 0.0395$], and hospital-acquired infection [OR 2.49; $p = 0.034$].

In the multivariate analysis, factors significantly associated with MDRO bacteraemia among colonized patient were only immunosuppression [OR = 2.96; $p = 0.0354$] and the hospital-acquired origin of bacteraemia [OR = 2.62; $p = 0.0427$].

**Conclusions:** According to our study, occurrence of bacteraemia due to MDRO among MDRO carriers was high. Factors associated with MDRO bacteraemia were severity of the episode and hospital-acquired origin of the bacteraemia. Thus, during bacteraemia among patients colonized with MDRO, if such characteristics are present, broad-spectrum antimicrobial treatment is recommended.

**Keywords:** Multidrug-resistant organism, Antimicrobial, Bacteraemia, Carriage

* Correspondence: aurelien.dinh@aphp.fr
[1]Infectious disease unit, Raymond Poincaré University Hospital, AP-HP, Versailles Saint-Quentin University, 104 Bd R. Poincaré, 92380 Garches, France
Full list of author information is available at the end of the article

## Background

There is currently an epidemiologic dramatic increase of multidrug-resistant organisms (MDRO) [1–5].

Infections caused by MDRO have been associated with severe adverse clinical outcomes, leading to increased mortality, prolonged hospital stay, and increased costs, mostly because of delayed effective therapy [6–9]. This dramatic spread takes place in both the community and hospital setting.

However, colonization and infection due to MDRO should be differentiated.

At this time, colonization with MDRO among patients is more frequent than infection.

But colonization with MDRO is a risk factor for infections due to MDRO, especially in transplanted patients and in intensive care unit [10–12].

If sepsis or sepsis-mimicking events occur among MDRO carriers, effective probabilistic broad-spectrum antibiotics are often prescribed in common practice [13]. Consequently, broad-spectrum antimicrobial treatments are increasingly used as empiric therapy among colonized patients. It could lead to unnecessary antibiotic exposure and selective pressure, creating more bacterial resistance.

This vicious circle is worryingly contributing to a rapid international dissemination of MDRO [14–16].

Physicians should therefore consider a prudent use of broad-spectrum antibiotics to limit new emergence of MDRO.

This requires updated studies to identify current risk factors for MDRO infection among MDRO carriers.

The primary objective of our study was to determine the occurrence of MDRO bacteraemia among bacteraemic patients colonized with MDRO, and which associated factors are predictive of bacteraemia due to MDRO among this population.

## Methods

### Settings and design

We performed a retrospective monocentric study among MDRO carriers (from any site: urine, respiratory, digestive, cutaneous), hospitalized with bacteraemia between January 2013 and August 2016 in our teaching hospital, according to STROBE statement [17]. We compared characteristics of patients with MDRO and non-MDRO bacteraemia.

Our university hospital is a disability referral centre for neurological impairment, including spinal cord injured patients. These patients are subject to high antimicrobial exposure because they might have a high rate of infections, especially urinary tract infections; they are also at increased risk of infection with multidrug-resistant bacteria [18–20]. The hospital has 255 acute-care facility beds (including 28 beds of intensive care unit) and 108 for rehabilitation, with around 8400 admissions annually.

Average hospital stays are 6.9 days for acute care and 36.5 days for rehabilitation.

An active surveillance policy for MDRO carriage among high-risk patients is implemented: nasal swab for methicillin-resistant Staphylococcus aureus (MRSA), and rectal swab for Gram negative resistant bacteria and vancomycin-resistant enterococci.

Systematic screening is performed at hospital admission for all patients coming from acute or long-term care facilities, and for community patients previously known as carriers.

Moreover, weekly screening is performed in our intensive care and surgery departments.

All hospitalized patients with positive blood cultures for bacteria were identified from the microbiology laboratory database, and microbiological data was obtained and reviewed. Patients with MDRO carriage (at least one site) during the last 3 months until day of sepsis were included.

Medical charts were reviewed using a standardized data set to collect: demographic characteristics (age, sex, comorbidities, risk factors, etc); clinical, biological, and microbiological data (clinical and severity signs, laboratory tests, organisms identified), and outcomes of each episode.

Blood cultures were performed using aerobic and anaerobic blood culture vials incubated in a Bactec FX instrument (Bactec Ped+ and Lytic/10 Anaerobic/F, BD Diagnostics, Le Pont de Claix, France). The positive blood culture vials were subcultured on blood and chocolate Polyvitex agar plates. All isolates were then identified using MALDI-TOF mass spectrometry (Maldi Biotyper 3.0, Bruker Daltonique, Marnes la Vallée, France).

Antimicrobial susceptibility testing was carried out using the agar disk diffusion method (Bio-Rad) or an automated broth microdilution method (Phoenix, BD Diagnostics, Oxford, UK). The breakpoints used were those defined by the French Committee for Antimicrobial Susceptibility Testing (http://www.sfm-microbiologie.org/UserFiles/files/casfm/CASFM%20V1_0%20FEV_2018.pdf).

### Definitions

**Bacteraemia** was defined as the association of at least one positive blood culture and a prescription of a systemic antibiotic treatment to treat bacteraemia. For common skin contaminants, such as coagulase-negative staphylococci or Corynebacterium sp., at least two different sets of blood cultures were required.

**Polymicrobial bacteraemia** was defined as having more than one organism found in the same bacteraemic episode.

**MDRO status** was determined for the Enterobacteriaceae group, Acinetobacter sp., Pseudomonas aeruginosa, and Enterococcus sp. as acquired non-susceptibility to at least one agent in three or more antimicrobial categories; for *Staphylococcus aureus* as resistance to methicillin [21].

**High zone of prevalence of MDRO** were southern Europe (Spain, Italy, Greece), North Africa and Asia according to European Centre for Disease Prevention and Control (ECDC) data (https://www.ecdc.europa.eu/en/home).

**Hospital-acquired infection** was determined as clinical signs of infection or infection arise at least 48 h after hospital admission.

**Prior colonization** was defined as isolation of MDRO from any site without any clinical signs of inflammation or sepsis, and antibiotic therapies targeting these MDRO, within a designated period of 3 months before the day of bacteraemia.

**Prior antibiotic use** was defined as the use of at least 1 dose of any antimicrobial treatment in a designated period of 3 months until the day before sepsis.

**Immunosuppression** included the following: diabetes mellitus, ongoing neoplasia, hemopathy, HIV, hypogamma globulinemia, immunosuppressive therapy (ie. corticotherapy > 20 mg/d, chemotherapy or immunosuppressive treatment such as cyclophosphamide, azathioprine and cyclosporine).

**Primary site of infection** were clinically suspected (by the physician in charge or reported on the medical chart) or bacteriologically documented with the same bacterial identification as that in the blood culture. Primary sites were categorized as urinary tract infection, catheter line-associated bacteraemia, osteoarticular infection, pulmonary tract infection, skin and soft tissue infection, intra-abdominal infection, and unknown when no primary site had been identified.

**Severity** was defined as the requirement of at least one of the following criteria: volume expansion, assisted (mechanical) ventilation, vasopressor requirement, and intensive care unit (ICU) admission during the episode.

**Cure** was defined as the absence of clinical and biological signs of infection at 1 month after end of antimicrobial treatment or at hospital discharge without any additional antimicrobial treatment.

**Mortality** was defined as dead status before 30 days after the end of antimicrobial treatment.

### Statistical analysis

All continuous variables are presented as mean and standard deviation, and the categorical variables are presented as frequencies. Correlations between risk factors and MDRO bacteraemia among patients colonized with MDRO were determined by Student's t-test for continuous variables and the Pearson's $\chi 2$ test for categorical variables.

Univariate analysis and multivariate analysis were performed. Variable for multivariate analysis were all associated risks that had a $p$-value $\leq 0.05$ and sex in the univariate analysis.

The relative risks of MDROs bacteraemia were estimated by calculating the adjusted odds ratios (OR) and corresponding 95% confidence intervals (CI).

All reported probability values ($P$-values) were based on two-sided tests, and a $P$-value of 0.05 was considered statistically significant. All analyses were performed using the Statistical Package for Social Science (SPSS) version 17.0 (SPSS, Chicago, IL, USA).

### Results

During the study period, a mean of $198 \pm 54$ screening per month was performed, and mean positive results for MDRO per patient was $23 \pm 5\%$, with 45% of extended-spectrum beta-lactamase (ESBL)-producers isolates.

In total, 368 episodes of bacteraemia were reviewed; 98 (26.6%) occurred among 77 MDRO carriers (Fig. 1). Eight bacteraemia episodes were plurimicrobial.

Considering the 98 episodes of bacteraemia among MDRO carriers, mean age was 55.8 years old, and sex ratio was 1.65. Prior antimicrobial treatment in the last 3 months occurred in 66 (67.3%) cases, 42 (42.9%) patients had an indwelling catheter, 33 (33.7%) were immunosuppressed, and 55 (56.1%) were considered as severe.

Main primary site of infections were urinary tract infections (25; 25.5%) and catheter-line associated infections (25; 25.5%); 12 (12.2%) patients presented primary bacteraemia.

Bacteraemia were hospital-acquired in 62 (63.3%) cases.

The rate of bacteraemia due to MDRO was 53.1% ($n = 52$) (Table 1). Among them, 41 (78.8%) episodes were due to multidrug-resistant *Enterobacteriaceae*, of which 22 (42.3%) were due to ESBL *Enterobacteriaceae*.

Overall, main colonizing bacteria were ESBL-producing *Escherichia coli* (EC) ($n = 40$; 40.8%), ESBL-producing *Klebsiella pneumoniae* (KP) ($n = 35$; 35.7%); MRSA ($n = 26$; 26.5%), and *Pseudomonas aeruginosa* (PA) ($n = 12$; 12.2%). Twenty-five patients (for 32 episodes) were carriers of several MDRO. Sites of carriage and microorganisms identified are presented in Table 2.

Among carriers with bacteraemia due to MDRO, a discordant identification between carriage and bacteraemia was found in 23 (44.2%) episodes (Table 3).

On the contrary, 29 (55.8%) episodes had a concordant identification, which were due to ESBL KP ($n = 10$), ESBL EC ($n = 7$), MRSA ($n = 4$), VIM-type carbapenemase-producing PA (n = 3), ESBL *Enterobacter cloacae* ($n = 2$), ceftaroline-resistant PA ($n = 1$), carbapenemase-producing *E. cloacae* ($n = 1$), and ceftaroline-resistant *Acinetobacter baumanii* ($n = 1$). Sites of carriage were rectal ($n = 18$), urinary ($n = 14$), respiratory ($n = 11$) and cutaneous ($n = 7$).

The global cure rate was 83/98 (84.6%).

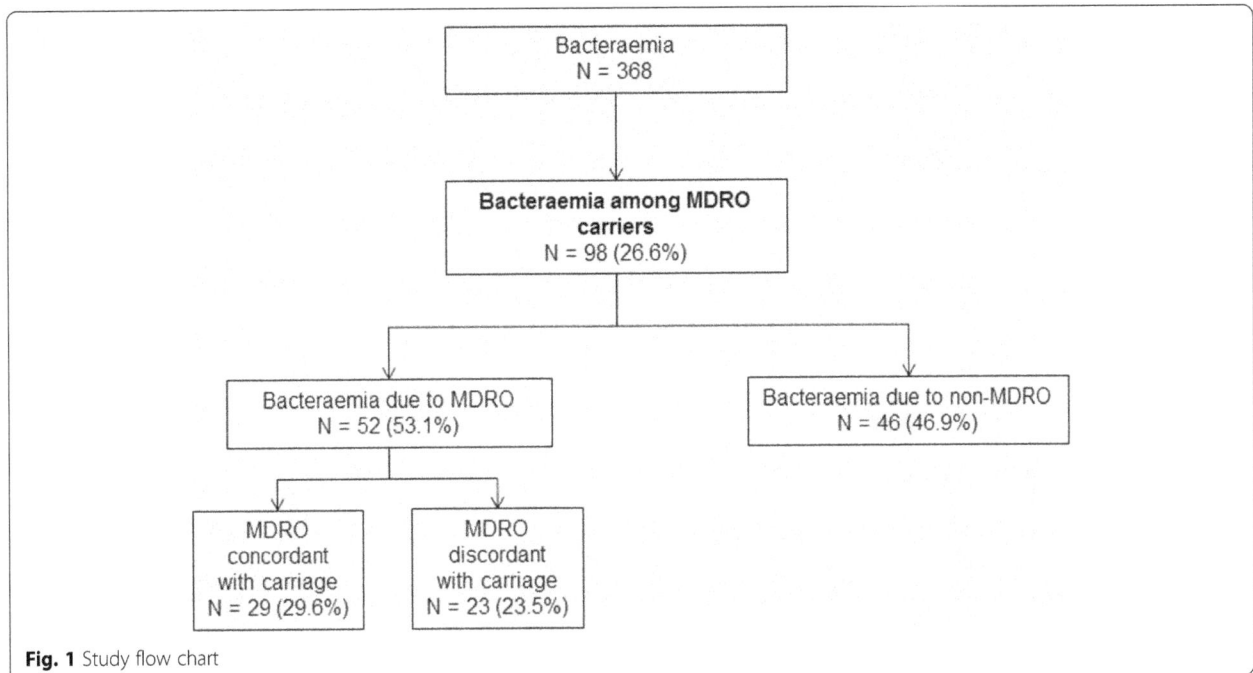

**Fig. 1** Study flow chart

**In univariate** analysis, there was no significant difference considering population with MDRO bacteraemia vs. non-MDRO bacteraemia, except for immunosuppression [OR 2.86; $p = 0.0207$], severity of the episode [OR 3.13; $p = 0.0232$], carriage of *Pseudomonas aeruginosa* [OR 5.24; $p = 0.0395$], and hospital-acquired infection [OR 2.49; $p = 0.034$] (Table 4).

**In the multivariate analysis** (Table 4), factors significantly associated with MDRO bacteraemia among colonized patient were only immunosuppression [OR = 2.96; $p = 0.0354$], and the nosocomial origin of bacteraemia [OR = 2.62; $p = 0.0427$].

## Discussion

In our study, the rate of MDRO bacteraemia among bacteraemic patients colonized with MDRO is high (53.1%).

Main factors associated with MDRO bacteraemia in those patients are immunosuppression, severity of the episode, colonization with *Pseudomonas aeruginosa*, and nosocomial infection in univariate analysis. In multivariate analysis, the only significant factors found are severity of the episode and the nosocomial origin of the infection.

The originality of our study is to focus on bacteraemic patient colonized with MDRO. Our main question is: when should we treat with probabilistic broad-spectrum antimicrobial treatment patients with known MDRO colonization and positive blood cultures?

### Risk factor for MDRO/ESBL infections

Most studies focused on colonization and infections due to multidrug-resistant *Enterobacteriaceae*, in ICU, or among immunosuppressed patients.

For example, in a 6-year prospective study, Razazi et al. screened 6303 patients admitted in ICU [22]; 843 (13.4%) had ESBL *Enterobacteriaceae* carriage detected. Among those carriers, 111 (13%) patients developed ICU-acquired pneumonia, of whom only 48 (43%) had ESBL *Enterobacteriaceae* pneumonia (6% of carriers). Moreover, considering ventilator-acquired pneumonia in ICU patients, Bruyère et al. noted in their retrospective study that the positive predictive value of digestive ESBL *Enterobacteriaceae* colonization for ESBL *Enterobacteriaceae* pneumonia was also low (41.5%) [23].

More generally, in a prospective multicenter cohort study in ICU, Barbier et al. demonstrated that ESBL *Enterobacteriaceae* infections increased carbapenem consumption, length of stay and day 28 mortality [24]. Also, ESBL *Enterobacteriaceae* infections (16.4%) were rather infrequent in carriers.

In Holland, a study focused on the predictive value of prior colonization for third-generation cephalosporin-resistant *Enterobacteriaceae* for infection due to the same microorganism [25]. This study was performed in all medical wards of an hospital, ICU included. The authors noted that, among 9422 episodes, 1657 (17.6%) of colonized patients were bacteraemic, and 64 (3.8%) were colonized with third-generation cephalosporin-resistant *Enterobacteriaceae*.

In this study, the occurrence of MDRO bacteraemia was low, corresponding to usual epidemiological data in Holland. In our study, the rate of infection due to MDRO is higher which may be due to local epidemiology.

Finally, an Israelian cohort study, with 431 carriers of carbapenem-resistant *Klebsiella pneumonia* (CRKP)

**Table 1** Main characteristics of multidrug-resistant organism carriers with bacteraemia

| Variable | Non MDR bacteraemia (n = 46) | MDR bacteraemia (n = 52) | Odds Ratio | P value |
|---|---|---|---|---|
| Sex (male) | 30 (65.2%) | 31 (59.6%) | 0.70 [0.35; 1.79] | 0.5683 |
| Recent (< 3 months) trip in zone with high MDRO prevalence[a] | 6 (13.0%) | 3 (5.8%) | 0.41 [0.10; 1.74] | 0.2250 |
| Prior antimicrobial treatment in last 6 months | 28 (60.9%) | 38 (73.1%) | 1.74 [0.74; 4.09] | 0.2004 |
| Urinary indwelling catheter | 19 (41.3%) | 23 (44.2%) | 1.13 [0.51; 2.51] | 0.7704 |
| Immunosuppression | 10 (21.7%) | 23 (44.2%) | 2.86 [1.17; 6.95] | *0.0207* |
| Severity | 7 (15.2%) | 19 (36.5%) | 3.13 [1.17; 8.36] | *0.0232* |
| Primary site of infection | | | | |
| UTI | 10 (21.7%) | 15 (28.8%) | 1.46 [0.58; 3.67] | 0.4218 |
| Intra abdominal infection | 6 (13.0%) | 5 (9.6%) | 0.71 [0.20; 2.50] | 0.5929 |
| Bone and joint infection | 4 (8.7%) | 0 (0.0%) | 0.00 [0.00; I] | 0.9710 |
| Respiratory tract infection | 2 (4.3%) | 6 (11.5%) | 2.87 [0.55; 14.98] | 0.2113 |
| Skin soft tissue infection | 7 (15.2%) | 4 (7.7%) | 0.46 [0.13; 1.70] | 0.2471 |
| Catheter line associated infcetion | 10 (21.7%) | 15 (28.8%) | 1.46 [0.58; 3.67] | 0.4218 |
| No primary site of infection | 5 (10.9%) | 7 (13.5%) | 1.28 [0.38; 4.33] | 0.6965 |
| Colonization MDR pathogen | | | | |
| Polymicrobial | 15 (32.6%) | 17 (32.7%) | | |
| CRE | 1 (2.2%) | 2 (3.8%) | | |
| ESBL *Escherichia coli* | 23 (50.0%) | 17 (32.7%) | 0.49 [0.22; 1.09] | 0.0814 |
| *Klebsiella* spp. | 18 (39.1%) | 25 (48.1%) | 1.44 [0.64; 3.22] | 0.3738 |
| ESBL *Klebsiella* spp. | 17 (37.0%) | 23 (44.2%) | | |
| Carba-R *Klebsiella* spp. | 1 (2.2%) | 1 (1.9%) | | |
| CASE *Klebsiella* spp. | 0 (0.0%) | 1 (1.9%) | | |
| *Citrobacter* spp. | 1 (2.2%) | 2 (3.8%) | 1.80 [0.16; 20.53] | 0.6360 |
| ESBL *Citrobacter* spp. | 1 (2.2%) | 2 (3.8%) | | |
| *Enterobacter* spp. | 5 (10.9%) | 8 (15.4%) | 1.63 [0.45; 5.98] | 0.4590 |
| ESBL *Enterobacter* spp. | 5 (10.9%) | 7 (13.5%) | | |
| Carba-R *Enterobacter* spp. | 0 (0.0%) | 1 (1.9%) | | |
| *Acinetobacter baumanii* | 2 (4.3%) | 3 (5.8%) | 0.43 [0.04; 4.92] | 0.4984 |
| ESBL *A. baumanii* | 1 (2.2%) | 1 (1.9%) | | |
| Carba-R *A. baumanii* | 1 (2.2%) | 1 (1.9%) | | |
| Cefta-R *A. baumanii* | 0 (0.0%) | 1 (1.9%) | | |
| *Pseudomonas aeruginosa* | 2 (4.3%) | 10 (19.2%) | 5.24 [1.08; 25.32] | *0.0395* |
| ESBL *P. aeruginosa* | 0 (0.0%) | 1 (1.9%) | | |
| Carba-R *P. aeruginosa* | 0 (0.0%) | 3 (5.8%) | | |
| Cefta-R *P. aeruginosa* | 2 (4.3%) | 6 (11.5%) | | |
| MRSA | 11 (23.9%) | 15 (28.8%) | 1.29 [0.52; 3.19] | 0.5814 |
| VRE | 1 (2.2%) | 0 (0.0%) | 0.88 [0.05; 14.51] | 0.9300 |
| Type of infections | | | | |
| Nosocomial | 24 (52.2%) | 38 (73.1%) | 2.49 [1.07; 5.78] | *0.0340* |
| Cure rate | 39 (84.8%) | 44 (84.6%) | 0.99 [0.33; 2.97] | 0.9817 |

[a]Geographic area with high incidence of extended-spectrum beta-lactamase-producing bacteria, CRE and VRE: Southern Europe (Spain, Italy, Greece), North Africa and Asia

*Carba-R* Carbapenem-resistant; *CASE* Cephalosporinase-producing; *Cefta-R* Ceftaroline-resistant; *CRE* Carbapenem-resistant Enterobacteriaceae; *ESBL* Extended-spectrum beta-lactamase; *MDR* Multidrug-resistant; *MRSA* Methicillin-resistant Staphylococcus aureus; *VRE* Vancomycin-resistant Enterococci italicised valued are statistically significant

**Table 2** Multidrug-resistant organism carriage according to site

|  | Urinary | Rectal | Respiratory | Cutaneous / Wound |
|---|---|---|---|---|
| ESBL *Enterobacteriaceae* | 30 | 59 | 2 | 13 |
| CRE (NDM + OXA types) | 1 | 2 | 0 | 0 |
| CASE *Enterobacteriaceae* | 0 | 1 | 0 | 0 |
| ESBL *Pseudomonas aeruginosa* | 1 | 0 | 0 | 3 |
| Carba-R *P. aeruginosa* | 0 | 2 | 0 | 2 |
| Cefta-R *P. aeruginosa* | 0 | 2 | 3 | 0 |
| ESBL *Acinetobacter baumanii* | 0 | 1 | 0 | 0 |
| OXA-23 *A. baumanii* | 0 | 2 | 0 | 0 |
| Cefta-R *A. baumanii* | 0 | 1 | 0 | 0 |
| MRSA | 3 | 0 | 19 | 4 |
| VRE | 0 | 1 | 0 | 0 |

*ESBL* Extended-spectrum beta-lactamase; *CRE* Carbapenem-resistant *Enterobacteriaceae*; *CASE* Cephalosporinase; *Carba-R* Carbapenem-resistant;
*Cefta-R* Ceftaroline-resistant; *MRSA* Methicillin-resistant *Staphylococcus aureus*; *VRE* Vancomycin-resistant Enterococci

**Table 3** Discordant identification between carriage and blood culture

| Carriage MDRO | Blood culture MDRO |
|---|---|
| ESBL *Escherichia coli* | MDR non-ESBL *E. coli* |
| ESBL *E. coli* | ESBL *K. pneumoniae* |
| ESBL *E. coli* | ESBL *K. pneumoniae* |
| CASE *Klebsiella pneumoniae* | MDR *K. pneumoniae* |
| ESBL *K. pneumoniae* | MDR non-ESBL *E. coli* |
| ESBL *K. pneumoniae* | MDR *K. pneumoniae* |
| ESBL *K. pneumoniae* | MDR *Proteus mirabilis* |
| ESBL *K. pneumoniae* | MDR *Serratia marcescens* |
| ESBL *K. pneumoniae* | Cefta-R *P. aeruginosa* |
| Cefta-R *Pseudomonas aeruginosa* | MDR non-ESBL *E. coli* |
| Cefta-R *P. aeruginosa* | MDR *Enterobacter cloacae* |
| ESBL *E. cloacae* | MDR *P. mirabilis* |
| ESBL *Acinetobacter baumanii* | MDR non-ESBL *E. coli* |
| Cefta-R *A. baumanii* | MDR *P. aeruginosa* |
| ESBL *Morganella morganii* | MDR Providencia stuartii |
| MRSA | MDR non-ESBL *E. coli* |
| MRSA | MDR non-ESBL *E. coli* |
| MRSA | ESBL *K. pneumoniae* |
| MRSA | MDR *Enterococcus faecium* |
| ESBL *E. coli*ESBL *K. pneumoniae*MRSA | MDR non-ESBL *E. coli* |
| ESBL *E. coli*ESBL *K. oxytoca* ESBL *Citrobacter* sp.ESBL *M. morganii* MRSA | MDR *P. mirabilis* |
| ESBL *E. coli*ESBL *K. pneumoniae* | MDR non-ESBL *E. coli* |
| ESBL *E. coli*MRSA | MDR non-ESBL *E. coli* |

*CASE* Cephalosporinase-producing; *Cefta-R* Ceftaroline-resistant; *ESBL* Extended-spectrum beta-lactamase; *MDRO* Multidrug-resistant organism;
*MRSA* Methicillin-resistant *Staphylococcus aureus*

**Table 4** Multivariate analysis associated with multidrug-resistant organism bacteraemia

| Variable | MDR bacteraemia | Univariate analysis | | Multivariate analysis | |
|---|---|---|---|---|---|
| | | Odds Ratio | P value | Odds Ratio | P value |
| Sex (male) | 31/61 (50.8%) | 0.70 [0.35; 1.79] | 0.5683 | 1.04 [0.40; 2.70] | 0.9403 |
| Immunosuppression | 23/33 (69.7%) | 2.86 [1.17; 6.95] | 0.0207 | 2.96 [1.08; 8.13] | 0.0354 |
| Severity | 19/26 (73.1%) | 3.13 [1.17; 8.36] | 0.0232 | 2.32 [0.78; 6.88] | 0.1303 |
| Colonization MDR Pseudomonas aeruginosa | 10/12 (83.3%) | 5.24 [1.08; 25.32] | 0.0395 | 2.95 [0.49; 17.77] | 0.2386 |
| Hospital-acquired | 38/62 (61.3%) | 2.49 [1.07; 5.78] | 0.034 | 2.62 [1.03; 6.64] | 0.0427 |

MDR Multidrug-resistant
italicised valued are statistically significant

included, noted that the rate of bloodstream infections (BSI) was 20% and rate of BSI due to Gram negative resistant bacteria was 80% (68/85) [26]. Among them, 19 BSI were due to CRKP and 20 to ESBL *Enterobacteriaceae*. However, in this study, no prognostic factors of CRKP BSI were identified.

The authors concluded that this raises the question regarding the use of probabilistic broad-spectrum antibiotic therapy for MDRO carriers who develop severe sepsis, as in our study.

Moreover, the authors also described frequent discordance between bacteria involved in carriage and in blood cultures [26].

Carriage of MDRO is generally the marker of high antibiotic exposure of the patient, which induces selective pressure on all flora. Yet, all MDRO are not screened, and usual screening techniques are not 100% sensitive. Therefore, a MDRO not identified during screening could be responsible for sepsis. But the indication of broad-spectrum antimicrobial treatment during sepsis among patients with MDRO carriage is still under debate, as patients do have a higher risk of MDRO infection, even if due to a different microorganism.

### Risks associated with infection due to MDRO

Regarding infection due to MRSA, colonization by MRSA is a well-known risk factor [27–29], especially in critically ill neonates children [30].

Thus, risk factors for infection due to MDRO is a complex phenomenon due to various microbiological, clinical, demographic and anamnestic characteristics [22, 23, 31, 32].

Use of algorithm to limit unnecessary use of broad-spectrum antimicrobial treatment should be encouraged [31, 32], as the one suggested by M. Basseti and J. Rodriguez Baño, which includes simple and easy to collect criteria: severity of the episode, community-acquired character, previous colonization to MDRO, indwelling device, age and previous exposure to antibiotic [33].

Lastly, new rapid diagnosis tests for bacterial resistance could help to avoid unnecessary broad-spectrum antimicrobial treatment among bacteraemic population known to be colonized by MDRO [34–37].

### Bias and weakness

The bias and weakness of our study are due to its monocentric and retrospective design, and limited sample size. Some data may be missing such as previous antimicrobial prescriptions due to memory bias. All patients were not systematically screened for MDRO at every site. Still, we studied several MDRO (ESBL bacteria, carbapenem-resistant *Enterobacteriaceae* and MRSA for example) and different sites of carriage which reflect every day practice in a tertiary care hospital. Finally, another limit of this work is that we were not able to identify patients with re-hospitalization or transferred from another hospital, which could imply an underestimation of the proportion of hospital-acquired infections.

Future research is needed to better understand the link between colonization and infection due to MDRO.

### Conclusions

According to our study, occurrence of bacteraemia due to MDRO among bacteraemic MDRO carriers was high. However, concordance between carried bacteria and blood culture bacteria was not always consistent.

Factors associated with MDRO bacteraemia were severity of the episode and nosocomial origin of the bacteraemia.

Thus, during bacteraemia among patients colonized with MDRO, if characteristics above described are present, broad-spectrum antimicrobial treatment is recommended.

### Abbreviations

BSI: bloodstream infections; CRKP: carbapenem-resistant *Klebsiella pneumonia*; EC: *Escherichia coli*; ECDC: European Centre for Disease Prevention and Control; ESBL: extended-spectrum beta-lactamase; HIV: human immunodeficiency virus; ICU: intensive care unit; KP: *Klebsiella pneumoniae*; MALDI-TOF: matrix assisted laser desorption ionisation - time of flight; MDRO: multidrug-resistant organisms; MRSA: methicillin-resistant *Staphylococcus aureus*; OR: odds ratio; PA: *Pseudomonas aeruginosa*.

### Acknowledgments

The authors would like to thank Elodie Choisy from the infectious disease unit of Raymond Poincaré Hospital for her help and support.

### Authors' contributions

ADi developed the study design. JLG and CL performed all laboratory tests. HM, CD and EMN were responsible for data collection. ADe performed statistical analysis. ADi and FBa were responsible for data analysis and data interpretation. CD, FBo, FBa and ADi drafted the first version of the manuscript. All authors revised and approved the final manuscript.

### Consent for publication
Not applicable.

### Competing interests
The authors declare that they have no competing interests.

### Author details
[1]Infectious disease unit, Raymond Poincaré University Hospital, AP-HP, Versailles Saint-Quentin University, 104 Bd R. Poincaré, 92380 Garches, France. [2]Pharmacy department, Raymond Poincaré University Hospital, AP-HP, Versailles Saint-Quentin University, 104 Bd R. Poincaré, 92380 Garches, France. [3]Microbiological laboratory, Raymond Poincaré University Hospital, AP-HP, Versailles Saint-Quentin University, 104 Bd R. Poincaré, 92380 Garches, France. [4]Intensive care unit, Orléans Hospital, 14 Avenue de l'Hôpital, 45067 Orléans, France.

### References

1. WHO. Antimicrobial resistance: global report on surveillance 2014 [Internet]. 2014 [cited 2018 Aug 21]. Available from: http://apps.who.int/iris/bitstream/handle/10665/112642/9789241564748_eng.pdf;jsessionid=99C1FBE19E0C74F2E8288949002DFE34?sequence=1

2. Drieux L, Brossier F, Duquesnoy O, Aubry A, Robert J, Sougakoff W, et al. Increase in hospital-acquired bloodstream infections caused by extended spectrum β-lactamase-producing Escherichia coli in a large French teaching hospital. Eur J Clin Microbiol Infect Dis. 2009;28:491–8.

3. Saurina G, Quale JM, Manikal VM, Oydna E, Landman D. Antimicrobial resistance in Enterobacteriaceae in Brooklyn, NY: epidemiology and relation to antibiotic usage patterns. J Antimicrob Chemother. 2000;45:895–8.

4. European Centre for Disease Prevention and Control (ECDC). Antimicrobial resistance surveillance in Europe 2016. Annual report of the European Antimicrobial Resistance Surveillance Network (EARS-Net) [Internet]. 2016 [cited 2018 Mar 26]. Available from: https://ecdc.europa.eu/sites/portal/files/documents/AMR-surveillance-Europe-2016.pdf

5. Centers for Disease Control and Prevention (CDC). Vital Signs: Carbapenem-Resistant Enterobacteriaceae. Morb Mortal Wkly Rep [Internet]. 2013 [cited 2018 Apr 2];62:165–70. Available from: https://www.cdc.gov/mmwr/preview/mmwrhtml/mm6209a3.htm

6. Lee SY, Kotapati S, Kuti JL, Nightingale CH, Nicolau DP. Impact of extended-Spectrum β-lactamase–producing Escherichia coli and Klebsiella species on clinical outcomes and hospital costs: a matched cohort study. Infect Control Hosp Epidemiol. 2006;27:1226–32.

7. Lautenbach E, Patel JB, Bilker WB, Edelstein PH, Fishman NO. Extended-Spectrum -lactamase-producing Escherichia coli and Klebsiella pneumoniae: risk factors for infection and impact of resistance on outcomes. Clin Infect Dis. 2001;32:1162–71.

8. Blot S, Depuydt P, Vogelaers D, Decruyenaere J, De WJ, Hoste E, et al. Colonization status and appropriate antibiotic therapy for nosocomial bacteremia caused by antibiotic-resistant gram-negative bacteria in an intensive care unit. Infect Control Hosp Epidemiol. 2005;26:575–9.

9. de Kraker MEA, Wolkewitz M, Davey PG, Koller W, Berger J, Nagler J, et al. Burden of antimicrobial resistance in European hospitals: excess mortality and length of hospital stay associated with bloodstream infections due to Escherichia coli resistant to third-generation cephalosporins. J Antimicrob Chemother. 2011;66:398–407.

10. Bonten MJ, Weinstein RA. The role of colonization in the pathogenesis of nosocomial infections. Infect Control Hosp Epidemiol. 1996;17:193–200.

11. Detsis M, Karanika S, Mylonakis E. ICU acquisition rate, risk factors, and clinical significance of digestive tract colonization with extended-Spectrum Beta-lactamase-producing Enterobacteriaceae: a systematic review and meta-analysis. Crit Care Med. 2017;45:705–14.

12. Gómez-Zorrilla S, Camoez M, Tubau F, Cañizares R, Periche E, Dominguez MA, et al. Prospective observational study of prior rectal colonization status

as a predictor for subsequent development of Pseudomonas aeruginosa clinical infections. Antimicrob Agents Chemother. 2015;59:5213–9.

13. Barbier F, Bailly S, Schwebel C, Papazian L, Azoulay É, Kallel H, et al. Infection-related ventilator-associated complications in ICU patients colonised with extended-spectrum β-lactamase-producing Enterobacteriaceae. Intensive Care Med. 2018;44:616–26.

14. Karah N, Haldorsen B, Hermansen NO, Tveten Y, Ragnhildstveit E, Skutlaberg DH, et al. Emergence of OXA-carbapenemase- and 16S rRNA methylase-producing international clones of Acinetobacter baumannii in Norway. J Med Microbiol. 2011;60:515–21.

15. Chen S, Hu F, Xu X, Liu Y, Wu W, Zhu D, et al. High prevalence of KPC-2-type carbapenemase coupled with CTX-M-type extended-spectrum beta-lactamases in carbapenem-resistant Klebsiella pneumoniae in a teaching hospital in China. Antimicrob agents Chemother. American Society for Microbiology (ASM). 2011;55:2493–4.

16. Munoz-Price LS, Hayden MK, Lolans K, Won S, Calvert K, Lin M, et al. Successful control of an outbreak of Klebsiella pneumoniae Carbapenemase—Producing K. pneumoniae at a long-term acute care hospital. Infect Control Hosp Epidemiol. 2010;31:341–7.

17. STROBE Statement [Internet]. [cited 2018 Sep 18]. Available from: https://www.strobe-statement.org/index.php?id=strobe-home

18. Dinh A, Saliba M, Saadeh D, Bouchand F, Descatha A, Roux ALL, et al. Blood stream infections due to multidrug-resistant organisms among spinal cord-injured patients, epidemiology over 16 years and associated risks: a comparative study. Spinal Cord [Internet]. 2016 [cited 2017 Mar 11];54:720–725. Available from: http://www.nature.com/doifinder/10.1038/sc.2015.234

19. Esposito S, Leone S, Noviello S, Lanniello F, Fiore M. Antibiotic resistance in long-term care facilities. New Microbiol. 2007;30:326–31.

20. Couderc C, Jolivet S, Thiébaut ACM, Ligier C, Remy L, Alvarez A-S, et al. Fluoroquinolone use is a risk factor for methicillin-resistant Staphylococcus aureus Acquisition in Long-term Care Facilities: a nested case-case-control study. Clin Infect Dis. 2014;59:206–15.

21. Magiorakos A-P, Srinivasan A, Carey RB, Carmeli Y, Falagas ME, Giske CG, et al. Multidrug-resistant, extensively drug-resistant and pandrug-resistant bacteria: an international expert proposal for interim standard definitions for acquired resistance. Clin Microbiol Infect. 2012;18:268–81.

22. Razazi K, Mekontso Dessap A, Carteaux G, Jansen C, Decousser J-W, de Prost N, et al. Frequency, associated factors and outcome of multi-drug-resistant intensive care unit-acquired pneumonia among patients colonized with extended-spectrum β-lactamase-producing Enterobacteriaceae. Ann Intensive Care. 2017;7:61.

23. Bruyère R, Vigneron C, Bador J, Aho S, Toitot A, Quenot J, et al. Significance of prior digestive colonization with extended-Spectrum β-lactamase–producing Enterobacteriaceae in patients with ventilator-associated pneumonia. Crit care med. Crit Care Med. 2016;44:699–706.

24. Barbier F, Pommier C, Essaied W, Garrouste-Orgeas M, Schwebel C, Ruckly S, et al. Colonization and infection with extended-spectrum β-lactamase-producing Enterobacteriaceae in ICU patients: what impact on outcomes and carbapenem exposure? J Antimicrob Chemother. 2016;71:1088–97.

25. Rottier WC, Bamberg YRP, Dorigo-Zetsma JW, van der Linden PD, Ammerlaan HSM, Bonten MJM. Predictive value of prior colonization and antibiotic use for third-generation cephalosporin-resistant Enterobacteriaceae bacteremia in patients with sepsis. Clin Infect Dis. 2015;60:1622–30.

26. Amit S, Mishali H, Kotlovsky T, Schwaber MJ, Carmeli Y. Bloodstream infections among carriers of carbapenem-resistant Klebsiella pneumoniae: etiology, incidence and predictors. Clin Microbiol Infect. 2015;21:30–4.

27. Simor AE, Loeb M, CIDS/CAMM guidelines committee. The management of infection and colonization due to methicillin-resistant Staphylococcus aureus: A CIDS/CAMM position paper. Can J Infect Dis. 2004;15:39–48.

28. Stenehjem E, Rimland D. MRSA nasal colonization burden and risk of MRSA infection. Am J Infect Control. 2013;41:405–10.

29. Garrouste-Orgeas M, Timsit J-F, Kallel H, Ben AA, Dumay MF, Paoli B, et al. Colonization with methicillin-resistant Staphylococcus aureus in ICU patients morbidity, mortality, and Glycopeptide use. Infect Control Hosp Epidemiol. 2001;22:687–92.

30. Milstone AM, Goldner BW, Ross T, Shepard JW, Carroll KC, Perl TM. Methicillin-resistant Staphylococcus aureus colonization and risk of subsequent infection in critically ill children: importance of preventing nosocomial methicillin-resistant Staphylococcus aureus transmission. Clin

Infect Dis. 2011;53:853–9.

31. Tumbarello M, Trecarichi EM, Bassetti M, De Rosa FG, Spanu T, Di Meco E, et al. Identifying patients harboring extended-Spectrum-β-lactamase-producing Enterobacteriaceae on hospital admission: derivation and validation of a scoring system. Antimicrob Agents Chemother. 2011;55:3485–90.

32. Goodman KE, Lessler J, Cosgrove SE, Harris AD, Lautenbach E, Han JH, et al. A clinical decision tree to predict whether a Bacteremic patient is infected with an extended-Spectrum β-lactamase–producing organism. Clin Infect Dis. 2016;63:896–903.

33. Bassetti M, Baño JR. Should we take into account ESBLs in empirical antibiotic treatment? Intensive Care Med. 2016;42:2059–2062.

34. Renvoisé A, Decré D, Amarsy-Guerle R, Huang T-D, Jost C, Podglajen I, et al. Evaluation of the βLacta test, a rapid test detecting resistance to third-generation cephalosporins in clinical strains of Enterobacteriaceae. J Clin Microbiol. American Society for Microbiology (ASM). 2013;51:4012–7.

35. Gallah S, Decré D, Genel N, Arlet G. The β-Lacta test for direct detection of extended-spectrum-β-lactamase-producing Enterobacteriaceae in urine. J Clin Microbiol American Society for Microbiology (ASM). 2014;52:3792–4.

36. Delport JA, Strikwerda A, Armstrong A, Schaus D, John M. MALDI-ToF short incubation identification from blood cultures is associated with reduced length of hospitalization and a decrease in bacteremia associated mortality. Eur J Clin Microbiol Infect Dis. 2017;36:1181–6.

37. Beganovic M, Costello M, Wieczorkiewicz SM. Effect of Matrix-Assisted Laser Desorption Ionization-Time of Flight Mass Spectrometry (MALDI-TOF MS) Alone versus MALDI-TOF MS Combined with Real-Time Antimicrobial Stewardship Interventions on Time to Optimal Antimicrobial Therapy in Patients with Positive Blood Cultures. Munson E, editor. J Clin Microbiol. 2017;55:1437–45.

# 22

# Extended-spectrum β-lactamase prevalence and virulence factor characterization of enterotoxigenic *Escherichia coli* responsible for acute diarrhea in Nepal from 2001 to 2016

Katie R. Margulieux[1]* (ID), Apichai Srijan[1], Sirigade Ruekit[1], Panida Nobthai[1], Kamonporn Poramathikul[1], Prativa Pandey[2], Oralak Serichantalergs[1], Sanjaya K. Shrestha[3], Ladaporn Bodhidatta[1] and Brett E. Swierczewski[1,4]

## Abstract

**Background:** Multidrug-resistant (MDR) Gram-negative bacterial species are an increasingly dangerous public health threat, and are now endemic in many areas of South Asia. However, there are a lack of comprehensive data from many countries in this region determining historic and current MDR prevalence. Enterotoxigenic *Escherichia coli* (ETEC) is a leading cause of both acute infant diarrhea and traveler's diarrhea in Nepal. The MDR prevalence and associated resistance mechanisms of ETEC isolates responsible for enteric infections in Nepal are largely unknown.

**Methods:** A total of 265 ETEC isolates were obtained from acute diarrheal samples (263/265) or patient control samples (2/265) at traveler's clinics or regional hospitals in Nepal from 2001 to 2016. Isolates were screened for antibiotic resistance, to include extended spectrum beta-lactamase (ESBL) production, via the Microscan Automated Microbiology System. ETEC virulence factors, specifically enterotoxins and colonization factors (CFs), were detected using multiplex PCR, and prevalence in the total isolate population was compared to ESBL-positive isolates. ESBL-positive isolates were assessed using multiplex PCR for genetic markers potentially responsible for observed resistance.

**Results:** A total of 118/265 (44.5%) ETEC isolates demonstrated resistance to ≥2 antibiotics. ESBL-positive phenotypes were detected in 40/265 isolates, with isolates from 2008, 2013, 2014, and 2016 demonstrating ESBL prevalence rates of 1.5, 34.5, 31.2, and 35.0% respectively. No difference was observed in overall enterotoxin characterization between the total ETEC and ESBL-positive populations. The CFs CS2 (13.6%), CS3 (25.3%), CS6 (30.2%), and CS21 (62.6%) were the most prevalent in the total ETEC population. The ESBL-positive ETEC isolates exhibited a higher association trend with the CFs CS2 (37.5%), CS3 (35%), CS6 (42.5%), and CS21 (67.5%). The primary ESBL gene identified was $bla_{CTX-M-15}$ (80%), followed by $bla_{SHV-12}$ (20%) and $bla_{CTX-M-14}$ (2.5%). The beta-lactamase genes $bla_{TEM-1}$ (40%) and $bla_{CMY-2}$ (2.5%) were also identified. It was determined that 42.5% of the ESBL-positive isolates carried multiple resistance genes.

**Conclusion:** Over 30% of ETEC isolates collected post-2013 and evaluated in this study demonstrated ESBL resistance. Persistent surveillance and characterization of enteric ETEC isolates are vital for tracking the community presence of MDR bacterial species in order to recommend effective treatment strategies and help mitigate the spread of resistant pathogens.

**Keywords:** ETEC, ESBL, Nepal

* Correspondence: katie.margulieux.ctr@afrims.org
[1]Department of Enteric Diseases, Armed Forces Research Institute of Medical Sciences, 315/6 Rajvithee Road, Bangkok 10400, Thailand
Full list of author information is available at the end of the article

## Background

Multidrug-resistant (MDR) Gram-negative bacterial species are an established prominent international public health threat [1]. MDR pathogens have an especially high prevalence in South Asia where bacterial infections are common and antibiotic use is widely unregulated [2–4]. A lack of comprehensive surveillance programs may result in the unchecked spread of MDR Gram-negative bacterial species and their associated resistance mechanisms. Developing countries with an established national surveillance network, such as Nepal, do not have the resources to perform in-depth isolate characterization to comprehensively identify resistance mechanisms carried by MDR bacterial isolates [5–7]. It is imperative that both archived and current bacterial isolates from underdeveloped regions undergo extensive MDR characterization to inform national strategies designed to halt the continuing spread of these dangerous pathogens.

Diarrheagenic *Escherichia coli* is a ubiquitous presence in the developing world and is responsible for a range of enteric infections [8–10]. Enterotoxigenic *E. coli* (ETEC) is defined by production of 1–3 enterotoxins, and is one of the leading causes of both acute infant diarrhea and traveler's diarrhea worldwide, including Nepal [11–14]. ETEC attaches to and colonizes cells in the small intestine along the epithelial surface through the interaction of bacterial colonization factors (CFs) with the intestinal cell wall [15, 16]. After the establishment of intestinal colonization, the bacterial cells produce heat-labile enterotoxins (LT) and/or heat-stable enterotoxins (STh or STp) that target vital cellular processes [8, 17, 18]. The production of these enterotoxins most commonly results in abdominal cramping and watery diarrhea, with more severe cases also presenting with fever and nausea. ETEC infections are typically self-limiting with resolution of symptoms 3–7 days after initial onset and a recommended treatment strategy of rest and oral rehydration therapy [8, 19]. In spite of ongoing efforts to develop an ETEC vaccine, no viable vaccine candidates have been produced thus far [20, 21]. ETEC virulence factors, such as enterotoxins and CFs, are potential targets for vaccines or therapeutic candidates, and determination of regional prevalence rates and specific virulence factors may serve to inform the development of globally effective vaccines [15, 18–21].

Severe ETEC cases presenting with cholera-like watery diarrhea that do not resolve through oral rehydration therapy may require treatment with antibiotics [8, 10]. Initial treatment has historically been administration of first-line beta-lactams and quinolones. However, the evolution and global dissemination of multiple classes of antimicrobial resistance mechanisms has led to an increase of MDR ETEC infections that are insensitive to first-line antibiotics [11, 22]. Beta-lactamases and Extended-spectrum β-lactamases

(ESBLs) confer resistance to a number of antibiotic classes, such as penicillins, extended-spectrum cephalosporins, and monobactams [23, 24]. Global dissemination of these mechanisms has occurred through clonal expansion and/or horizontal transfer of genetic resistance mechanisms between bacterial species [24]. Bacterial pathogens carrying ESBL resistance mechanisms are commonly associated with, and detected in, hospital-acquired infections. However, these antibiotic resistance mechanisms have spread to community-acquired isolates, and are increasingly identified in acute diarrhea and other enteric infections [12, 25–30]. ETEC infections are a large cause of acute diarrhea cases in Nepal, but prevalence rates of MDR ETEC isolates, both from a historic or current perspective, are unknown.

The current study determined antibiotic resistance and virulence factors of ETEC isolates previously identified from clinical acute diarrheal samples (263/265) or patient control samples (2/265) collected in Nepal between 2001 and 2016. The ETEC isolates were assayed to determine antimicrobial resistance profiles (including ESBL production) and virulence factor characterization, specifically enterotoxins and colonization factors. Antimicrobial resistance studies that encompass retrospective and current clinical isolates are vital to understanding the regional emergence of ESBL producing organisms, the existing treatment challenges, and the potential for ongoing dissemination. This study serves as a thorough investigation of antibiotic resistance in ETEC isolates from acute diarrheal samples in Nepal, and highlights the need for interventions that may address and stem the continual spread of MDR mechanisms in community settings.

## Methods

### Bacterial strains, media, and chemicals

A total of 265 ETEC isolates were previously isolated and identified from clinical acute diarrheal samples (263/265) or patient control samples (2/265) collected from hospitals and travel clinics in Nepal from 2001 to 2016. The isolates were archived for long-term storage at – 20 °C in Luria Bertani (LB) broth + 20% glycerol at the Armed Forces Research Institute of Medical Sciences (AFRIMS) in Bangkok, Thailand. The archived ETEC isolates were grown from frozen glycerol stocks on MacConkey agar (MAC) plates overnight at 37 °C. Isolated colonies were re-streaked on tryptic soy agar (TSA) plates, blood agar plates (BAP), or colonization factor agar (CFA) plates in preparation for further phenotypic analysis or DNA isolation.

### Antimicrobial susceptibility testing

All ETEC isolates were screened for ESBL production using the Microscan, Walkaway 40 automated system with Negative Breakpoint Combo 34 panels as per manufacturer's instructions (Beckman Coulter, West Sacramento, CA, USA).

ESBL-positive isolates were identified by automatic suscepti-bility testing panel results by assessing bacterial susceptibility to cefotaxime and ceftazidime with or without clavulanic acid. ESBL-positive ETEC isolates were confirmed through disk diffusion assay against beta-lactam combination agents using both cefotaxime (30 μg) and ceftazidime (30 μg) with or without clavulanic acid (10 μg) following Clinical and La-boratory Standards Institute guidelines [31]. A $\geq 5$ mm in-crease in zone diameter for either antimicrobial agent tested in combination with clavulanate and the zone diameter of the agent when tested along indicated ESBL production.

### Multiplex PCR for ETEC virulence factors

The previously identified and archived ETEC isolates were re-tested to confirm the presence of ETEC entero-toxin genes (*lt*, *sth*, and *stp*) using multiplex PCR as pre-viously described in detail [32]. ETEC colonization factors (CFA/1, CS1, CS2, CS3, CS4, CS5, CS6, CS7, CS8, CS12, CS13, CS14, CS15, CS17, CS18, CS19, CS20, CS21, and CS22) were identified using multiplex PCR as previously described in detail [32].

### Multiplex PCR for ESBL gene identification and DNA sequencing

ETEC isolates that tested positive for ESBL production were further characterized to determine potential genetic elements responsible for the observed antimicrobial resist-ance through multiplex PCR as described previously [33]. All PCR primers and conditions used for beta-lactamase or ESBL characterization were listed previously [33]. The genes identified from the multiplex PCR assays were se-quenced to determine variant type. Genetic sequencing services were contracted through AITbiotech (Singapore) or First BASE (Selangor, Malaysia). The PCR products were prepared and sent for sequencing according to com-pany instruction. The nucleotide sequences were analyzed with Sequencher software version 5.3 and BLAST software (http://www.Ncbi.nlm.nih.gov/BLAST).

### Statistics

Statistical analyses were performed using GraphPad QuickCalcs. Experimental groups were analyzed using a chi-square with Fisher's exact test with a two-tailed *p* value of $\leq 0.05$ considered statistically significant.

## Results

### Antibiotic resistance characterization of ETEC isolates

A total of 117/265 (44.1%) ETEC isolates demonstrated full susceptibility to all antibiotics tested, with an add-itional 30/265 (11.3%) resistant to only a single antibiotic tested. The remaining 118/265 (44.5%) isolates demon-strated resistance to $\geq 2$ antibiotics tested (Table 1). Anti-biotic resistance to ampicillin was most common (113/265, 42.6%), followed by trimethoprim/sulfamethoxazole

(77/265, 29.1%), tetracycline (74/265, 27.9%), and ampi-cillin/ sulbactam (32/265, 12.1%). A lesser number of isolates were shown to be resistant to ciprofloxacin (15/265, 5.7%) and no isolates showed antibiotic resistance to ertapenem. Of the 118 isolates with increased drug-resistance, 40 demonstrated phenotypic production of ESBLs with resistance to the extended-spectrum β-la ctams cefotaxime (40/40, 100%), ceftazidime (39/40, 97.5%), and/or ceftriaxone (35/40, 87.5%) (Table 1). ESBL-production in all positive ETEC isolates was con-firmed through a disk diffusion test. A single isolate from 2008 was positive for ESBL production (1/62, 1.5%). The remaining ESBL-positive ETEC isolates were collected during 2013 (8/21), 2014 (10/32), and 2016 (21/60), resulting in yearly prevalence rates of 34.5, 31.2, and 35.0%, respectively (Table 1). Of the ESBL-positive ETEC isolates, the majority were recovered from acute diarrheal samples (39/40, 97.5%), however, 1/40 (2.5%) was recovered from a patient control sample.

### ETEC enterotoxin gene characterization and prevalence

Detection of the ETEC enterotoxin genes *lt*, *sth*, and/or *stp* was performed for all isolates. The enterotoxin gene *lt* was detected in a total of 132/265 (49.8%) isolates, *sth* was detected in a total of 152/265 (57.3%) isolates, and *stp* was detected in a total of 72/265 (27.5%) isolates. Multiple enterotoxin genes were detected in 88/265 (33.2%) isolates, and enterotoxin gene combinations prevalence are described in Table 2. The enterotoxin combination of *sth* only was significantly detected less frequently in ESBL-positive isolates compared to ESBL-negative isolates (15% vs. 30.9%; *p* = 0.0156). No other enterotoxin gene (by total percent detected or by combi-nations) demonstrated a statistically significant differ-ence in prevalence rates between the two populations.

### ETEC CF characterization and prevalence

CFs were detected in 222/265 (83.8%) of the total ETEC isolates, and multiple CFs were detected in 162/265 (61.1%) isolates. CS2 (13.6%), CS3 (25.3%), CS6 (30.2%), and CS21 (62.6%) were the most preva-lent CFs identified in the total ETEC population. The ESBL-positive ETEC isolates showed a trend of higher association with CS2 (37.5%), CS3 (35%), CS6 (42.5%), and CS21 (67.5%) compared to the total population. The ESBL-positive ETEC population had a statistically significant higher prevalence rate compared to the ESBL-negative population for CS2 (37.5.0% vs. 9.3%; *p* = 0.0002). Conversely, the ESBL-negative population had a statistically significant higher prevalence of CS1 compared to the ESBL-positive population (10.2% vs 0.0%; *p* = 0.0311). The multiple CF combinations CS6/CS21 and CS2/CS3/CS21 were the most preva-lent in both the total population and ESBL-positive

**Table 1** Total number of ETEC isolates, isolates resistant to ≥2 antibiotics, and isolates that display ESBL-positive phenotypes per year

| Year | Total # of Isolates | Isolates $R \geq 2$ Antibiotics (%) | ESBL Positive Isolates (%) |
|---|---|---|---|
| 2001 | 12 | 9 (75) | 0 |
| 2002 | 30 | 5 (16.7) | 0 |
| 2003 | 5 | 3 (60) | 0 |
| 2007 | 34 | 8 (23.5) | 0 |
| 2008 | 62 | 25 (40.3) | 1 (1.5) |
| 2009 | 8 | 4 (50) | 0 |
| 2012 | 1 | 0 | 0 |
| 2013 | 21 | 11 (52.4) | 8 (35.6) |
| 2014 | 32 | 14 (43.8) | 10 (31.2) |
| 2016 | 60 | 39 (65) | 21 (35) |
| Total | 265 | 118 (44.5) | 40 (15.1) |

population (Table 3). The CF combination CS2/CS3/CS21 was statistically significantly higher in the ESBL-positive ETEC population when compared to the ESBL-negative ETEC population (25.0% vs. 7.1%; $p$ = 0.0018). No other CFs or CF combinations were statistically significant between the two populations, despite overall higher prevalence trends demonstrated in the ESBL-positive ETEC population for many CFs and CF combinations.

### ESBL gene identification

ESBL-positive ETEC isolates were screened for carriage of known prevalent ESBL and/or beta-lactamase genes using a multiplex PCR assay [33]. The most prevalent ESBL gene detected was $bla_{CTX-M}$ group 1 with 32/40 (80%) of isolates harboring this gene. This gene was further identified as $bla_{CTX-M-15}$ through PCR sequencing analysis (Table 4). Additionally, the ESBL genes $bla_{SHV-12}$ and $bla_{CTX-M-14}$ were identified with prevalence rates of 20% (8/40) and 2.5% (1/40), respectively.

The beta-lactamase genes $bla_{TEM-1}$ (16/40, 40%) and $bla_{CMY-2}$ (1/40, 2.5%) were also shown to be carried in the ESBL-positive ETEC population. A total of 17/40 (42.5%) isolates were shown to carry multiple ESBL and/or beta-lactamase genes (Table 4). Notably, the multiplex PCR screen did not identify any ESBL or beta-lactamase genes in one phenotypically ESBL-positive ETEC isolate. The multiplex PCR assay performed in this study screens for prevalent resistance genes, but is not a comprehensive

**Table 2** Enterotoxin gene detection within total ETEC population and ESBL-positive population

| Enterotoxin(s) | Total $n$ = 265 (%) | ESBL Positive $n$ = 40 (%) |
|---|---|---|
| *lt* | 132 (49.8) | 23 (57.5) |
| *sth* | 152 (57.3) | 21 (52.5) |
| *stp* | 73 (27.5) | 13 (32.5) |
| Multiple | 88 (33.2) | 17 (42.5) |
| Combinations | | |
| *lt* only | 44 (16.6) | 6 (15) |
| *sth* only | 82 (30.9) | 6 (15) |
| *stp* only | 51 (19.2) | 11 (27.5) |
| *lt/sth* | 66 (24.9) | 15 (37.5) |
| *lt/stp* | 18 (6.8) | 2 (5) |
| *lt/sth/stp* | 4 (1.5) | 0 |

**Table 3** Colonization factor characterization within total ETEC population and ESBL-positive ETEC population

| Colonization Factor | Total $n$ = 265 (%) | ESBL Positive $n$ = 40 (%) |
|---|---|---|
| CFA/1 | 18 (6.8) | 3 (7.5) |
| CS1 | 23 (8.7) | 0 |
| CS2 | 36 (13.6) | 15 (37.5) |
| CS3 | 67 (25.3) | 14 (35) |
| CS4 | 8 (3) | 0 |
| CS6 | 80 (30.2) | 17 (42.5) |
| CS7 | 5 (1.9) | 0 |
| CS8 | 11 (4.2) | 0 |
| CS12 | 6 (2.3) | 2 (5) |
| CS13 | 1 (0.4) | 0 |
| CS14 | 5 (1.9) | 0 |
| CS17 | 10 (3.8) | 0 |
| CS20 | 5 (1.9) | 0 |
| CS21 | 166 (62.6) | 27 (67.5) |
| None Detected | 43 (16.2) | 3 (7.5) |
| Multiple CFs | 162 (61.1) | 30 (75) |
| Combinations | | |
| CS6/CS21 | 55 (20.8) | 12 (30) |
| CS2/CS3/CS21 | 26 (9.8) | 10 (25) |
| CS1/CS3/CS21 | 22 (8.3) | 0 |

**Table 4** Determination of ESBL and beta-lactamase gene type

| Year | No. of Isolates | No. of Isolates with Gene(s) Detected (%) | | | | | No Genes Detected | Multiple Genes |
|---|---|---|---|---|---|---|---|---|
| | | $bla_{CTX-M-15}$ | $bla_{CTX-M-14}$ | $bla_{SHV-12}$ | $bla_{TEM-1}$ | $bla_{CMY-2}$ | | |
| 2008 | 1 | 1 (100) | 0 | 0 | 0 | 0 | 0 | 0 |
| 2013 | 8 | 8 (100) | 0 | 1 (12.5) | 6(75) | 0 | 0 | 7 (87.5) |
| 2014 | 10 | 8 (80) | 1 (10) | 1 (10) | 4(40) | 0 | 0 | 4 (40) |
| 2016 | 21 | 15 (71.4) | 0 | 6 (28.6) | 6(28.6) | 1 (4.8) | 1 (4.8) | 6 (23.8) |
| Total | 40 | 32 (80) | 1 (2.5) | 8 (20) | 15(37.5) | 1 (2.5) | 1 (2.5) | 17 (42.5) |

investigation of ESBL genes. As such, additional analysis of this isolate may identify the presence of less prevalent or novel ESBL genes.

## Discussion

MDR Gram-negative bacterial pathogens are a global public health threat [1, 6]. ESBL-producing bacterial strains were first detected in, and were mostly limited to, hospital-associated infections, but began being detected in community-associated infections beginning in the early 2000's [25, 27, 28, 34]. Initial reports of community-associated ESBL-producing *E. coli* strains, including reports originating from Nepal, are mainly comprised of pathogens isolated from urinary tract or blood stream infections [35–39]. However, community-associated infections isolated from enteric MDR pathogens are being increasingly reported in South and Southeast Asia [8, 11, 12, 22, 26, 30].

ETEC is an enteric pathogen that results in both acute infant diarrhea and traveler's diarrhea [8, 10, 15]. ESBL-producing ETEC may result in treatment failures for infections that were previously easily treatable with first-line antibiotic administration. In the current study, only a single ESBL-positive ETEC isolate was identified from isolates archived in 2001–2009 from Nepal. However, over 30% of the ETEC isolates collected after 2013 phenotypically display ESBL production. This suggests that ESBL resistance mechanisms in Nepal have expanded relatively recently into community-associated bacterial pathogens, and represents a new threat to both the community as well as international travelers in the region. Notably, international travelers have been shown to be a potential vector for the spread of resistant bacterial pathogens through acquisition during travel, contributing to the global dissemination of MDR enteric pathogens [40]. The combination of established community prevalence and additional spread by infected travelers may contribute to local and global dissemination of ESBL-positive ETEC isolates.

ETEC virulence factors, such as enterotoxins and CFs, are of particular interest as potential targets for infection intervention as vaccine or therapeutic targets [15, 18, 21]. The expression of enterotoxins and CFs are essential for ETEC colonization of the small intestine and resulting pathogenesis. Blocking bacterial cell adhesion to the

small intestine and/or neutralizing enterotoxins results in a limited ETEC infection and significantly reduces infection morbidity [15, 18, 21]. The currently reported prevalence of the enterotoxins LT, STh, and STp in this study were comparative to previous studies reviewed and analyzed by Isidean, et al. [18]. The most prevalent CFs in the current study were CS21, CS6, CS3, and CS2, while the most prevalent CFs in previously conducted studies reviewed by Isidean et al were CFA/1, CS6, and CS21 [18]. Notably, CFA/1 was detected at a lower rate in the current study than previously reported (6.8 vs 20%), indicating CFA/1 may not be a priority target for ETEC interventions in South Asia [18]. Overall, the current study suggests vaccines and therapeutics targeting the enterotoxins LT and STh, and the CF's CS21, CS6, CS2, and CS3 would likely be most efficacious against ETEC infections in South Asia. This study demonstrated that these virulence factors are also prevalent in the ESBL-positive ETEC population, a group that is important to target for vaccine efficacy as MDR ETEC continues to emerge and spread throughout the region. It is important that ongoing studies characterizing virulence factors in MDR ETEC populations are performed to determine relevant intervention strategies against currently circulating strains.

Many ESBL genes have been reported as actively circulating in South Asia in hospital- and community-associated infections, including $bla_{CTX-M}$ group 1 and group 9, $bla_{PER}$, $bla_{VEB}$, $bla_{GES}$, and $bla_{SHV}$ [41]. Within the gene family $bla_{CTX-M}$, $bla_{CTX-M-15}$ and $bla_{CTX-M-14}$ are the most common type of ESBL found worldwide [27, 42]. Aligning with the global findings of gene prevalence, previous studies conducted in Nepal have identified $bla_{CTX-M-15}$ as prevalent in hospital-associated *E. coli* infections, while $bla_{TEM}$ and $bla_{SHV}$ were also detected at a lower frequencies [43, 44]. In the current study, $bla_{CTX-M-15}$ was detected in the majority of ESBL-positive ETEC isolates. The genes $bla_{SHV-12}$, $bla_{CTX-M-14}$, $bla_{TEM-1}$, and $bla_{CMY-2}$ were also identified at lower rates, and multiple resistance genes were detected in 40% of the characterized isolates. Importantly, ESBL resistance mechanisms are often located on mobile plasmids [42, 45, 46]. As such, enteric ETEC strains that are ESBL-positive may potentially serve as a community reservoir in Nepal for the dissemination of ESBL resistance mechanisms via clonal expansion and/or horizontal transfer to other bacterial species that do not result in enteric infections. A large percentage of ETEC isolates identified in the current study contain multiple resistance mechanisms, suggesting that horizontal transfer of ESBL genes is actively occurring within enteric bacterial pathogens. Interestingly, this study identified an ESBL-positive ETEC isolate from a patient control sample, absent of diarrheal symptoms, indicating the established presence of asymptomatic MDR pathogens in the community that may contribute to gene dissemination. Additional studies are necessary to observe the source and spread of ESBL resistance mechanisms in community-associated infections in Nepal.

Limitations of the current study include small sample sizes per year and the lack of clinical patient information. These limitations serve to highlight the need for additional long-term, comprehensive enteric pathogen surveillance to track ongoing MDR emergence and spread in community settings. ESBL-positive *E. coli* often have limited treatment options, such as carbapenem antibiotics. However, the efficacy of these treatment options are compromised by increased prevalence of carbapenemase resistance mechanisms, such as $bla_{NDM-1}$, $bla_{KPC}$, and $bla_{IMP}$. No carbapenemase-producing ETEC were identified in the current study, but continued surveillance is imperative for tracking if, or more likely when, community-associated MDR ETEC isolates acquire carbapenem-resistance mechanisms in Nepal.

## Conclusions

MDR Gram-negative bacterial species pose a dangerous threat to global public health, including community-associated MDR enteric infections that are increasingly prevalent. The current study demonstrated that ESBL resistance mechanisms have spread to community-associated pathogens in Nepal, with over 30% of ETEC isolates collected after 2013 demonstrating ESBL production. Both retrospective and recent surveillance studies of ETEC isolates identified from acute diarrheal clinical samples are vital for tracking the community presence of emerging antibiotic resistance mechanisms. Consistent, long-term surveillance may lead to better informed treatment options, alternative therapeutic development, and community-based interventions to mitigate the spread of resistant bacterial strains beyond hospital environments.

## Abbreviations
AFRIMS: Armed Forces Research Institute of Medical Sciences; CFs: Colonization factors; ESBL: Extended spectrum beta-lactamase; ETEC: Enterotoxigenic *Escherichia coli*; LT: Heat-labile enterotoxin; MDR: Multidrug resistance; ST: Heat-stabile enterotoxin

## Acknowledgements
The authors would like to thank Dr. John Crawford, members of the AFRIMS Department of Enteric Diseases, Walter Reed/AFRIMS Research Unit Nepal, Bharatpur Hospital, Kanti Children's Hospital, Sukraraj Tropical and Infectious Disease Hospital, and CIWEC Hospital and Travel Medicine Clinic for assistance, advice, and helpful discussion throughout the project and during manuscript preparation.
Material has been reviewed by the Walter Reed Army Institute of Research. There is no objection to its presentation and/or publication. The opinions or assertions contained herein are the private views of the author, and are not to be construed as official, or as reflecting true views of the Department of the Army or the Department of Defense.

## Funding
This work was funded by the Armed Forces Health Surveillance Branch – Global Emerging Infections Surveillance and Response System (AFHSB-GEIS). The funding source had no role in the design, performance, or interpretation and analysis of this study.

## Authors' contributions
KRM and KP performed the experiments presented in this work. KRM and BES wrote the manuscript. KRM, AS, SR, PN, KP, PP, OS, SS, LB, and BES designed the experiments, analyzed the resulting data, and reviewed, revised and approved the final manuscript.

## Consent for publication
Not applicable.

## Competing interests
The authors have no competing interests to declare.

## Author details
[1]Department of Enteric Diseases, Armed Forces Research Institute of Medical Sciences, 315/6 Rajvithee Road, Bangkok 10400, Thailand. [2]CIWEC Hospital and Travel Medicine Clinic, Kathmandu, Nepal. [3]Walter Reed/AFRIMS Research Unit Nepal, Kathmandu, Nepal. [4]Present Address: Bacterial Diseases Branch, Walter Reed Army Institute of Research, Silver Spring, MD, USA.

## References
1. Centers for Disease Control and Prevention. Antibiotic resistance threats in the United States, 2013. 2013. https://www.cdc.gov/drugresistance/threat-report-2013/index.html.
2. Lai CC, Lee K, Xiao Y, Ahmad N, Veeraraghavan B, Thamlikitkul V, Tambyah PA, Nelwan RHH, Shibl AM, Wu J-J, et al. High burden of antimicrobial drug resistance in Asia. J Glob Antimicrob Resist. 2014;2:141–7.
3. Hawkey PM. Prevalence and clonality of extended-spectrum β-lactamases in Asia. Clin Microbiol Infect. 2008;14:159–65.
4. Jean SS, Hsueh PR. High burden of antimicrobial resistance in Asia. Int J Antimicrob Agents. 2011;37:291–5.
5. Basnyat B, Pokharel P, Dixit S, Giri S. Antibiotic use, its resistance in Nepal and recommendations for action: a situation analysis. J Nepal Health Res Counc. 2015;13:102–11.
6. Ayukekbong JA, Ntemgwa M, Atabe AN. The threat of antimicrobial resistance in developing countries: causes and control strategies. Antimicrob Resist Infect Control. 2017;6:47.
7. Vernet G, Mary C, Altmann DM, Doumbo O, Morpeth S, Bhutta ZA, Klugman KP. Surveillance for antimicrobial drug resistance in under-resourced countries. Emerg Infect Dis. 2014;20:434–41.
8. Qadri F, Svennerholm A-M, Faruque ASG, Sack RB. Enterotoxigenic *Escherichia coli* in developing countries: epidemiology, microbiology, clinical features, treatment, and prevention. Clin Microbiol Rev. 2005;18:465–83.
9. Vila J, Saez-Lopez E, Johnson JR, Romling U, Dobrindt U, Canton R, Giske CG, Naas T, Carattoli A, Martinez-Medina M, et al. *Escherichia coli*: an old friend with new tidings. FEMS Microbiol Rev. 2016;40:437–63.
10. Croxen MA, Law RJ, Scholz R, Keeney KM, Wlodarska M, Finlay BB. Recent advances in understanding enteric pathogenic *Escherichia coli*. Clin Microbiol Rev. 2013;26:822–80.
11. Pandey P, Bodhidatta L, Lewis M, Murphy H, Shlim DR, Cave W, Rajah R, Springer M, Batchelor T, Sornsakrin S, Mason CJ. Travelers' diarrhea in Nepal: an update on the pathogens and antibiotic resistance. J Travel Med. 2011;18:102–8.

12. Murphy H, Pandey P. Pathogens for travelers' diarrhea in Nepal and resistance patterns. Curr Infect Dis Rep. 2012;14:238–45.

13. Turner SM, Scott-Tucker A, Cooper LM, Henderson IR. Weapons of mass destruction: virulence factors of the global killer enterotoxigenic *Escherichia coli*. FEMS Microbiol Lett. 2006;263:10–20.

14. Shah N, DuPont HL, Ramsey DJ. Global etiology of travelers' diarrhea: systematic review from 1973 to the present. Am J Trop Med Hyg. 2009;80:609–14.

15. Madhavan TPV, Sakellaris H. Colonization factors of enterotoxigenic *Escherichia coli*. Adv Appl Microbiol. 2015;90:155–97.

16. Fleckenstein JM, Munson GM, Rasko DA. Enterotoxigenic *Escherichia coli*: orchestrated host engagement. Gut Microbes. 2013;4:392–6.

17. Sears CL, Kaper JB. Enteric bacterial toxins: mechanisms of action and linkage to intestinal secretion. Microbiol Rev. 1996;60:167–215.

18. Isidean SD, Riddle MS, Savarino SJ, Porter CK. A systematic review of ETEC epidemiology focusing on colonization factor and toxin expression. Vaccine. 2011;29:6167–78.

19. Fleckenstein JM, Hardwidge PR, Munson GP, Rasko DA, Sommerfelt H, Steinsland H. Molecular mechanisms of enterotoxigenic *Escherichia coli* infection. Microbes Infect. 2010;12:89–98.

20. Zhang W, Sack DA. Progress and hurdles in the development of vaccines against enterotoxigenic *Escherichia coli* in humans. Expert Rev Vaccines. 2012;11:677–94.

21. Zhang W, Sack DA. Current progress in developing subunit vaccines against Enterotoxigenic *Escherichia coli*-associated diarrhea. Clin Vaccine Immunol. 2015;22:983–91.

22. Tribble DR. Resistant pathogens as causes of traveller's diarrhea globally and impact(s) on treatment failure and recommendations. J Travel Med. 2017;24:S6–S12.

23. Rossolini GM, D'Andrea MM, Mugnaioli C. The spread of CTX-M-type extended-spectrum β-lactamases. Clin Microbiol Infect. 2008;14:33–41.

24. Bajaj P, Singh NS, Virdi JS. *Escherichia coli* β-lactamases: what really matters. Front Microbiol. 2016; https://doi.org/10.3389/fmicb.2016.00417.

25. Kassakian SZ, Mermel LA. Changing epidemiology of infections due to extended spectrum β-lactamase producing bacteria. Antimicrob Resist Infect Control. 2014;3:9.

26. Kumar P, Bag S, Ghosh TS, Dey P, Dayal M, Saha B, Verma J, Pant A, Saxena S, Desigamani A, et al. Molecular insights into antimicrobial resistance traits of multidrug resistant enteric pathogens isolated from India. Sci Rep. 2017;7:14468.

27. Pitout JD, Laupland KB. Extended-spectrum β-lactamase-producing *Enterobacteriaceae*: an emerging public-health concern. Lancet Infect Dis. 2008;8:159–66.

28. Pitout JD. *Enterobacteriaceae* that produce extended-spectrum β-lactamases and AmpC β-lactamases in the community: the tip of the iceberg? Curr Pharm Des. 2013;19:257–63.

29. Pan H, Zhang J, Kuang D, Yang X, Ju W, Huang Z, Guo J, Li Y, Zhang P, Shi W, et al. Molecular analysis and antimicrobial susceptibility of enterotoxigenic *Escherichia coli* from diarrheal patients. Diagn Microbiol Infect Dis. 2015;81:126–31.

30. Mendez Arancibia E, Pitart C, Ruiz J, Marco F, Gascón J, Vila J. Evolution of antimicrobial resistance in enteroaggregative *Escherichia coli* and enterotoxigenic *Escherichia coli* causing traveller's diarrhoea. J Antimicrob Chemother. 2009;64:343–7.

31. Clinical and Laboratory Standards Institute. Performance standards for antimicrobial susceptiblity testing - 28th edition. Wayne: Clinical and Laboratory Standards Institute; 2017.

32. Rodas C, Iniguez V, Qadri F, Wiklund G, Svennerholm AM, Sjoling A. Development of multiplex PCR assays for detection of enterotoxigenic *Escherichia coli* colonization factors and toxins. J Clin Microbiol. 2009;47: 1218–20.

33. Dallenne C, Da Costa A, Decre D, Favier C, Arlet G. Development of a set of multiplex PCR assays for the detection of genes encoding important beta-lactamases in Enterobacteriaceae. J Antimicrob Chemother. 2010;65:490–5.

34. Pitout JD, Nordmann P, Laupland KB, Poirel L. Emergence of Enterobacteriaceae producing extended-spectrum β-lactamases (ESBLs) in the community. J Antimicrob Chemother. 2005;56:52–9.

35. Baral P, Neupane S, Marasini BP, Ghimire KR, Lekhak B, Shrestha B. High prevalence of multidrug resistance in bacterial uropathogens from Kathmandu, Nepal. BMC Res Notes. 2012;5:38.

36. Khadgi S, Timilsina U, Shrestha B. Plasmid profiling of multidrug resistant *Escherichia coli* strains isolated from urinary tract infection patients. BMC Res Notes. 2013;5:38.

37. Parajuli NP, Maharjan P, Parajuli H, Joshi G, Paudel D, Sayami S, Khanal PR. High rates of multidrug resistance among uropathogenic *Escherichia coli* in children and analyses of ESBL producers from Nepal. Antimicrob Resist Infect Control. 2017;6:9.

38. Ansari S, Nepal HP, Gautam R, Shrestha S, Neopane P, Gurung G, Chapagain ML. Community acquired multi-drug resistant clinical isolates of *Escherichia coli* in a tertiary care center of Nepal. Antimicrob Resist Infect Control. 2015;4:15.

39. Sharma AR, Bhatta DR, Shrestha J, Banjara MR. Antimicrobial susceptibility pattern of *Escherichia coli* isolated from urinary tract infected patients attending Bir hospital. Nepal J Sci Technol. 2013;14:177–84.

40. Arcilla MS, van Hattem JM, Haverkate MR, Bootsma MCJ, van Genderen PJJ, Goorhuis A, Grobusch MP, Lashof AMO, Molhoek N, Schultsz C, et al. Import and spread of extended-spectrum beta-lactamase-producing *Enterobacteriaceae* by international travellers (COMBAT study): a prospective, multicentre cohort study. Lancet Infect Dis. 2017;17:78–85.

41. Hijazi SM, Fawzi MA, Ali FM, Abd El Galil KH. Prevalence and characterization of extended-spectrum β-lactamases producing Enterobacteriaceae in healthy children and associated risk factors. Ann Clin Microbiol Antimicrob. 2016;15:3.

42. Cantón R, González-Alba JM, Galán JC. CTX-M enzymes: origin and diffusion. Front Microbiol. 2012;3:110.

43. Sherchan JB, Hayakawa K, Miyoshi-Akiyama T, Ohmagari N, Kirikae T, Nagamatsu M, Tojo M, Ohara H, Sherchand JB, Tandukar S. Clinical epidemiology and molecular analysis of extended-spectrum-beta-lactamase-producing *Escherichia coli* in Nepal: characteristics of sequence types 131 and 648. Antimicrob Agents Chemother. 2015;59:3424–32.

44. Pokhrel RH, Thapa B, Kafle R, Shah PK, Tribuddharat C. Co-existence of β-lactamases in clinical isolates of *Escherichia coli* from Kathmandu, Nepal. BMC Res Notes. 2014;7:694.

45. Sidjabat HE, Paterson DL. Multidrug-resistant *Escherichia coli* in Asia: epidemiology and management. Expert Rev Anti-Infect Ther. 2015;13: 575–91.

46. Carattoli A. Plasmids and the spread of resistance. Int J Med Microbiol. 2013; 303:298–304.

# 23

# Costs of outpatient and inpatient MRSA screening and treatment strategies for patients at elective hospital admission - a decision tree analysis

Luise Hutzschenreuter[1]* iD, Steffen Flessa[1], Kathleen Dittmann[2] and Nils-Olaf Hübner[2,3]

## Abstract

**Background:** Nosocomial infections are among the most common complications in hospitals. A major part is caused by multidrug-resistant organisms (MDRO). MRSA is still the most prominent and frequent MDRO. The early detection of carriers of multidrug-resistant bacteria is an effective measure to reduce nosocomial infections caused by MDRO. For patients who are planning to go to the hospital, an outpatient screening for MDRO and pre-hospital decolonization is recommended. However, the effectiveness of such pre-admission MDRO management in preparation for a planned hospital stay has not yet been sufficiently scientifically examined from an economic perspective.

**Methods:** A decision tree will be used to develop scenarios for MDRO screening and treatment in the context of the outpatient and inpatient sectors using MRSA-positive patients as an example. Subsequently, the expected costs for the respective strategy are presented.

**Results:** The decision tree analysis shows that the expected costs of outpatient MRSA management are €8.24 and that of inpatient MRSA management are €672.51.

**Conclusion:** The forward displacement of the MRSA screening to the ambulatory sector and any subsequent outpatient decolonization for patients with a planned hospitalization is the most cost-effective strategy and should become a standard benefit. Excluding opportunity costs, the expected costs of inpatient MRSA management are €54.94.

**Keywords:** Methicillin-resistant *Staphylococcus aureus*, Outpatient screening, Decolonization, Admission screening, Costs, Expected costs, Decision tree analysis

## Background

Nosocomial infections are among the most common complications in German hospitals, and are caused by an increasing proportion of multidrug-resistant organisms (MDRO) [1]. A key measure for the control of MDRO is the early detection of carriers (screening) to initiate appropriate infection control measures, suppression therapy and adequate antibiotic therapy. MDRO screening has the potential to increase patient safety and reduce the transmission risk of the pathogen to fellow patients, thus reducing the cost of hospitalized MRSA treatment. So far, sectoral boundaries between health care providers have been a major barrier to efficient solutions. Screening for MDRO carriers in preparation for a planned hospital stay (e.g. for elective surgery) is not performed in Germany, since the necessary structures are missing and the effects are not sufficiently scientifically proven. Studies in ambulatory surgery shows benefits of preventative MRSA measures [2].

Using the multidrug-resistant organism MRSA (Methicillin-Resistant *Staphylococcus aureus*) as an representative of MDRO, a large number of studies have shown that inpatient decolonization treatments of high-risk patients lead to additional financial burdens of hospitals, for example, by extending the length of stay and higher costs for hygiene management. Studies describes MRSA-attributed

---

* Correspondence: luise.hutzschenreuter@uni-greifswald.de
[1]Institute of Health Care Management, University of Greifswald, Friedrich-Loeffler-Str. 70, 17489 Greifswald, Germany
Full list of author information is available at the end of the article

costs of €6000 to €10,000 per patient case. [3–5]. Due to the paucity of literature on the costs of outpatient MRSA screening and a possible subsequent outpatient decolonization in preparation for inpatient hospitalization a comparison of outpatient and inpatient screening has to date been impossible. Due to reimbursement problems pre-admission MRSA-screening is usually not performed and a good calculation of costing data is required to perform an economic screening. The present study is intended to close this gap. From a health-economics perspective, the aim of the study is to calculate the expected costs of pre-admission MRSA treatment and inpatient MRSA management.

The study is part of the PRIME project initiated by the MDRO-network KOMPASS e. V., which introduced pre-admission MRDO screening using the example of MRSA as a model in the north-eastern part of Germany (Mecklenburg-Vorpommern). The project is funded by the Ministry of Economics, Construction and Tourism Mecklenburg-Vorpommern.

## Methods

The purpose of this study was to calculate the expected costs of the outpatient and inpatient MRSA treatment strategy for elective hospital admission using a decision tree analysis. Therefor a mixed methods were used for collecting all the necessary data. The first step of developing the decision tree was to collect data during inpatient and subsequently outpatient MRSA screenings in an own survey. The data of outpatient and inpatient MRSA decolonization treatments used were obtained from previously published studies. A decision tree developed thereafter was backed by these values.

### Definition of screening and successful decolonization

In the context of this research study, MRSA screening means a targeted anamnesis of risk factors (for all patients) and, if one or more risk factors were present, a microbiological analysis by means of a swab test. It is therefore a two-stage screening process.

The definition of risk factors are guided by the recommendations of the german Commission for Hospital Hygiene and Infection Prevention (KRINKO). Following risk factors were defined for MRSA colonization:

- *patients with known MDRO history*
- *hospitalization abroad*
- *moving from elderly-care facility or chronically care dependency*
- *patients with contact to MDRO carrier during a preceding hospital stay (e.g. as a room-mate)*
- *patients with hospitalization (> 3 days) or treatment in an intensive care unit in the preceding 12 months*
- *antibiotic treatment in the preceding 12 months*

- *patients with work-related contact to animals in agricultural animal fattening*
- *presence of a catheter, tracheal cannula etc.*
- *dialysis patients*
- *patients with skin ulceration, gangrene, chronic wound, deep tissue infection*
- *patient is not able to provide information*

If patients have risk factors, swabs were taken from the nose and throat combined and possibly from existing wounds.

A successful decolonization means that after the completion of a decolonization cycle (eradication with local antiseptic treatment of nose (Mupirocin) and throat, whole antiseptic body wash, etc.) and two days break, swabs are taken of all defined predilection sites at three consecutive days and all findings are negative. The decolonization is carried out according to a standardized procedure. The procedure is the same in both outpatient and inpatient settings.

### Collection of real data

In a general hospital, personnel and material costs for MRSA screening were collected over a two-week period as part of the admission screening of patients. A second MRSA screening was carried out in the outpatient sector. Based on this, the cost calculation for the screening took place.

### Personnel costs

In the first step all MRSA-attributed screening processes were identified. Afterwards the costs per minute were calculated by dividing annual personnel costs (average gross wage in accordance with the collective agreement plus employer contributions) by annual working time. This resulted in carer staff costs of €0.41 per minute.

### Material costs

The cost of personal protective equipment (disposable gloves) was based on the average consumption amount, which was valued at the hospital's purchase price. The costs of the swabs were not included in the analysis. These were provided by the external laboratory and are part of the laboratory's service.

### Laboratory costs

For this cost analysis, the calculation of laboratory costs was based on the scale of charges (GOP) of the German uniform valuation standard for outpatient physician services (EBM), as the laboratory services were provided by an external laboratory. GOP 30954 (targeted MRSA detection on chromogenic selective medium) was used with a value of €5.32 per test. It was assumed that the hospital and the doctor's office incurred costs of this amount for laboratory services per screening.

## Decision tree analysis

The basis of the analysis is a multi-level decision tree with the expected costs of alternative MRSA screening and decolonization strategies in patients who are faced with a planned hospitalization. The first and most authoritative decision is whether the MRSA screening takes place on an outpatient basis, meaning at the referring physician's office, or upon hospital admission of the patient. In this study, a two-stage MRSA screening (step 1: screening for risk factors; step 2: swab in high-risk patients) is assumed. To detect MRSA, conventional cultural cultivation of the test material was chosen.

The decision tree analysis is based on the following assumptions:

- The probability of exhibiting MRSA risk factors or being MRSA carriers is the same for patients admitted to hospital admission and before being admitted to the outpatient area.
- Patients who have been screened at hospital admission are preemptively isolated for 48 h until the findings are available.
- The unit has a high occupancy rate and two-bed rooms for the calculation of the costs per locked bed (opportunity costs).
- In the absence of risk factors for MRSA or a negative result, the path of the decision tree ends and there are no additional costs.
- In this model we supposed that one decolonization cycle is necessary for successful MRSA eradication.

The decision tree contains rectangles for decisions, circles for possibilities (these are to be placed with probabilities) and triangles for the end of a branch (path). To determine the optimal strategy in the decision tree, the rollback method was chosen. Accordingly, the optimal strategy comprises that sequence of alternative courses of action which leads to the minimum expected value. The strategy with the lowest expected costs will be sought.

The expected costs were calculated in 2 steps. All of the parameters collected and used are defined in Table 1.

First, the respective costs per path were calculated for the scenarios of MRSA management (paths A to F) presented in the decision tree. The respective formulae are shown in Table 2.

In a second step, the expected costs E(x) of the outpatient (out) and inpatient (hos) MRSA management alternatives were calculated using the rollback method. Based on the costs per path, the following formulae were used:

$$E_{out} = \left[C_B \cdot (1 - p_{MRSA+}) + C_C \cdot p_{MRSA+}\right] \cdot p_{R+} + C_A \cdot (1 - p_{R+})$$

$$E_{hos} = \left[C_E \cdot (1 - p_{MRSA+}) + C_F \cdot p_{MRSA+}\right] \cdot p_{R+} + C_D \cdot (1 - p_{R+})$$

## Level of analysis

The level of analysis examines the effects caused by the variation of an input parameter. In this study, the influence of the parameter rate of spatial isolation on the expected costs of the inpatient MRSA management strategy was evaluated. A given parameter was varied in three steps:

Scenario 1: This is the baseline scenario in the decision tree, meaning that the costs of preemptive isolation and the isolation while decolonization were considered.
Scenario 2: The preemptive isolation of screened patients until the results are available has been omitted. In case of positive MRSA findings, the patient was isolated while decolonization. This means that only a part of the isolation costs have been included in the calculation of the expected costs.
Scenario 3: The calculation of the expected costs was done without isolation costs. There were no opportunity

**Table 1** Description and quantification of parameters

| Parameter | Description | Value | References |
|---|---|---|---|
| $p_{R+}$ | Probability of having risk factors for MRSA | 72.5% | own elicitation |
| $p_{MRSA+}$ | MRSA prevalence in high-risk patients | 3.94% | [8] |
| $C_{ris}$ | Costs of screening for risk factors | €0.48 | own elicitation |
| $C_{sc}$ | Costs for swabs, documentation and laboratory testing as part of the screening (swab test) | €7.09 | own elicitation |
| $C_{pre\_iso}$ | Opportunity costs for a locked bed during preemptive isolation per day | €328.36 | own elicitation |
| $T_{pre\_iso}$ | Time in which the patient is preemptively isolated (in days) | 2 days | see assumption |
| $C_{dec\_hos}$ | Costs for decolonization (hygienic management (workload + materials) and laboratory) in the hospital per case | €1726.66 | [4] |
| $C_{iso\_hos}$ | Opportunity costs for a locked bed during decolonization per day | €328.36 | own elicitation |
| $T_{iso\_hos}$ | Time in which the patient is isolated during decolonization (in days) | 15.08 days | [8] |
| $C_{dec\_out}$ | Costs of outpatient decolonization per case | €91.77 | [10] |

**Table 2** Formulas to calculate the total cost per path in the decision tree

| Path | Description | Formula |
|---|---|---|
| A | Patient without risk factors (outpatient) | $C_A = C_{ris}$ |
| B | Risk patient with negative MRSA findings (outpatient) | $C_B = C_{ris} + C_{sc}$ |
| C | Patients screened and decolonized on an outpatient basis, followed by inpatient admission | $C_C = C_{ris} + C_{sc} + C_{dec\_out}$ |
| D | Patient without risk factors (inpatient) | $C_D = C_{ris}$ |
| E | Patient screened in hospital, preemptive isolation to findings, result: MRSA negative | $C_E = C_{ris} + C_{sc} + C_{pre\_iso} \cdot T_{pre\_iso}$ |
| F | Patient screened in hospital, preemptive isolation, result: MRSA positive, then isolated and decolonized in hospital | $C_F = C_{ris} + C_{sc} + C_{pre\_iso} \cdot T_{pre\_iso} + C_{dec\_hos} + C_{iso\_hos} \cdot T_{iso\_hos}$ |

Legend: $C_A$ = Costs of path A in the decision tree, $C_B$ = Costs of path B in the decision tree, $C_C$ = Costs of path C in the decision tree, $C_D$ = Costs of path D in the decision tree, $C_E$ = Costs of path E in the decision tree, $C_F$ = Costs of path F in the decision tree

costs associated with the MRSA management, because the patient was not spatially isolated.

Using the rollback method, the expected costs of inpatient MRSA management were calculated by varying the isolation cost parameter.

## Results
### Screening costs
Due to the equivalent procedure of inpatient and outpatient MRSA screening, the time and material effort for this is approximately the same. The calculated costs for MRSA screening are shown in Table 3. The risk factor survey takes on average 1:10 min. This results in personnel costs of €0.48 per screening of risk factors. The second step of the screening, both in the hospital and in the doctor's office, consists of swabbing, labeling of the swab tubes, documentation and packaging of the samples for the laboratory. These activities are part of the process "swab test". This process requires an average of 4:05 min both in the doctor's office and in the hospital. The personnel costs are €1.67. The swabbing itself takes an average of 0:55 min. The material costs for the use of a pair of disposable gloves are €0.10. According to the GOP, costs of €5.32 are incurred for the laboratory examination. Overall, the costs of the swab test are €7.09.

**Table 3** Screening costs

| | $C_{ris}$ | $C_{sc}$ |
|---|---|---|
| Staff | | |
| duration [min] | 01:10 | 04:05 |
| costs [€] | 0.48 | 1.67 |
| Material | | |
| gloves [piece] | 0 | 2 |
| costs [€] | 0 | 0.10 |
| Laboratory | | |
| costs [€] | 0 | 5.32 |
| Total costs [€] | 0.48 | 7.09 |

### Decision tree paths
The decision tree developed is shown in Fig. 1. Following six paths (A to F) of outpatient and inpatient MRSA management of patients with a planned hospital admission were described:

Path A (outpatient): Patient with planned hospital admission were screened of risk factors for MRSA at an outpatient medical office. No risk factors are present, the MRSA screening is finished and hospital admission is possible.

Path B (outpatient): Risk factors for MRSA are recorded. One or more risk factors are present. Swabs are taken from the nose and throat and if present, from wounds. Evidence is provided by culturing the material in the laboratory. After 48 h, the findings are available. The result is negative. No further measures are induced and the patient can be hospitalized.

Path C (outpatient): Screening of MRSA and laboratory test such as path B. The findings are positive. An outpatient eradication of MRSA was implemented.

Path D (inpatient): Patient will be screened of risk factors for MRSA at hospital admission. There are no risk factors.

Path E (inpatient): Risk factors for MRSA are collected at hospital admission. One or more risk factors are present. Swabs are taken from defined predilection sites and microbiologically examined. Until the findings are available (after approximately 48 h), the patient is preemptively isolated on ward. The findings are negative. No further measures are induced and the patient can go to ward.

Path F (inpatient): Screening of MRSA, laboratory test and preemptive isolation such as path E. The findings are positive. The isolation continues and in addition to initiating basic hygiene barrier measures, eradicative treatment is carried out.

In total, six possible scenarios (Paths A to F) from MRSA screening to eradication were developed (Fig. 1).

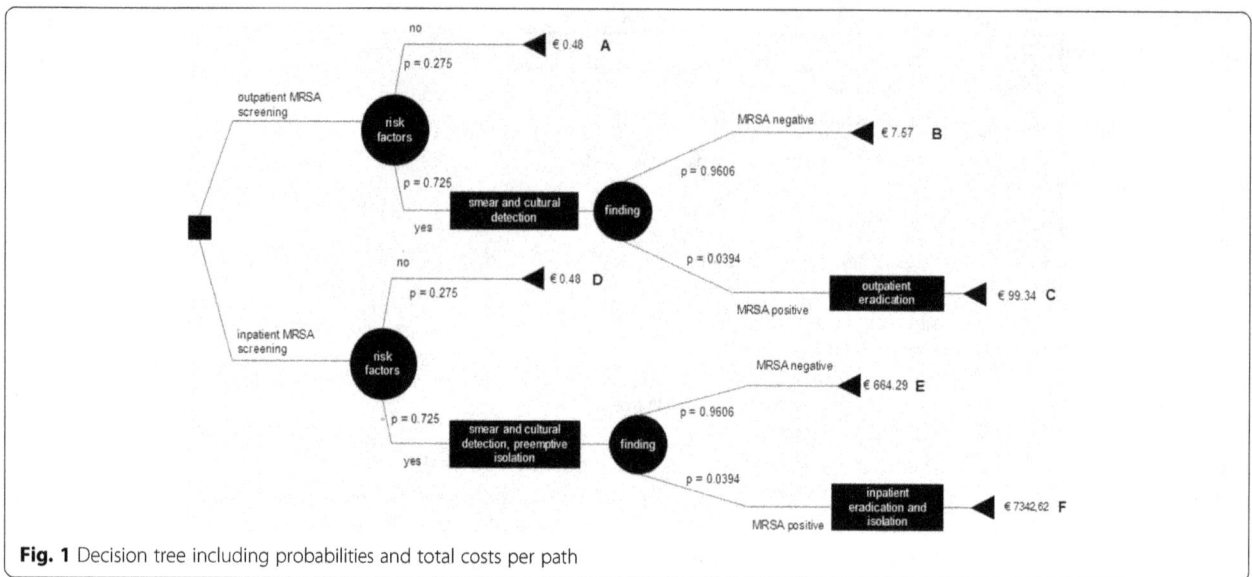

**Fig. 1** Decision tree including probabilities and total costs per path

In scenarios A, B and C, MRSA management takes place in the outpatient sector. Scenarios D, E and F relate to inpatient MRSA management.

## Costs calculation of paths

The decision tree also shows the costs that were calculated per path. The lowest costs are incurred with paths A and D (patient without risk factor), at €0.48. From an economic point of view, it does not matter whether the assessment of the risk factors is carried out on an outpatient or inpatient basis, as the same personnel costs arise for the collection of the risk factors in both contexts. If a follow-up examination is carried out after the identification of risk factors with a subsequent negative result, the costs in the ambulatory area (path B/€7.57) are significantly lower than those in the inpatient area (path E/€664.29). The greatest cost factor in the hospital is the two-day preemptive isolation of the patient (opportunity costs through a locked bed) until the findings are available.

If a patient is tested outpatient positive for the sponsorship of MRSA and then carried out an outpatient decolonization (path C) costs incurred by a registered doctor in the amount of €99.34. The highest costs are found in path F (patient inpatient positive for MRSA tested and then decolonized stationary) with €7342.62.

## Expected costs of the strategies

The calculation of the expected costs for outpatient and inpatient MRSA management by means of the rollback method has shown that when practicing MRSA management, the attending physician generates expected costs ($E_{out}$) per patient of €8.24. The expected costs of the inpatient MRSA management strategy ($E_{hos}$) are €672.51.

## Level of analysis

In the scenarios where the patient is isolated in the hospital (paths E and F), the initial situation creates opportunity costs by locking beds while isolating the patient. If the opportunity costs are ignored in whole or in part, as expected, the expected costs for the considered inpatient MRSA management strategy change. In the basic scenario (preemptive isolation and isolation given a positive finding), expected costs were €672.51 for inpatient MRSA management. If preemptive isolation of the patient is not performed until the lab results are ready (unclear MRSA status), the expected costs of the inpatient MRSA management strategy are reduced to €196.39 per patient. If a procedure is chosen without spatial isolation of the patient, the expected costs of inpatient MRSA management are €54.94 (Table 4).

## Discussion

The decision tree analysis shows that the expected costs of outpatient MRSA management (€8.24 per case) are far below those of inpatient MRSA management (€672.51 per case). Diller et al. (2008) show that pre-admission MRSA screening is cost-effective [6]. In their study, they had discovered 5 MRSA-positive patients by pre-admission screening and decolonized them before hospitalization. As a result, they could avoided costs for MRSA-treatment and isolation of approximately €30,000 to €50,000. Also Wernitz et al. (2005) demonstrated that precocious screening and if necessary decolonization of MRSA reduce costs [7]. Giese et al. (2013) calculated that a pre-admission decolonization at home in 22 cases saved a total of about €134,000 to €205,000 [8]. In conclusion, pre-admission screening and if necessary decolonization before hospital treatment is advantageous from an economic perspective.

**Table 4** Expected costs of the inpatient MRSA management strategy with variable opportunity costs

| Scenario | Description | Expected costs of inpatient MRSA management |
|---|---|---|
| 1 | Basic scenario (preemptive isolation and isolation if MRSA positive) | €672.51 |
| 2 | No preemptive isolation of the screened patient, but isolation if MRSA positive while decolonization | €196.39 |
| 3 | Inpatient MRSA management without isolation of the patient (no opportunity costs) | €54.94 |

If only MRSA screening is initially considered, a significant cost difference between outpatient (path B / €7.57) and inpatient MRSA screening (path E / €664.29) can be seen. The cost of determining the risk factors and performing the smear are identical. The enormously higher costs of inpatient MRSA screening can be explained by the costs for preemptive isolation of all patients, where were taken swabs (48 h til presence of laboratory results) in hospital. An outpatient MRSA screening does not require isolation of the patient. Therefore, there are no costs for isolation in the outpatient sector. The costs of MRSA screening are determined by the method of laboratory test. In our study a conventional cultural cultivation of the test material was chosen, which imply a preemptive isolation. If a polymerase chain reaction (PCR) method were chosen, preemptive isolation is not necessary and no additional costs for isolation are incurred [9].

The level of analysis has shown that the expected costs of inpatient MRSA management are still higher than those in the outpatient setting, if patient isolation is excluded. When considering MRSA decolonization, the different levels of costs can be attributed primarily to the extent of expenses incurred by the service provider for eradication therapy of an MRSA patient. For example, in the case of outpatient MRSA decolonization, the personnel, material and laboratory costs incurred arise when the patient has contact with the doctor's office during eradication therapy (for example control smears, counseling session). The actual decolonization is carried out by the patient independently at home. The cost of the necessary decontamination set, consisting of antiseptic preparations such as mouthwash, washing lotion and surface disinfectant cannot be charged to statutory health insurance (SHI); this is funded by the patient him- or herself. Only the antibacterial nasal ointment can be prescribed as an authorized medicinal product covered by the SHI. The costs of an MRSA decolonization in the hospital arise from the extra work required for hygiene management (e.g., increased personnel and material costs for changing clothes), the implementation of eradication therapy, including all the preparations used to decolonize the patient, the laboratory costs and the opportunity cost of blocking beds during isolation of the patient [6]. All preparations and protective equipment necessary for treatment are provided and financed by the hospital, and no costs will be charged to the patient.

The greatest expense factor of hospital MRSA management are the opportunity costs. These arise both in the preemptive isolation of all screened patients and in the isolation of MRSA-positive patients while decolonization. However, there are also indications that in the reality of German hospitals, hardly any patients are rejected and therefore no opportunity costs are incurred [10]. This depends on the hospital's bedload. Additional costs arise for organizing the room change when patients requiring isolation are admitted to the ward. These costs for preparing a suitable room, relocating other patients, and the related space management cannot be illustrated in this study, but should be mentioned.

**Current settlement situation of outpatient MRSA services**

Until now, outpatient MRSA coverage is only provided by statutory health insurance if it concerns the further treatment of an MRSA-colonized patient after hospital discharge (on the settlement of GOP 30949 to 30952 in section 30.12 of the EBM). Expansion of the billable positions in the EBM by pre-admission screening and subsequent outpatient decolonization before hospital admission should be targeted from an economic perspective.

*Demands for pre-admission screening*

The Commission for Hospital Hygiene and Infection Prevention at the Robert Koch Institute considers an advanced MRSA screening in planned hospital admissions useful for reducing the transmission and infection risk [11]. Since 2015, the National Association of Statutory Health Insurance Physicians has also been calling for the compensation of outpatient services that are associated with pre-admission MRSA screening [12]. The aim is to curb the spread of the pathogen. Specifically, this requirement refers to a smear test in patients with risk factors who are about to undergo surgery. Several studies have proven that MRSA screening and subsequent decolonization of MRSA-positive patients prior to surgery reduces the number of postoperative wound infections and leads to cost savings [13, 14].

**Strengths and limitations**

The strengths and limitations of this study should not go unmentioned. The collection of real data for MRSA screening enabled real costs to be calculated for the scenarios presented in the decision tree. For the development of the decision tree and the calculation of the expected costs of the MRSA management strategies, only a few assumptions had to be made due to the extensive data collection in MRSA screenings and the resulting data. A strength of the study is that the expected cost were calculated in dependent on the probability of occurrence. The method of roll-back analysis enables to generalize the costs of the outpatient and inpatient strategy. The use of secondary data for the cost calculation for MRSA eradication is justified in the scope of the project, which has primarily introduced a pre-admission MRSA screening and has not additionally examined the subsequent decolonization. The decision tree can only use for planned hospital admission. This decision tree cannot be applied to patients admitted as an emergency in the hospital. Another limitation is that individual characteristics of planned hospital admissions or patients cannot be taken into account in this model (eg., whether the individual patient can carry out the decolonization at home independently or needs help from a community nurse). The main strength of our study is that the developed decision tree and the cost calculation can be a decision-making aid, whether from an economic perspective a pre-admission MRSA screening or MRSA decolonization should be introduced in preparation for a planned hospitalization.

## Conclusion

The expected costs of an outpatient MRSA strategy are always lower than those of an inpatient strategy, as there is no isolation of the patient and the decolonization is performed independently by the patient at home. From the point of view of this cost analysis, pre-admission MRSA management is recommended before a planned hospital stay.

### Abbreviations
EBM: German uniform valuation standard for outpatient physician services; GOP: Scale of charges; KRINKO: The Commission for Hospital Hygiene and Infection Prevention; MDRO: Multidrug resistant organisms; MRSA: Methicillin-Resistant *Staphylococcus aureus*; SHI: Statutory health insurance

### Acknowledgements
(not applicable)

### Funding
This study is integrated in the PRIME-Project, which is co-financed by the European Union and the European Regional Development Fund (ERDF), operational program Mecklenburg-Vorpommern 2014–2020.

### Authors' contributions
LH was responsible for conception and design of the study, acquisition of data and interpretation of data. KD supported the study. SF and NH supervised conception and design of the study. LH drafted the manuscript. All authors revised the paper and approved the final manuscript.

### Consent for publication
(not applicable)

### Competing interests
The authors declare that they have no competing interests.

### Author details
[1]Institute of Health Care Management, University of Greifswald, Friedrich-Loeffler-Str. 70, 17489 Greifswald, Germany. [2]Institute of Hygiene and Environmental Health, University Medicine of Greifswald, Walther-Rathenau-Straße 49a, 17489 Greifswald, Germany. [3]IMD Laboratory Greifswald MVZ GmbH, Vitus-Bering-Straße 27a, 17493 Greifswald, Germany.

### References

1. Geffers C, Gastmeier P. Nosokomiale Infektionen und multiresistente Erreger in Deutschland: Epidemiologische Daten aus dem Krankenhaus-Infektions-Surveillance-System. Dtsch Arztebl Int. 2011;108(6):87–93. https://doi.org/10.3238/arztebl.2011.0087 PubMed PMID: 21373275 .

2. Kavanagh KT, Calderon LE, Saman DM, Abusalem SK. The use of surveillance and preventative measures for methicillin-resistant staphylococcus aureus infections in surgical patients. Antimicrob Resist Infect Control. 2014;3:18. https://doi.org/10.1186/2047-2994-3-18 PubMed PMID: 24847437 .

3. Popp W, Hilgenhöner M, Leisebein T, Müller H. Personalkosten durch Isolierungsmaßnahmen von MRSA-Patienten. Gesundh ökon Qual manag. 2003;8(3):187–90. https://doi.org/10.1055/s-2003-40481 .

4. Hübner C, Hübner N-O, Hopert K, Maletzki S, Flessa S. Analysis of MRSA-attributed costs of hospitalized patients in Germany. Eur J Clin Microbiol Infect Dis. 2014;33(10):1817–22. https://doi.org/10.1007/s10096-014-2131-x PubMed PMID: 24838677 .

5. Herr CEW, Heckrodt TH, Hofmann FA, Schnettler R, Eikmann TF. Additional costs for preventing the spread of methicillin-resistant Staphylococcus aureus and a strategy for reducing these costs on a surgical ward. Infect Control Hosp Epidemiol. 2003;24(9):673–8. https://doi.org/10.1086/502274 PubMed PMID: 14510250 .

6. Diller R, Sonntag AK, Mellmann A, Grevener K, Senninger N, Kipp F, et al. Evidence for cost reduction based on pre-admission MRSA screening in general surgery. Int J Hyg Environ Health. 2008;211(1–2):205–12. https://doi.org/10.1016/j.ijheh.2007.06.001 PubMed PMID: 17692566 .

7. Wernitz MH, Keck S, Swidsinski S, Schulz S, Veit SK. Cost analysis of a hospital-wide selective screening programme for methicillin-resistant Staphylococcus aureus (MRSA) carriers in the context of diagnosis related groups (DRG) payment. Clin Microbiol Infect. 2005;11(6):466–71. https://doi.org/10.1111/j.1469-0691.2005.01153.x PubMed PMID: 15882196 .

8. Giese A, Bous J, Werner S, Lemm F, Wilhelm M, Henning BF. Postponing elective hospitalizations for pre-admission MRSA screening and decolonization. A study evaluating eligibility and acceptance among patients of a German university hospital. Int J Hyg Environ Health. 2013;216(2):126–31. https://doi.org/10.1016/j.ijheh.2012.04.005 PubMed PMID: 22683064 .

9. Tübbicke A, Hübner C, Hübner N-O, Wegner C, Kramer A, Fleßa S. Cost comparison of MRSA screening and management - a decision tree analysis. BMC Health Serv Res. 2012;12:438. https://doi.org/10.1186/1472-6963-12-438 PubMed PMID: 23198880 .

10. Schwendler M. Ambulante MRSA-Sanierungsbehandlung bei Patienten mit chronischen Wunden: Durchführbarkeit, Akzeptanz, Fallerlöse und Kosten [Inaugural-Dissertation]. Greifswald: Universitätsmedizin Greifswald; 2017.

11. KRINKO. Empfehlungen zur Prävention und Kontrolle von Methicillin-resistenten Staphylococcus aureus-Stämmen (MRSA) in medizinischen und pflegerischen Einrichtungen. Bundesgesundheitsbl. 2014;57(6):695–732. https://doi.org/10.1007/s00103-014-1980-x .

12. Hillienhof A. Infektionsschutz: Prästationäres MRSA-Screening gefordert. Deutsches Ärzteblatt. 2015;112:33–4.

13. Humphreys H, Becker K, Dohmen PM, Petrosillo N, Spencer M, van Rijen M, et al. Staphylococcus aureus and surgical site infections: benefits of screening and decolonization before surgery. J Hosp Infect. 2016;94(3):295–304. https://doi.org/10.1016/j.jhin.2016.06.011 PubMed PMID: 27424948 .

14. Bode LGM, Kluytmans JAJW, Wertheim HFL, Bogaers D, Vandenbroucke-Grauls CMJE, Roosendaal R, et al. Preventing surgical-site infections in nasal carriers of Staphylococcus aureus. N Engl J Med. 2010;362(1):9–17. https://doi.org/10.1056/NEJMoa0808939 PubMed PMID: 20054045 .

# 24

# Prevalence of methicillin resistant *Staphylococcus aureus*, multidrug resistant and extended spectrum β-lactamase producing gram negative bacilli causing wound infections at a tertiary care hospital of Nepal

Narbada Upreti[1*], Binod Rayamajhee[2,3*] (iD), Samendra P. Sherchan[4], Mahesh Kumar Choudhari[5] and Megha Raj Banjara[1]

## Abstract

**Background:** Treatment and prevention of wound infection continues to be a challenging issue in clinical settings of Nepal especially in the context of globally growing problem of antimicrobial resistance. Study on opportunistic pathogens and sensitivity to commonly prescribed local antimicrobial agents are cardinal to reduce the disease burden of wound infections. The aim of this study was to determine the prevalence and antimicrobial susceptibility pattern of methicillin resistant *Staphylococcus aureus* (MRSA) and extended spectrum β-lactamase (ESBL) producing bacteria from wound infections of patients at a tertiary care hospital in Nepal.

**Methods:** Pus specimens were processed using standard microbiological procedures. Antimicrobial susceptibility test was performed following the modified Kirby Bauer disc diffusion technique. Clinical information of patients was obtained from preformed questionnaire and hospital record.

**Results:** One hundred eighty two pus specimens from wounds of different body parts: leg, hand, backside, abdominal part, foot, breast and chest, head and neck region were collected and analyzed; 113 bacterial isolates were isolated showing the overall bacterial growth rate of 62%, where the highest rate was among patients of ≤10 years age group (82.1%). A higher rate (68.5%) of bacterial isolates were from inpatients ($p < 0.05$). Among 116 bacterial isolates, *Staphylococcus aureus* was the most predominant bacteria (56.9%) followed by *Escherichia coli* (8.6%), coagulase negative staphylococci (7.8%), *Acinetobacter* spp. (5.2%), *Klebsiella pneumoniae* (5.2%), *Pseudomonas aeruginosa* (4.3%), *Enterococcus* spp. (4.3%), *Citrobacter freundii* (2.6%), *Proteus vulgaris* (1.6%) and *P. mirabilis* (0.9%). Both Gram positive (73.3%) and negative (78.8%) isolates showed high frequency of sensitive to gentamycin.

**Conclusion:** Among *S. aureus* isolates, 60.6% were MRSA strains, whereas 40% of *K. pneumoniae* and 33.3% of *C. freundii* were ESBL producing bacteria followed by *E. coli* (25%). It is thus paramount to address the burden of silently and speedily increasing infections caused by drug resistant strains of MRSA and ESBL in Nepal.

**Keywords:** Wound infection, Methicillin resistant *Staphylococcus aureus*, ESBL, Multidrug resistant, Nepal

* Correspondence: upreti.naru@gmail.com; rayamajheebinod@gmail.com
[1]Central Department of Microbiology, Tribhuvan University, Kirtipur, Nepal
[2]National College (Tribhuvan University), Khusibu, Kathmandu, Nepal
Full list of author information is available at the end of the article

## Background

Wound infections result after the active interactions that takes place between a host, a potential pathogen and the surrounding extrinsic factors. The intensity of wound infections may range from a simple self-healing to a severe and life threatening [1]. Tissue invasion by bacterial pathogens is determined by the location of wound [2]. The common bacterial pathogens isolated from wound infections are *Staphylococcus aureus*, *S. epidermidis*, *S. pyogenes*, coagulase negative staphylococci (CoNS), *Acinetobacter* spp., *Pseudomonas* spp., *Escherichia coli*, *Klebsiella* spp., *Proteus* spp., *Enterobacter* spp., *Citrobacter* spp., and anaerobes such as *Clostridium* spp. and *Peptostreptococcus* spp. [3, 4]. Acquisition of drug resistance by these pathogenic strains has posed serious challenges for the remedy and management of wound infections around the world [5]. Wound infections can be monomicrobial or polymicrobial [6]. The presence of bacterial pathogens in wound infections is not uncommon but all wounds do not support the same range and number of species [7]. Hospital-acquired wound infections are the leading cause of morbidity hence, proper management of wound infection in clinical settings is paramount [8]. The treatment of wound infections is being more challenging due to methicillin resistant *S. aureus* (MRSA), involvement of polymicrobial flora and fungi [9]. In addition, antimicrobial resistance (AMR) is creating a serious problem in all clinical settings and AMR has become the biggest public health threat globally [10].

MRSA, a leading strain of wound infections, involves significant areas of skin or deeper soft tissues like abscesses, cellulitis, burns or infected deep ulcers [11]. Extended spectrum β- lactamase (ESBL) producing Enterobacteriaceae are also in frontline of wound infections. In ESBL, positive strains plasmid mediated AmpC enzymes, and carbapenem hydrolyzing β- lactamase (carbapenemases) conferred resistance to the newer β- lactam antimicrobials [12]. ESBL have been reported most frequently in *Escherichia coli* and *Klebsiella* spp. including other bacterial species such as *Salmonella enterica*, *P. aeruginosa*, and *Serratia marcescens* [13]. This surge in antimicrobial resistance further delays wound healing and the infection becomes more worst which increases hospital stay, prolongs trauma care, and high medical costs [14]. On the other hand, most of the clinical laboratories in underdeveloped countries are not equipped with testing facilities to detect ESBL producing bacteria. In Nepal, there is scanty data on the prevalence of ESBL-producing bacteria causing wound infections. The goal of this study was to determine the prevalence of MRSA, multidrug resistant and ESBL producing Gram negative bacilli from wound infections of patients visiting KIST Medical College and Teaching Hospital, Lalitpur, Nepal. Early reporting of drug resistant pathogens and evidence-based treatment algorithm can control the wound infections.

## Methods

### Study site and population

A descriptive cross-sectional study was designed and carried out to determine the bacteriological profile of wound infections. MRSA, MDR and ESBL producing bacteria were identified from the pus samples of patients with wound infection visiting KIST Medical College and Teaching Hospital, Kathmandu, Nepal from November 2014 to August 2015. A total of 182 pus and Fine Needle Aspirate specimens were collected from patients with clinical features of wound infection like patients with pain, complaints of regular discharge, foul smelling and red swelling. During the study, patients of all age groups and both genders from out-patients (39/182) and in-patients (143/182) were included. Patients who were admitted in the hospital for more than 3 days and/or in prior antibiotic treatment and anaerobic wound infections were excluded from this study.

### Sampling procedure

Pus specimens were collected from elective surgery wounds of hospital wards [surgical, post- operative, trauma, orthopedic, ENT (eye-nose-throat), gynecology wards], open and dressed wounds. Sterile cotton swabs and fine needle syringes (FNS) were used to collect pus samples from open wounds then each sample was labeled properly with date/time of sample collection, collection method and the patient's details. Swabs from open wounds were aseptically collected after cleaned off while pus from dressed wounds were collected after removing the dressing items. The information of each patient was recorded such as site of infection, signs and symptoms, other underlying diseases, and prior antibiotics administration. Before collecting the sample, the area was rinsed with sterile normal saline and then a sterile cotton swab was gently rolled over the surface of the wound. The swab with pus was kept in a sterile test tube with cap where details was labeled properly. For the collection of pus sample from deep wounds, FNS was used. Specimens were collected from wounds of different body parts: leg, hand, back part of body, abdominal part, foot region, breast and chest part, head and neck region. Amies transport medium was used to transport the collected specimens. For Fine Needle Aspiration Cytology (FNAC), the syringe was properly capped, labeled and dispatched to the laboratory immediately.

### Processing of samples

#### Macroscopic examination of samples

Among 182 pus specimens collected, 56 (30.8%) were from the leg region, 43 (23.6%) from hand, 15 (8.2%)

from back part of body, 14 (7.8%) from abdominal part, 15 (8.2%) from foot region, 6 (3.3%) from breast and chest part, and 33 (18.1%) were from head and neck region wounds. All the specimens were visually examined for consistency, color, turbidity, presence or absence of blood depending upon the type and site of wound. Additionally, pus swabs were observed whether they were labeled correctly or not.

### Microscopic examination of samples

After transportation of specimens to the laboratory, Gram staining of each specimens was performed [15].

### Culture of specimens and identification of isolated bacteria

Pus specimens were inoculated into Chocolate agar, Blood agar, MacConkey agar, Nutrient agar and Potato Dextrose agar plates as per the clinical laboratory guidelines [16]. The preliminary identification of the isolated bacteria was done based on colony form, size, shape, pigmentation, margin, and elevation. The isolated organisms were identified by performing different biochemical tests and Gram staining then antimicrobial susceptibility tests were performed. In case of no growth after 24 h of incubation further incubation was done up to 48 h at 37 C. After proper incubation period, the culture plates were examined for microbial growth. In every case, each plate was carefully observed. Then, biochemical tests were performed in sterile media for the identification of bacterial isolates. Identification of Staphylococci spp. was done by Gram staining, catalase test, slide coagulase and tube coagulase test. Similarly, Gram negative strains were identified based on result of different biochemical tests; Oxidase, Catalase, Methyl Red (MR), Voges Proskauer (VP), Citrate utilization, Urea Hydrolysis, Triple Sugar Iron agar (TSI), Sulfide Motility and Indole test. Colony morphology and microscopic observation were taken in account for identification of *Candida* spp.

### Examination of antimicrobial susceptibility pattern of isolated organism

Antimicrobial susceptibility pattern was performed for isolated and identified bacteria from pus samples following the modified Kirby Bauer disc diffusion technique. A dilution of the identified organism was prepared comparing with the standard 0.5 McFarland turbidity which was used to swab over the Mueller Hinton agar (MHA) medium for the antimicrobial susceptibility test (AST). Discs of antibiotic used for Gram positive bacteria were ampicillin (10 μg), cefotaxime (30 μg), gentamycin (10 μg), ciprofloxacin (5 μg), trimethoprim + sulfamethoxazole (25 μg), cefoxitin (30 μg), amikacin (30 μg) and tetracycline (30 μg) whereas antibiotics used for Gram negative organisms were ampicillin (10 μg), trimethoprim + sulfamethoxazole (25 μg), gentamycin (10 μg), ciprofloxacin

(5 μg), cefazolin (30 μg), ceftriaxone (30 μg), cefotaxime (30 μg), amikacin (30 μg), piperacillin (100 μg), tobramycin (10 μg), imipenem (10 μg), and meropenem (10 μg). After 24 h of incubation period at 37 C, the zone of inhibition (ZOI) was measured then the results were analyzed according to the guidelines issued by the Clinical Laboratory Standard Institute (CLSI - M100-S25, 2015) [16]. Isolates resistant to two or more antimicrobial classes were reported as multi drug resistant (MDR) strains. Antimicrobials and their doses were selected based on prescription frequency by physician and availability in the study setting. Minimum inhibitory and bactericidal concentration (MIC and MBC) of used antimicrobials were not determined due to unavailability of all antimicrobials powder at the time of study period.

### Screening and confirmation for ESBL producers

Enterobacteriaceae isolates were screened for possible ESBL producing bacteria using antibiotic discs of cefotaxime (30 μg), ceftazidime (30 μg), ceftriaxone (30 μg) and aztreonam (30 μg) [17]. According to the guidelines, bacterial isolates showing ceftazidime < 22 mm, and cefotaxime < 27 mm are the possible ESBL producer. The suspected ESBL producer strains were subjected to double disc synergy test (DDST) for the confirmation of ESBL producing Enterobacteriaceae [18].

### Statistical analysis

All data were examined using iBM SPSS version 21.0. Frequencies were calculated for categorical variables. Chi-square test was calculated to analyze significant difference at 95% of confidence level, $p$ value of < 0.05 was considered significant, unless otherwise noted.

### Quality control

All prepared biochemical and streaking media were checked for their sterility. Strains of *E. coli* ATCC 25922 and *S. aureus* ATCC 25923 were used as reference strains for quality control of AST and biochemical tests. The same strain of *E. coli* was also considered as a negative control during the screening and phenotypic confirmation (DDST) tests of ESBL producing Gram-negative bacilli.

## Results
### Bacterial growth

A total of 182 samples were collected and examined from hospital patients with clinical features of wound infection, 113 (62%) specimens were positive for aerobic bacterial growth. Out of 116 bacterial isolates obtained from 113 positive samples, 83 (71.6%) bacterial isolates were Gram positive and 33 (28.4%) isolates were Gram negative. Among processed specimens, 64% (100/156) of pus swabs and 50% (13/26) of aspirated pus specimens have shown aerobic bacterial growth (Fig. 1). Out of 113

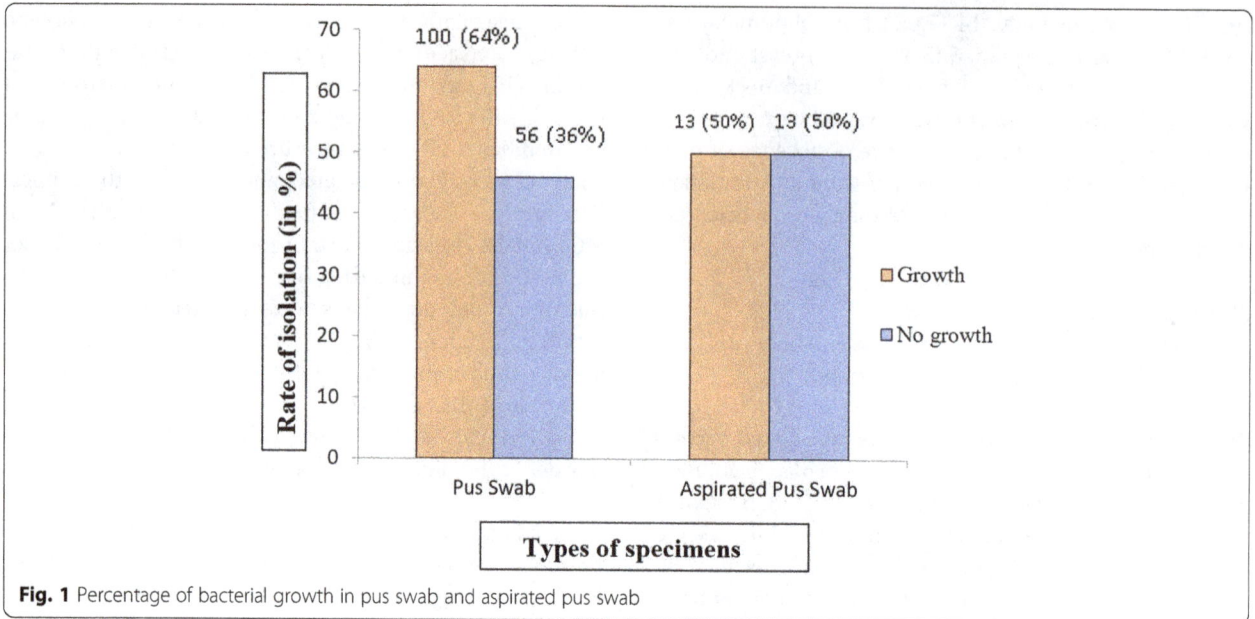

**Fig. 1** Percentage of bacterial growth in pus swab and aspirated pus swab

specimens positive for aerobic bacterial culture, polymicrobial growth was observed in 3 (2.7%) specimens where combinations of *S. aureus - Acinetobacter* spp., *S. aureus - Citrobacter freundii* and *Enterococcus* spp. - *Candida* spp. were reported. High incidence of MRSA 60.6% (40/66), MDR (80% of *E. coli*, 68.2% of *S. aureus*, 80% of *P. aeruginosa*, 77.7% of CoNS and 50% of *Proteus* spp.) and ESBL (25% of *E. coli*, 40% of *K. pneumoniae*, and 33.3% of *C. freundii*) producing isolates were reported in this study.

Sixty two (34.1%) specimens processed were collected from the leg, 36 (19.8%) from hand, 16 (8.8%) from backside, 15 (8.2%) from abdominal, 22 (12.1%) from foot, 13 (7.1%) from breast and chest, 18 (9.9%) from head and neck part. Majority of patients (86%) were presented with fever, lethargy and muscle pain at the time of sample collection. None of the patients were reported with any underlying diseases. Patients who had other infections and antibiotic treatment were excluded from the study subject.

**Wound infection in relation with demographic characteristics of the patients**
Eighty one (44.5%) samples were from male patients and among them 45 (55.5%) samples showed aerobic bacterial growth, while 101 (55.5%) samples were from female patients, and 68 (68.3%) samples were positive for aerobic bacterial growth but there was no significant difference in between aerobic bacterial growth and gender of patients ($p > 0.05$) (Table 1). Highest rate of wound infection was observed among patients of age group ≤10 years (82.1%), followed by patients of age group 71–80 years (77.8%).

**Growth pattern in outpatient and inpatient departments**
One hundred forty three samples were from inpatient department (from different wards) and 39 samples were from outpatient department. Out of 143 samples from inpatient, 98 (68.5%) were positive and out of 39 samples from outpatient, 15 (38.5%) were positive for bacterial growth. Type of patients based on department had a positive correlation with aerobic bacterial growth ($p < 0.05$).

Pus specimens were collected from inpatient departments/wards (such as surgical wards, post- operative

**Table 1** Socio-demographic features of the patients and ratio of wound infection

| Demographic features | Infected [No. (%)] | Not infected [No. (%)] | Total [No. (%)] |
|---|---|---|---|
| Sex | | | |
| Male | 45 (55.6) | 36 (44.4) | 81 (44.5) |
| Female | 68 (67.3) | 33 (32.7) | 101 (55.5) |
| Total | 113 (62.1) | 69 (37.9) | 182 (100) |
| Age in years | | | |
| ≤ 10 | 23 (82.1) | 5 (17.9) | 28 (15.4) |
| 11–20 | 18 (60.0) | 12 (40.0) | 30 (16.5) |
| 21–30 | 12 (44.4) | 15 (55.6) | 27 (14.9) |
| 31–40 | 21 (65.6) | 11 (34.4) | 32 (17.6) |
| 41–50 | 9 (40.9) | 13 (59.1) | 22 (12.0) |
| 51–60 | 15 (68.2) | 7 (31.8) | 22 (12.0) |
| 61–70 | 8 (66.7) | 4 (33.3) | 12 (6.6) |
| 71–80 | 7 (77.8) | 2 (22.2) | 9 (5.0) |
| Total | 113 (62.00) | 69 (38.00) | 182 (100) |

wards, orthopedic ward, ENT (eye-nose-throat), gynecology wards) and from outpatient department. Eighty nine (48.9%) specimens were from traumatic cases, followed by 57 (31.3%) specimens which were from postoperative cases. The most common bacterial isolate was *S. aureus* followed by *E. coli*. Out of 116 microbial isolates, 83 (71.6%) were Gram-positive and among them, *S. aureus* 66 (79.6%) was the most common isolate followed by CoNS 9 (10.8%), *Enterococcus* spp. 5 (6%) and *Candida* spp. 3 (3.6%). On the other hand, 33 (28.4%) were Gram-negative of which *E. coli* 10 (30.3%) was predominant isolate followed by *K. pneumoniae* 6 (18.2%), *Acinetobacter* spp. 6 (18.2%), *P. aeruginosa* 5 (15.1%), *C. freundii* 3 (9.1%), *P. vulgaris* 2 (6.1%) and *P. mirabilis* 1 (3%). In pus swab, *S. aureus* (58%) was the predominant isolate followed by *E. coli* (10%) and CoNS (9%). Similarly, in case of aspirates pus samples, *S. aureus* (50%) was the highest followed by *K. pneumoniae* (18.7%) (Table 2 and Additional file 1).

### Antibiogram result of gram negative bacteria isolated from patients at KIST Hospital, November 2014 to august 2015

A total of 10 *E. coli* were isolated from wound specimens and 80% (8/10) of isolates were sensitive to gentamicin, 60% were sensitive to ciprofloxacin, 50% were sensitive to cefotaxime and 40% were sensitive to cotrimoxazole. All isolates of *E. coli* (100%) were resistant to ampicillin followed by cefazolin (80%) and ceftriaxone (70%). All the isolates of *P. aeruginosa* (100%) were susceptible to amikacin, tobramycin and imipenem while 80% of the *P. aeruginosa* isolates were sensitive to ciprofloxacin. In contrast, 40% and 60% of *P. aeruginosa* isolates were resistant to ceftazidime and piperacillin respectively. Similarly, 83.3% (6/5) of *K. pneumoniae* were sensitive to meropenem while 66.7% of isolates were susceptible to ciprofloxacin,

gentamycin and amikacin. A total of 50% of the *K. pneumoniae* isolates were sensitive to cotrimoxazole and ceftriaxone. All the isolates (100%) of both *Proteus vulgaris* and *P. mirabilis* were susceptible to cefotaxime and amikacin. There was 100% resistant of *P. mirabilis* to cotrimoxazole and cefazolin while 50% and 100% of *P. vulgaris* isolates were resistant to cotrimoxazole and cefazolin respectively. All isolates (100%) of *C. freundii* were resistant to ampicillin and cefazolin while 33.3% (1/3) were sensitive to ciprofloxacin, cotrimoxazole, cefotaxime, gentamycin and ceftriaxone (Table 3).

### Antibiogram result of gram positive S. aureus, CoNS, and Enterococcus species

Among total isolated *S. aureus*, 77.3% of *S. aureus* were susceptible to gentamycin, where 75.8% of the isolates were susceptible to cefotaxime. Similarly, 45.5% of *S. aureus* were susceptible to ciprofloxacin while 39.4% of *S. aureus* isolates were susceptible to cefoxitin. Eighty percent of *Enterococcus* spp. were sensitive to tetracycline. (Table 4). Among 66 *S. aureus* isolated from pus swab and aspirated pus, 40 (60.6%) isolates of *S. aureus* were MRSA.

### ESBL producers among Enterobacteriaceae isolates

Among 10 isolates of *E. coli*, 2 (25%) were positive for ESBL and among 6 isolates of *K. pneumoniae*, 2 (40%) were positive for ESBL. Additionally, among 3 isolates of *C. freundii*, 1 (33.3%) was ESBL positive whereas *Proteus* spp. were negative for ESBL (Table 5).

### Antibiogram result of isolates

Eighty percent (80%) of *E. coli* and 68.2% of *S. aureus* were MDR (resistant to two or more than two antimicrobial classes) strains. Similarly, 80% of *P. aeruginosa* and 77.7% of CoNS were MDR strains. Additionally, 83.3% of *K. pneumoniae* isolates were resistant to at least two different classes of used antibiotics. In this study, 50% of *Proteus* spp. isolates were MDR (Table 6).

### Discussion

Aerobic bacteria causing wound infections were isolated and identified from pus specimens by series of biochemical tests and their antimicrobial susceptibility patterns to commonly used antibiotics in study area were examined. Enterobacteriaceae isolates were further processed for confirmation of ESBL producer. In this study, 60.4% of culture positive specimens showed monomicrobial growth, 1.7% showed polymicrobial and 37.9% were negative for aerobic bacterial growth. This finding is consistent with previous studies conducted by Egbe et al. and Kumari et al. [19, 20]. Bhatta et al., [21] have reported 60% of bacterial wound infection from Nepal in 2008. Out of 182 non-repeated samples analyzed, 143 (78.6%) samples were from inpatients, where 98 (68%) were positive for aerobic

**Table 2** Pattern of microbial isolates in wound samples

| Type of organism | Type of Specimens | | | | Total | |
| --- | --- | --- | --- | --- | --- | --- |
| | Pus swab | | Aspirated pus | | | |
| | No. | % | No. | % | No. | % |
| S. aureus | 58 | 58 | 8 | 50 | 66 | 56.9 |
| E. coli | 10 | 10 | – | – | 10 | 8.6 |
| P. aeruginosa | 5 | 5 | – | – | 5 | 4.3 |
| CoNS | 9 | 9 | – | – | 9 | 7.8 |
| Acinetobacter spp. | 6 | 6 | – | – | 6 | 5.2 |
| Enterococcus spp. | 3 | 3 | 2 | 12.5 | 5 | 4.3 |
| C. freundii | 1 | 1 | 2 | 12.5 | 3 | 2.6 |
| K. pneumoniae | 3 | 3 | 3 | 18.7 | 6 | 5.2 |
| P. vulgaris | 2 | 2 | – | – | 2 | 1.6 |
| P. mirabilis | 1 | 1 | – | – | 1 | 0.9 |
| Candida spp. | 2 | 2 | 1 | 6.3 | 3 | 2.6 |
| Total | 100 | 100 | 16 | 100 | 116 | 100 |

**Table 3** Antibiotic susceptibility test result of Gram negative bacteria isolated from pus specimens

| Isolates | Antimicrobial agents | | | | | | | | | |
|---|---|---|---|---|---|---|---|---|---|---|
| | RXN | AMP | AK | CIP | COT | GEN | CTX | CTR | CZ | MRP |
| E.. coli (10) | S | 0 | Nt | 6 (60) | 4 (40) | 8 (80) | 5 (50) | 3 (30) | 2 (20) | Nt |
| | R | 10 (100) | Nt | 4 (40) | 6 (60) | 2 (20) | 5 (50) | 7 (70) | 8 (80) | Nt |
| P. aeruginosa (5) | S | Nt | 5 (100) | 4 (80) | Nt | Nt | Nt | Nt | Nt | Nt |
| | R | Nt | 0 | 1 (20) | Nt | Nt | Nt | Nt | Nt | Nt |
| K. pneumoniae (6) | S | Nt | 4 (66.7) | 4 (66.7) | 3 (50) | 4 (66.7) | Nt | 3 (50) | Nt | 5 (83.3) |
| | R | Nt | 2 (33.3) | 2 (33.3) | 3 (50) | 2 (33.3) | Nt | 3 (50) | Nt | 1 (16.7) |
| P. vulgaris (n = 2) | S | 0 | 2 (100) | 1 (50) | 1 (50) | Nt | 2 (100) | Nt | 0 | Nt |
| | R | 2 (100) | 0 | 1 (50) | 1 (50) | Nt | 0 | Nt | 2 (100) | Nt |
| P. mirabilis (n = 1) | S | 1 (100) | 1 (100) | 1 (100) | 0 | Nt | 1 (100) | Nt | 0 | Nt |
| | R | 0 | 0 | 0 | 1 (100) | Nt | 0 | Nt | 1 (100) | Nt |
| C. freundii (3) | S | 0 | Nt | 1 (33.3) | 1 (33.3) | 1 (33.3) | 1 (33.3) | 1 (33.3) | 0 | Nt |
| | R | 3 (100) | Nt | 2 (66.7) | 2 (66.7) | 2 (66.7) | 2 (66.7) | 2 (66.7) | 3 (100) | Nt |
| Acinetobacter spp. (n = 6) | S | 2 (33.3) | 4 (66.7) | 4 (66.7) | 3 (50) | 4 (66.7) | 3 (50) | Nt | 3 (50) | Nt |
| | R | 4 (66.7) | 2 (33.3) | 2 (33.3) | 3 (50) | 2 (33.3) | 3 (50) | Nt | 3 (50) | Nt |

| Isolates | Antimicrobial agents | | | | | | | | | |
|---|---|---|---|---|---|---|---|---|---|---|
| | RXN | AMP | AK | CIP | CAZ | TOB | IMP | PI | CZ | MRP |
| P. aeruginosa (5) | S | Nt | 5 (100) | 4 (80) | 2 (40) | 5 (100) | 5 (100) | 3 (60) | Nt | Nt |
| | R | Nt | 0 | 1 (20) | 3 (60) | 0 | 0 | 2 (40) | Nt | Nt |
| Total (n = 38) | S | 3 (13.6) | 21 (84) | 25 (65.7) | 14 (42.4) | 22 (73.3) | 17 (63) | 10 (41.7) | 5 (22.7) | 5 (83.3) |
| | R | 19 (86.4) | 4 (16) | 13 (34.3) | 19 (57.6) | 8 (26.7) | 10 (37) | 14 (58.3) | 17 (77.3) | 1 (16.7) |

Nt not tested, S Sensitive, R Resistant, RXN Reaction, AMP Ampicillin, AK Amikacin, CIP Ciprofloxacin, COT trimethoprim + sulfamethoxazole (cotrimoxazole), GEN Gentamicin, CTX Cefotaxime, Caz Ceftazidime, TOB Tobramycin, IMP Imipenem, PI Piperacillin, CTR Ceftriaxone, CZ Cefazolin, MRP Meropenem

bacterial growth. Our finding shows higher rate of wound infection in inpatients (68%) as compare to outpatients (39%) and the result was statistically significant ($p < 0.05$). Similar finding was reported by Stephen et al. [19]. Among 182 specimens collected, 156 (85.7%) were pus swabs with 64% (100/156) aerobic bacterial growth and 26 (14.3%) were aspirated pus where 13 (50%) were positive for aerobic bacterial growth. Shrestha et al., [21] have

found the similar prevalence rate in Nepal before. Pus aspiration is generally taken as sample of choice from deep seated and closed wound infections [22, 23].

Eighty one (44.5%) pus specimens were collected from male patients, while 101 (55.5%) specimens were from female patients and the result was statistically insignificant ($p > 0.05$). In this study, female patients outnumbered the male patients [24] but other studies showed wound

**Table 4** Antibiotic susceptibility test result of Gram positive bacteria isolated from pus specimens

| Isolates | Antimicrobial agents | | | | | | | |
|---|---|---|---|---|---|---|---|---|
| | RXN | AMP | AK | CIP | COT | GEN | CTX | CX | TE |
| S. aureus (n = 66) | S | 5 (7.6) | Nt | 37 (56.1) | 26 (39.4) | 54 (81.8) | 53 (80.3) | 26 (39.4) | 29 (43.9) |
| | R | 61 (92.4) | Nt | 29 (43.9) | 40 (60.6) | 12 (18.2) | 13 (19.7) | 40 (60.6) | 37 (56.1) |
| CoNS (n = 9) | S | 1 (11.1) | Nt | 3 (33.3) | 4 (44.4) | 6 (66.7) | 2 (22.2) | 4 (44.4) | 5 (55.6) |
| | R | 8 (88.9) | Nt | 6 (66.7) | 5 (55.6) | 3 (33.3) | 7 (77.8) | 5 (55.6) | 4 (44.4) |
| Enterococcus spp. (n = 5) | S | 3 (60) | 2 (40) | 3 (60) | 3 (60) | 3 (60) | 3 (60) | Nt | 4 (80) |
| | R | 22 (40) | 3 (60) | 2 (40) | 2 (40) | 2 (40) | 2 (40) | Nt | 1 (20) |
| Total (n = 80) | S | 9 (11.25) | 2 (40) | 43 (53.75) | 33 (41.25) | 63 (78.75) | 58 (72.5) | 30 (40) | 38 (47.5) |
| | R | 71 (88.75) | 3 (60) | 37 (46.25) | 47 (58.75) | 17 (21.25) | 22 (27.5) | 45 (60) | 42 (52.5) |

Nt not tested, S Sensitive, R Resistant, RXN Reaction, AMP Ampicillin, AK Amikacin, CIP Ciprofloxacin, COT trimethoprim + sulfamethoxazole (cotrimoxazole), GEN Gentamicin, CTX Cefotaxime, CX Cefoxitin, TE Tetracycline

**Table 5** ESBL producers among Enterobacteriaceae

| Bacterial isolates | Total | ESBL producer | |
|---|---|---|---|
| | | No. | % |
| E. coli | 10 | 2 | 25.0 |
| K. pneumoniae | 6 | 2 | 40.0 |
| P. vulgaris | 2 | 0 | 0 |
| P. mirabilis | 1 | 0 | 0 |
| C. freundii | 3 | 1 | 33.3 |

infection was higher in male as compared to female [25, 26]. In our study, lower number of male patients (44.5%) might be due to small sample size as compared to other studies. In this study, monomicrobial growth (97.3%) was higher than polymicrobial growth (2.7%) both in pus swab and aspirated pus. Multiple studies carried out in wound infections have shown higher rate of monomicrobial infection than polymicrobial infection [27]. Similarly a high rate (86–100%) of monomicrobial wound infection was reported from different states of India [28, 29].

Among different age groups, the prevalence of wound infections was highest among age group ≤10 years (82.1%) followed by age group 70–80 years (77.8%). This is in agreement with study carried by Lakhey et al. where higher prevalence of wound infection was reported among patients of age group 60–80 years [20]. Similarly, in a study done by Mohammedaman et al., [5] in South Ethiopia, 87.5% wound infection was in patients with age ≥ 60 years. Since old individuals and children have weak immunity,

that might be the reason for them being more prone to wound infections. Ranjan et al. have reported more pathogenic strains from patients of age group 21–40 years in post-operative wound infections in India [30].

Among 116 bacterial isolates, 11 different species were identified. S. aureus (56.9%) was the most common isolate followed by E. coli (8.6%) and CoNS (7.8%). Other identified bacteria from pus specimens included P. aeruginosa (4.3%), Acinetobacter spp. (5.2%), Enterococcus spp. (4.3%), C. freundii (2.6%), K. pneumoniae (5.2%), P. vulgaris (1.6%), and P. mirabilis (0.9%). The predominance of S. aureus in wound infection is supported by different studies [21, 30]. As being a normal flora of human skin, it can get access into the wound easily. Kansakar et al., [32] have reported that 82.5% of bacterial growth in pus samples and 13 different bacterial species were isolated where S. aureus was predominant (57.7%) species followed by E. coli (11%) and CoNS (3%). According to Mumtaz et al., [33] S. aureus was the most common bacteria (49%) found in wound infections followed by E. coli (25.9%), Klebsiella spp. (9.5%), P. aeruginosa (8.6%), Proteus spp. (4%) and Acinetobacter (2.7%) spp. S. aureus is the most common strain (25%) as a commensal organism of human skin and nasal passage. Hence, most frequent isolation of S. aureus from pus specimens might also be due to contamination of collected specimens with skin normal flora [31]. Contribution of multidrug resistant Acinetobacter spp. to nosocomial infections has increased over the past decade, and many outbreaks involving this bacterium have been reported worldwide [32].

**Table 6** Antibiogram result of isolates

| Isolated organisms | Antibiogram | | | | | Total MDR [N(%)] |
|---|---|---|---|---|---|---|
| | No. (%) of resistance | | | | | |
| | R2 | R3 | R4 | R5 | | |
| Gram positive | | | | | | |
| S. aureus (n = 66) | 20 (30.3) | 18 (27.3) | 3 (4.5) | 4 (6.1) | | 45 (68.2) |
| CoNS (n = 9) | 4 (44.4) | 1 (11.1) | 2 (22.2) | 0 | | 7 (77.7) |
| Enterococcus spp. (n = 5) | 3 (60) | 0 | 1 (20) | 0 | | 4 (80) |
| Total (n = 80) | 27 (33.75) | 19 (23.75) | 6 (7.5) | 4 (5) | | 56 (70) |
| Gram negative | | | | | | |
| E. coli (n = 10) | 6 (60) | 1 (10) | 0 | 1 (10) | | 8 (80) |
| P. aeruginosa (n = 5) | 2 (40) | 1 (20) | 1 (20) | 0 | | 4 (80) |
| Acinetobacter spp. (n = 6) | 2 (33.3) | 1 (16.7) | 1 (16.7) | 0 | | 4 (66.7) |
| C. freundii (n = 3) | 2 (66.7) | 0 | 0 | 0 | | 2 (66.7) |
| K. pneumoniae (n = 6) | 2 (33.3) | 1 (16.7) | 0 | 2 (33.3) | | 5 (83.3) |
| P. vulgaris (n = 2) | 1 (50) | 0 | 0 | 0 | | 1 (50) |
| P. mirabilis (n = 1) | 1 (50) | 0 | 0 | 0 | | 1 (50) |
| Total (n = 33) | 10 (30.3) | 3 (9.1) | 2 (6.1) | 2 (6.1) | | 17 (51.5) |

R2-R5 number of antibiotics class where an isolate was resistant

Shrestha et al., [21] have found that 85% of *S. aureus* isolates were sensitive to ciprofloxacin, 83% and 82% were sensitive to cephalexin and cotrimoxazole respectively. In this study, 60.6% of Staphylococci isolates were resistant to cefoxitin. *S. aureus* which was resistant to cefoxitin antibiotic was reported as MRSA species. Rajbhandari et al., [36] have also reported 61.6% of MRSA prevalence in wound infection. The second common isolate of this study was *E. coli* where 80%, 60%, 50% and 40% of the isolates were susceptible to gentamycin, ciprofloxacin, cefotaxime and cotrimoxazole respectively. All the isolates of *E. coli* (100%) were resistant to ampicillin where 30% and 20% were resistant to ceftriaxone and cefazolin respectively. Similarly, 60% and 40% of *E. coli* isolates were susceptible to ciprofloxacin and cotrimoxazole respectively. This study showed low sensitivity rate as compared to other studies [33]. Hence, increased antimicrobial resistant rate of *E. coli* depicts its important role in nosocomial infections.

All the isolates of *P. aeruginosa* (100%) were sensitive to amikacin, tobramycin and imipenem while 80% and 60% were sensitive to ciprofloxacin and piperacillin respectively. Only 40% of the *P. aeruginosa* were susceptible to the antibiotic ceftazidime. In a study conducted by Shrestha et al., [21] 93% of isolates were sensitive to amikacin and 66.7% of isolates were sensitive to ciprofloxacin. Our finding in this context is similar with other results where *P. aeruginosa* isolated from pus samples has shown least resistance to ciprofloxacin (6.2–24%) [34]. More prevalence of antimicrobial resistant *P. aeruginosa* in wound infection is being a challenging issue especially in resource limited countries [26].

*K. pneumoniae* was most sensitive to meropenem (83.3%) and 66.7% of *K. pneumoniae* isolates were equally resistant to gentamycin, ciprofloxacin, and amikacin where 50% of isolated *K. pneumoniae* were resistant to cotrimoxazole and ceftriaxone. In a study reported by Mohammedaman et al., [5] 35.7% of *K. pneumoniae* were resistant to ciprofloxacin and doxycycline. Furthermore, Rajput et al., [24] had reported that 45.5% and 80% of *K. pneumoniae* strains were resistant to ciprofloxacin and cotrimoxazole respectively. All isolates (100%) of *P. vulgaris* were susceptible to amikacin, and cefotaxime but 100% of *P. vulgaris* isolates were resistant to ampicillin and cefazolin while 50% of isolated *P. vulgaris* were resistant to ciprofloxacin and cotrimoxazole. All isolates (100%) of *P. mirabilis* were sensitive to ciprofloxacin, amikacin and cefotaxime whereas 100% were resistant to ampicillin, cotrimoxazole and cefazolin. This result is comparable with study carried by Bhatta et al. [20].

Among Enterobacteriaceae isolates, 25% of *E. coli*, 40% of *K. pneumoniae* and 33.3% of *C. freundii* were ESBL producer. But none of the *Proteus* species were ESBL producer. Chander et al., [35] have reported 13.51% and 16.55% of *E. coli* and *K. pneumoniae* as ESBL producer

respectively. The prevalence rate may vary based on sample collection method, site of sample collection, microbial detection technique, antimicrobial agents used, and geographical location. In this study, 68.2% of *S. aureus* and 80% of *E. coli* isolates were MDR strains. The highest rate (83.3%) of MDR was observed in *K. pneumoniae*. This finding is in agreement with the study conducted in South-West Ethiopia by Mohammedaman et al. [5]. Most of the Gram negative isolates were resistant to ampicillin (86.4%) and cefazolin (77.3%) while 88.6% and 60% of Gram positive bacteria were resistant to ampicillin and amikacin respectively. In Nepal, oral administration of antibiotics is common practice which may reduce absorption of antibiotics by blood stream. Long term use of antibiotics via oral route could contribute to bacteria developing resistance.

Wound infection is a burning public health issue especially in developing countries. Severe wound infection can cause great loss including higher rate of morbidity and mortality; longer hospital stays, delay in wound healing, increase economic burden and increase discomfort which in turn increases disease burden significantly. Wound infection is being a common nosocomial infections which accounts for 0–80% of patient's mortality [35, 36].

Modernization in control and prevention of infections has not completely controlled wound infection due to increasing problem of antimicrobial resistance [37]. As compared to previous studies, antimicrobial resistance pattern is increasing at high rate. Multiple factors may contribute to rapid development of antimicrobial resistance by pathogens including misuse, overuse, and underuse of antimicrobials by both clinicians and patients. In Nepal, people purchase antimicrobials without physician's prescription, which is a common practice. This leads to misuse of antimicrobials that contributes to the emergence and spread of antimicrobial resistant strain. MRSA and ESBL producing bacteria are creating a serious problem in wound treatment in different parts of the country.

## Conclusion

In this study, the most common isolate was *S. aureus* in pus specimens. Among *S. aureus* isolates, 60.6% were MRSA strains, whereas 40% of *K. pneumoniae* and 33.3% *C. freundii* were ESBL producer followed by *E. coli* (25%). Eighty percent (80%) of *E. coli*, *P. aeruginosa*, and 68.2% of *S. aureus* were MDR strains. This study emphasizes the importance of strict nosocomial infection control strategies and careful prescription of antimicrobials should be implemented by the health care centres. It should be mandatory to screen out ESBL, MRSA, and MDR pathogens and regular monitoring of their antimicrobial susceptibility pattern for prevention and control of wound infections. Early reporting of drug resistant pathogens and evidence-based treatment algorithm can control the wound infections. Research on AMR is in its infancy stage in Nepal, but it is paramount to establish surveillance programs to reduce burden of wound infections.

## Abbreviations
AMR: Antimicrobial resistance; AST: Antibiotic susceptibility test; ATCC: American type culture collection; CDC: Centers for disease control and prevention; CLSI: Clinical laboratory standard institute; CoNS: Coagulase negative Staphylococci; DDST: Double disc synergy test; ENT: Eye-Nose-Throat; ESBL: Extended spectrum β-lactamase; FNAC: Fine needle aspiration cytology; MDR: Multi-drug resistant; MHA: Mueller Hinton agar; MRSA: Methicillin resistant Staphylococcus aureus; SPSS: Statistical package for the social sciences; WHO: World health organization; ZOI: Zone of inhibition; μg: Micro gram

## Acknowledgements
We would like to acknowledge KIST Medical College and Teaching Hospital, and all the staff of pathology department for guiding the study and Hi Media Pvt. Ltd., India- who provided antibiotic discs for the antimicrobial susceptibility tests.

## Authors' contributions
First author: NU is primary author who designed the study methodology, performed laboratory investigations and prepare the manuscript. Second authors: MRB and MKC helped for design the study, analysis of results, proof reading of article, manage necessary arrangements during laboratory investigations and supervised the complete study. BR and SS edited, proof read, helped in data analysis and revised the complete manuscript for submission. All authors approved the final manuscript before submission to the Antimicrobial Resistance & Infection Control.

## Consent for publication
Not applicable.

## Competing interests
The authors declare they do not have any competing interests.

## Author details
[1]Central Department of Microbiology, Tribhuvan University, Kirtipur, Nepal. [2]National College (Tribhuvan University), Khusibu, Kathmandu, Nepal. [3]Department of Infectious Diseases and Immunology, Kathmandu Research Institute for Biological Sciences (KRIBS), Lalitpur, Nepal. [4]Department of Global Environmental Health Sciences, School of Public Health and Tropical Medicine, Tulane University, New Orleans, LA, USA. [5]KIST Medical College and Teaching Hospital, Imadole, Lalitpur, Nepal.

## References
1. Moet GJ, Jones RN, Biedenbach DJ, Stilwell MG, Fritsche TR. Contemporary causes of skin and soft tissue infections in North America, Latin America, and Europe: report from the SENTRY antimicrobial surveillance program (1998–2004). Diagn Microbiol Infect Dis. 2007;57(1):7–13.
2. Oluwatosin OM. Surgical wound infection: a general overview. Ann Ibadan Postgrad Med. 2005;3(2):26–31.
3. Collier M. Wound-bed management: key principles for practice. Professional nurse (London, England) 2002;18(4):221–225.
4. Forbes BA, Sahm DF, Weissfeld AS. Overview of bacterial identification methods and strategies. Bailey and Scott's Diagnostic Microbiology. 12. Mosby Elsevier, Missouri. 2007:216–247.
5. Mama M, Abdissa A, Sewunet T. Antimicrobial susceptibility pattern of bacterial isolates from wound infection and their sensitivity to alternative topical agents at Jimma University specialized hospital, south-West Ethiopia. Ann Clin Microbiol Antimicrob. 2014;13(1):14.
6. Brook IT, Frazier EH. The aerobic and anaerobic bacteriology of perirectal abscesses. J Clin Microbiol. 1997;35(11):2974–6.
7. Liu SS, Richman JM, Thirlby RC, Wu CL. Efficacy of continuous wound catheters delivering local anesthetic for postoperative analgesia: a quantitative and qualitative systematic review of randomized controlled trials. J Am Coll Surg. 2006;203(6):914–32.
8. Centers for Disease Control and Prevention (CDC). Soft tissue infections among injection drug users-San Francisco, California, 1996-2000. MMWR Morb Mortal Wkly Rep. 2001;50(19):381.
9. Steed LL, Costello J, Lohia S, Jones T, Spannhake EW, Nguyen S. Reduction of nasal Staphylococcus aureus carriage in health care professionals by treatment with a nonantibiotic, alcohol-based nasal antiseptic. Am J Infect Control. 2014;42(8):841–6.
10. Cohen ML. Changing patterns of infectious disease. Nature. 2000;406(6797):762.
11. Weigelt J, Itani K, Stevens D, Lau W, Dryden M, Knirsch C. Linezolid CSSTI study group. Linezolid versus vancomycin in treatment of complicated skin and soft tissue infections. Antimicrob Agents Chemother. 2005;49(6):2260–6.
12. Jacoby GA. AmpC β-lactamases. Clin Microbiol Rev. 2009;22(1):161–82.
13. Bush K. Extended-spectrum β-lactamases in North America, 1987–2006. Clinical Microbiology and Infection. 2008;14:134–43.
14. Magiorakos AP, Srinivasan A, Carey RB, Carmeli Y, Falagas ME, Giske CG, Harbarth S, Hindler JF, Kahlmeter G, Olsson-Liljequist B, Paterson DL. Multidrug-resistant, extensively drug-resistant and pandrug-resistant bacteria: an international expert proposal for interim standard definitions for acquired resistance. Clin Microbiol Infect. 2012;18(3):268–81.
15. Smith, A.C., Hussey, M.A., 2005. Gram stain protocols.
16. Wayne PACLSI. Performance standards for antimicrobial susceptibility testing; twenty-fifth informational supplement. CLSI document M100-S25. In: Clinical and laboratory standards institute; 2015.
17. Wayne PA. Clinical and laboratory standards institute. Performance standards for antimicrobial susceptibility testing, vol. 17; 2007.
18. Harwalkar A, Sataraddi J, Gupta S, Yoganand R, Rao A, Srinivasa H. The detection of ESBL-producing Escherichia coli in patients with symptomatic urinary tract infections using different diffusion methods in a rural setting. J Infect Public Health. 2013;6(2):108–14.
19. Mshana SE, Kamugisha E, Mirambo M, Chakraborty T, Lyamuya EF. Prevalence of multiresistant gram-negative organisms in a tertiary hospital in Mwanza, Tanzania. BMC Res Notes. 2009;2(1):49.
20. Kumari K. Pattern of bacterial isolates and antibiogram from open wound infection among the indoor patients of Bir Hospital (Doctoral dissertation, M. Sc. Dissertation, Central Department of Microbiology, Tribhuvan University, Kirtipur, Kathmandu, Nepal).
21. CPa B, Mb L. The distribution of pathogens causing wound infection and their antibiotic susceptibility pattern. J Nepal Health Res Counc. 2008;5(1):22–6.
22. Parikh AR, Hamilton S, Sivarajan V, Withey S, Butler PE. Diagnostic fine-needle aspiration in postoperative wound infections is more accurate at predicting causative organisms than wound swabs. Ann R Coll Surg England. 2007;89(2):166–7.
23. Bowler PG, Duerden BI, Armstrong DG. Wound microbiology and associated approaches to wound management. Clin Microbiol Rev. 2001;14(2):244–69.
24. Rajput A, Singh KP, Kumar V, Sexena R, Singh RK. Antibacterial resistance pattern of aerobic bacteria isolates from burn patients in tertiary care hospital. Biomedical research. 2008;19(1). http://www.alliedacademies.org/biomedical-research/archive/aabmr-volume-19-issue-1-year-2008.html.
25. Gelaw A, Gebre-Selassie S, Tiruneh M, Mathios E, Yifru S. Isolation of bacterial pathogens from patients with postoperative surgical site infections and possible sources of infections at the University of Gondar Hospital, Northwest Ethiopia. J Environ Occup Sci. 2014;3(2):103–8.
26. Goswami NN, Trivedi HR, Goswami AP, Patel TK, Tripathi CB. Antibiotic sensitivity profile of bacterial pathogens in postoperative wound infections at a tertiary care hospital in Gujarat, India. J Pharmacol Pharmacother. 2011;2(3):158.
27. Komolafe OO, James J, Kalongolera L, Makoka M. Bacteriology of burns at the queen elizabeth central hospital, Blantyre, Malawi. Burns. 2003;29(3):235–8.
28. Sanjay KR, Prasad MN, Vijaykumar GS. A study on isolation and detection of drug resistance gram negative bacilli with special importance to post operative wound infection. J Microbiol Antimicrob. 2011;3(9):68–75.
29. Lakshmidevi N. Surgical site infections: assessing risk factors, outcomes and antimicrobial sensitivity patterns. Afr J Microbiol Res. 2009;3(4):175–9.
30. Mulu W, Kibru G, Beyene G, Damtie M. Postoperative nosocomial infections and antimicrobial resistance pattern of bacteria isolates among patients

admitted at Felege Hiwot referral hospital, Bahirdar, Ethiopia. Ethiop J Health Sci. 2012;22(1):7–18.

31. Adegoke AA, Komolafe AO. Nasal colonization of school children in Ile-Ife by multiple antibiotic resistant *Staphylococcus aureus*. Int J Biotechnol Allied Sci. 2008;3(1):317–22.

32. Forster, D.H. and Daschner, F.D., 1998. *Acinetobacter* species as nosocomial pathogens.

33. Biadglegne F, Abera B, Alem A, Anagaw B. Bacterial isolates from wound infection and their antimicrobial susceptibility pattern in Felege Hiwot referral Hospital North West Ethiopia. Ethiop J Health Sci. 2009;19(3):173–177.

34. Manyahi J. Bacteriological spectrum of post operative wound infections and their antibiogram in a Tertiary Hospital, Dar Es Salaam, Tanzania (Doctoral dissertation, Muhimbili University of Health and Allied Sciences).

35. Gottrup F, Melling A, Hollander DA. An overview of surgical site infections: aetiology, incidence and risk factors. EWMA J. 2005;5(2):11–5.

36. Howell-Jones RS, Wilson MJ, Hill KE, Howard AJ, Price PE, Thomas DW. A review of the microbiology, antibiotic usage and resistance in chronic skin wounds. J Antimicrob Chemother. 2005;55(2):143–9.

37. Heinzelmann M, Scott M, Lam T. Factors predisposing to bacterial invasion and infection. Am J Surg. 2002;183(2):179–90.

# Permissions

# List of Contributors

**Pooja Maharjan, Hridaya Parajuli, Govardhan Joshi and Deliya Paudel**
Department of Clinical Laboratory Services, Manmohan Memorial Medical College and Teaching Hospital, Swayambhu, Kathmandu, Nepal

**Narayan Prasad Parajuli**
Department of Clinical Laboratory Services, Manmohan Memorial Medical College and Teaching Hospital, Swayambhu, Kathmandu, Nepal
Department of Laboratory Medicine, Manmohan Memorial Institute of Health Sciences, Kathmandu, Nepal

**Sujan Sayami**
Department of Pediatrics, Manmohan Memorial Medical College and Teaching Hospital, Kathmandu, Nepal

**Puspa Raj Khanal**
Department of Laboratory Medicine, Manmohan Memorial Institute of Health Sciences, Kathmandu, Nepal

**Elisabetta Nucleo, Mariasofia Caltagirone, Vittoria Mattioni Marchetti and Roberta Migliavacca**
Department of Clinical Surgical Diagnostic and Pediatric Sciences, Laboratory of Microbiology and Clinical Microbiology, University of Pavia, Via Brambilla 74, 27100 Pavia, Italy

**Roberto D'Angelo and Elena Fogato**
Laboratory of Clinical Microbiology, ASP "Golgi-Redaelli", via Bartolomeo d'Alviano 78, 20146 Milan, Italy

**Massimo Confalonieri and Camilla Reboli**
O.U. of Microbiology, Azienda Sanitaria Locale di Piacenza, Piacenza, Italy

**Albert March, Ferisa Sleghel and Gertrud Soelva**
Geriatric Unit, Comprensorio Sanitario di Bolzano, Bolzano, Italy

**Elisabetta Pagani and Richard Aschbacher**
Microbiology and Virology Laboratory, Comprensorio Sanitario di Bolzano, Bolzano, Italy

**Teysir Halaby and Roel Verkooijen**
Laboratory for Medical Microbiology and Public Health, Boerhaavelaan 59, 7555, BB, Hengelo, The Netherlands

**Nashwan al Naiemi**
Laboratory for Medical Microbiology and Public Health, Boerhaavelaan 59, 7555, BB, Hengelo, The Netherlands
Department of Medical Microbiology & Infection Control, VU University Medical Center, Amsterdam, The Netherlands
Medical Microbiology and Infection Control, Ziekenhuisgroep Twente, Almelo, The Netherlands

**Rob Klont**
Laboratory for Medical Microbiology and Public Health, Boerhaavelaan 59, 7555, BB, Hengelo, The Netherlands
Department of intensive care, Medisch Spectrum Twente, Enschede, The Netherlands

**Christina vandenbroucke-Grauls**
Department of Medical Microbiology & Infection Control, VU University Medical Center, Amsterdam, The Netherlands

**Bert Beishuizen**
Department of intensive care, Medisch Spectrum Twente, Enschede, The Netherlands

**José A. Ferreira**
Department of Statistics, Informatics and Modelling, National Institute for Public Health and the Environment, RIVM, Bilthoven, The Netherlands

**Maha Al Ammari and Abdulrahman Al Turaiki**
King Abdullah International Medical Research Center (KAIMRC)/King Abdulaziz Medical City(KAMC), Ministry of National Guard - Health Affairs, Riyadh, Saudi Arabia

**Mohammed Al Essa**
King Abdullah International Medical Research Center (KAIMRC)/King Abdulaziz Medical City(KAMC), Ministry of National Guard - Health Affairs, Riyadh, Saudi Arabia
College of Pharmacy, King Saud bin Abdulaziz University for Health Sciences, Riyadh, Saudi Arabia

**Abdulhameed M. Kashkary and Sara A. Eltigani**
Ministry of Health Kingdom of Saudi Arabia, Riyadh, Saudi Arabia

**Anwar E. Ahmed**
College of Public Health and Health Informatics, King Saud bin Abdulaziz University for Health Sciences, Riyadh, Saudi Arabia

**Jade E. McLellan and Joshua I. Pitcher**
Department of Medicine, Austin Health, University of Melbourne, Melbourne, VIC, Australia

**M. Lindsay Grayson**
Department of Medicine, Austin Health, University of Melbourne, Melbourne, VIC, Australia
Infectious Diseases & Microbiology Departments, Austin Health, Melbourne, VIC, Australia
Department of Epidemiology and Preventive Medicine, Monash University, Melbourne, VIC, Australia

**Susan A. Ballard and Elizabeth A. Grabsch**
Infectious Diseases & Microbiology Departments, Austin Health, Melbourne, VIC, Australia

**Jan M. Bell**
Infectious Diseases and Microbiology, SA Pathology, Adelaide, South Australia, Australia

**Mary Barton**
School of Pharmacy and Medical Sciences, University of South Australia, Adelaide, South Australia, Australia

**I-Wen Lin**
Department of Family Medicine, National Taiwan University Hospital, Bei-Hu Branch, No.87, Neijiang Street, Taipei City 10845, Taiwan

**Chiao-Yu Huang**
Department of Family Medicine, Renai Branch, No.10, Sec. 4, Ren'ai Rd., Da'an Dist, Taipei City 106, Taiwan, Republic of China
Institute of Health Policy and Management, National Taiwan University, No. 1, Sec. 4, Roosevelt Rd, Taipei 10617, Taiwan, Republic of China

**Sung-Ching Pan**
Department of Internal Medicine, National Taiwan University Hospital, No.7, Zhongshan S. Rd., Zhongzheng Dist, Taipei City 100, Taiwan, Republic of China

**Yng-Chyi Chen**
Department of Nursing, National Taiwan University Hospital, Bei-Hu Branch, No.87, Neijiang Street, Taipei City 10845, Taiwan

**Chia-Ming Li**
Department of Family Medicine, National Taiwan University Hospital, Bei-Hu Branch, No.87, Neijiang Street, Taipei City 10845, Taiwan

**Bothyna Ghanem and Randa Nayef Haddadin**
Department of Pharmaceutics and Pharmaceutical Technology, School of Pharmacy, The University of Jordan, Amman 11942, Jordan

**Wei Guo, Shao-Chun Guo, Min Li, Li-Hong Li and Yan Qu**
Department of Neurosurgery, Tangdu Hospital, Fourth Military Medical University, Xi'an, Shaanxi 710038, China

**Qingchun Li, Gang Zhao, Limin Wu, Min Lu, Wei Liu, Yifei Wu, Le Wang, Ke Wang and Li Xie**
Hangzhou Center for Disease Control and Prevention, Mingshi Road, Hangzhou City 310021, Zhejiang Province, China

**Han-ZhuQian**
Department of Biostatistics, Yale School of Public Health, New Haven, Connecticut, USA

**Ralph Tayyar and Jad Sfeir**
Department of Internal Medicine, Division of Infectious Diseases, American University of Beirut, Cairo Street Riad El Solh, Beirut 1107 2020, Lebanon

**Zeina A. Kanafani and Souha S. Kanj**
Department of Internal Medicine, Division of Infectious Diseases, American University of Beirut, Cairo Street Riad El Solh, Beirut 1107 2020, Lebanon
Infection Control and Prevention Program, American University of Beirut, Cairo Street Riad El Solh, Beirut 1107 2020, Lebanon

**Nada Zahreddine**
Infection Control and Prevention Program, American University of Beirut, Cairo Street Riad El Solh, Beirut 1107 2020, Lebanon

**George F. Araj**
Department of Pathology and Laboratory Medicine, American University of Beirut, Cairo Street Riad El Solh, Beirut 1107 2020, Lebanon

**Ghassan M. Matar**
Department of Experimental Pathology, Microbiology and Immunology, American University of Beirut, Cairo Street Riad El Solh, Beirut 1107 2020, Lebanon

**Ines Zollner-Schwetz, Elisabeth Zechner and Robert Krause**
Department of Internal Medicine, Section of Infectious Diseases and Tropical Medicine, Medical University of Graz, Auenbruggerplatz 15, A-8036 Graz, Austria

**Elisabeth Ullrich, Josefa Luxner and Eva Leitner**
Institute of Hygiene, Microbiology and Environmental Medicine, Medical University of Graz, Graz, Austria

**Christian Pux, Gerald Pichler and Walter Schippinger**
Geriatric Health Centers of the City of Graz, Graz, Austria

**Andreas F. Widmer**
Department of Infectious Diseases and Hospital Epidemiology, University Hospital Basel, 4051 Basel, Switzerland

**Danielle Vuichard Gysin**
Department of Infectious Diseases and Hospital Epidemiology, University Hospital Basel, 4051 Basel, Switzerland
Department of Internal Medicine, Cantonal Hospital Thurgau, Muensterlingen, Switzerland

**Barry Cookson**
Division of Infection and Immunity, University College London, London, UK

**Henri Saenz**
ESCMID Executive Office, Basel, Switzerland

**Markus Dettenkofer**
Institute of Hospital Hygiene and Infection Prevention, Gesundheitsverbund Landkreis Konstanz, Radolfzell, Germany

**Xiaofang Huang, Yesong Wang, Wei Cui and Gensheng Zhang**
Department of Critical Care Medicine, Second Affiliated Hospital, Zhejiang University School of Medicine, Hangzhou, Zhejiang 310009, People's Republic of China

**Sijun Pan**
Department of Critical Care Medicine, Second Affiliated Hospital, Zhejiang University School of Medicine, Hangzhou, Zhejiang 310009, People's Republic of China
Department of Critical Care Medicine, Anji County People's Hospital, Huzhou, Zhejiang Province 313300, China

**Zhongxiang Yao**
Department of Critical Care Medicine, Anji County People's Hospital, Huzhou, Zhejiang Province 313300, China

**Li Li and Changyun Zhao**
Department of Critical Care Medicine, Zhejiang Hospital, Hangzhou 310013, China

**Jean Uwingabiye, Abdelhay Lemnouer, Mohammed Frikh, Bouchra Belefquih, Fatna Bssaibis, Adil Maleb, Yassine Benlahlou, Jalal Kassouati, Lhoussain Louzi and Mostafa Elouennass**
Department of Clinical Bacteriology, Mohammed V Military Teaching Hospital, Research Team of Epidemiology and Bacterial Resistance, Faculty of Medicine and Pharmacy, Mohammed V University, Rabat, Morocco

**Ignasi Roca and Jordi Vila**
Department of Clinical Microbiology and ISGlobal-Barcelona Ctr. Int. Health Res. CRESIB, Hospital Clínic - Universitat de Barcelona, Barcelona, Spain

**Tarek Alouane and Azeddine Ibrahimi**
Medical Biotechnology Laboratory (Medbiotech), Faculty of Medicine and Pharmacy, Mohammed V University, Rabat, Morocco

**Nawfal Doghmi, Abdelouahed Bait and Charki Haimeur**
Department of Intensive Care Units, Mohammed V Military Teaching Hospital, Faculty of Medicine and Pharmacy, Mohammed V University, Rabat, Morocco

**Nicholas Agyepong, Usha Govinden and Sabiha Yusuf Essack**
Antimicrobial Research Unit, Discipline of Pharmaceutical Sciences, University of Kwa-Zulu Natal, Durban, South Africa

**Alex Owusu-Ofori**
School of Medical Sciences, Kwame Nkrumah University of Science and Technology, Kumasi, Ghana

**Fithamlak Bisetegen Solomon**
School of Medicine, Wolaita Sodo University, Sodo, Ethiopia

**Fiseha Wadilo**
Wolaita Sodo University, School of Medicine, Sodo, Ethiopia

**Efrata Girma Tufa**
Department of medical laboratory, Wolaita Sodo University, Sodo, Ethiopia

**Meseret Mitiku**
College of health science and medicine, school of medicine, MaddaWalabu University, Bale Goba, Ethiopia

**Gowri Raman, Esther E. Avendano and Jeffrey Chan**
Center for Clinical Evidence Synthesis, Tufts Medical Center, 800 Washington Street, Boston, MA 02111, USA

**Sanjay Merchant and Laura Puzniak**
Merck & Co., Inc., Kenilworth, NJ, USA

**Melkamu Berhane**
Department of Pediatrics and Child Health, Jimma University, Jimma, Ethiopia

**Sisay Bekele**
Department of Ophthalmology, Jimma University, Jimma, Ethiopia

**Yonas Yilma**
Department of Surgery, Jimma University, Jimma, Ethiopia

**Netsanet Fentahun**
Department of Health Education and Behavioral Health, Jimma University, Jimma, Ethiopia

**Henok Assefa**
Department of Epidemiology and Statistics, Jimma University, Jimma, Ethiopia

**Aina Gomila, Evelyn Shaw and Miquel Pujol**
Department of Infectious Diseases, Hospital Universitari de Bellvitge, Institut Català de la Salut (ICS-HUB), Feixa Llarga s/n, L'Hospitalet de Llobregat, 08907 Barcelona, Spain
Spanish Network for Research in Infectious Diseases (REIPI RD12/0015), Instituto de Salud Carlos III, Madrid, Spain

Institut d'Investigació Biomèdica de Bellvitge (IDIBELL), Feixa Llarga s/n, L'Hospitalet de Llobregat, 08907 Barcelona, Spain

**Jordi Carratalà**
Department of Infectious Diseases, Hospital Universitari de Bellvitge, Institut Català de la Salut (ICS-HUB), Feixa Llarga s/n, L'Hospitalet de Llobregat, 08907 Barcelona, Spain
Spanish Network for Research in Infectious Diseases (REIPI RD12/0015), Instituto de Salud Carlos III, Madrid, Spain
Institut d'Investigació Biomèdica de Bellvitge (IDIBELL), Feixa Llarga s/n, L'Hospitalet de Llobregat, 08907 Barcelona, Spain
University of Barcelona, Barcelona, Spain

**Cristian Tebé**
Institut d'Investigació Biomèdica de Bellvitge (IDIBELL), Feixa Llarga s/n, L'Hospitalet de Llobregat, 08907 Barcelona, Spain

**Leonard Leibovici and Noa Eliakim-Raz**
Department of Medicine E, Beilinson Hospital, Rabin Medical Center, Petah Tikva; Sackler Faculty of Medicine, Tel Aviv University, Tel Aviv, Israel

**Irith Wiegand, Christiane Vank, Cuong Vuong and Ibironke Addy**
AiCuris Anti-infective Cures GmbH, Wuppertal, Germany

**Laura Vallejo-Torres and Stephen Morris**
UCL Department of Applied Health Research, University College London, London, UK

**Joan M. Vigo**
Informatics Unit, Fundació Institut Català de Farmacologia, Barcelona, Spain

**Margaret Stoddart, Sally Grier and Alasdair MacGowan**
Department of Medical Microbiology, Southmead Hospital, North Bristol NHS Trust, Bristol, UK

**Nienke Cuperus and Leonard Van den Heuvel**
Julius Center for Health Sciences and Primary Care, University Medical Center Utrecht, Utrecht, Netherlands

**Shraddha Siwakoti, Abhilasha Sharma, Ratna Baral, Narayan Raj Bhattarai and Basudha Khanal**
Department of Microbiology, B. P. Koirala Institute of Health Sciences, Dharan 56700, Nepal

**Asish Subedi**
Department of Anaesthesiology and Critical care, B. P. Koirala Institute of Health Sciences, Dharan, Nepal

**Hélène Mascitti, Clara Duran, Elisabeth-Marie Nemo, Ruxandra Câlin, Alexis Descatha, Benjamin Davido and Aurélien Dinh**
Infectious disease unit, Raymond Poincaré University Hospital, AP-HP, Versailles Saint-Quentin University, 104 Bd R. Poincaré, 92380 Garches, France

**Frédérique Bouchand**
Pharmacy department, Raymond Poincaré University Hospital, AP-HP, Versailles Saint-Quentin University, 104 Bd R. Poincaré, 92380 Garches, France

**Jean-Louis Gaillard and Christine Lawrence**
Microbiological laboratory, Raymond Poincaré University Hospital, AP-HP, Versailles Saint-Quentin University, 104 Bd R. Poincaré, 92380 Garches, France

**François Barbier**
Intensive care unit, Orléans Hospital, 14 Avenue de l'Hôpital, 45067 Orléans, France

**Katie R. Margulieux, Apichai Srijan, Sirigade Ruekit, Panida Nobthai, Kamonporn Poramathikul, Oralak Serichantalergs and Ladaporn Bodhidatta**
Department of Enteric Diseases, Armed Forces Research Institute of Medical Sciences, 315/6 Rajvithee Road, Bangkok 10400, Thailand

**Brett E. Swierczewski**
Department of Enteric Diseases, Armed Forces Research Institute of Medical Sciences, 315/6 Rajvithee Road, Bangkok 10400, Thailand
Present Address: Bacterial Diseases Branch, Walter Reed Army Institute of Research, Silver Spring, MD, USA

**Prativa Pandey**
CIWEC Hospital and Travel Medicine Clinic, Kathmandu, Nepal

**Sanjaya K. Shrestha**
Walter Reed/AFRIMS Research Unit Nepal, Kathmandu, Nepal

**Luise Hutzschenreuter and Steffen Flessa**
Institute of Health Care Management, University of Greifswald, Friedrich-Loeffler-Str. 70, 17489 Greifswald, Germany

**Kathleen Dittmann**
Institute of Hygiene and Environmental Health, University Medicine of Greifswald, Walther-Rathenau-Straße 49a, 17489 Greifswald, Germany

**Nils-Olaf Hübner**
Institute of Hygiene and Environmental Health, University Medicine of Greifswald, Walther-Rathenau-Straße 49a, 17489 Greifswald, Germany
IMD Laboratory Greifswald MVZ GmbH, Vitus-Bering-Straße 27a, 17493 Greifswald, Germany

**Narbada Upreti and Megha Raj Banjara**
Central Department of Microbiology, Tribhuvan University, Kirtipur, Nepal

**Binod Rayamajhee**
National College (Tribhuvan University), Khusibu, Kathmandu, Nepal
Department of Infectious Diseases and Immunology, Kathmandu Research Institute for Biological Sciences (KRIBS), Lalitpur, Nepal

**Samendra P. Sherchan**
Department of Global Environmental Health Sciences, School of Public Health and Tropical Medicine, Tulane University, New Orleans, LA, USA

**Mahesh Kumar Choudhari**
KIST Medical College and Teaching Hospital, Imadole, Lalitpur, Nepal

# Index

www.ingramcontent.com/pod-product-compliance
Lightning Source LLC
Chambersburg PA
CBHW082016190326
41458CB00010B/3203